MEDICAL MASTERCLASS

Cardiology and Respiratory Medicine

Disclaimer

Although every effort has been made to ensure that drug doses and other information are presented accurately in this publication, the ultimate responsibility rests with the prescribing physician. Neither the publishers nor the authors can be held responsible for any consequences arising from the use of information contained herein. Any product mentioned in this publication should be used in accordance with the prescribing information prepared by the manufacturers.

The information presented in this publication reflects the opinions of its contributors and should not be taken to represent the policy and views of the Royal College of Physicians of London, unless this is specifically stated.

Every effort has been made by the contributors to contact holders of copyright to obtain permission to reproduce copyright material. However, if any have been inadvertently overlooked, the publisher will be pleased to make the necessary arrangements at the first opportunity.

Medical Masterclass

EDITOR-IN-CHIEF

John D. Firth DM FRCP
Consultant Physician and Nephrologist
Addenbrooke's Hospital
Cambridge

Cardiology and Respiratory Medicine

EDITORS

Michael I. Polkey MRCP PhD
Consultant Physician
Royal Brompton Hospital
London

Paul R. Roberts MB ChB MRCP MD
Specialist Registrar, Cardiology
Southampton General Hospital
Southampton

Blackwell
Science

© 2001 Royal College of Physicians of London, 11 St Andrews Place, London NW1 4LE, Registered Charity No. 210508

Published by:
Blackwell Science Ltd
Editorial Offices:
Osney Mead, Oxford OX2 0EL
25 John Street, London WC1N 2BS
23 Ainslie Place, Edinburgh EH3 6AJ
350 Main Street, Malden
    MA 02148-5018, USA
54 University Street, Carlton
    Victoria 3053, Australia
10, rue Casimir Delavigne
    75006 Paris, France

Other Editorial Offices:
Blackwell Wissenschafts-Verlag GmbH
Kurfürstendamm 57
10707 Berlin, Germany

Blackwell Science KK
MG Kodenmacho Building
7–10 Kodenmacho Nihombashi
Chuo-ku, Tokyo 104, Japan

Iowa State University Press
A Blackwell Science Company
2121 S. State Avenue
Ames, Iowa 50014-8300, USA

First published 2001

Set by Graphicraft Limited, Hong Kong
Printed and bound in Italy by
Rotolito Lombarda SpA, Milan

The Blackwell Science logo is a trade mark of Blackwell Science Ltd, registered at the United Kingdom Trade Marks Registry

The right of the Authors to be identified as the Authors of this Work has been asserted in accordance with the Copyright, Designs and Patents Act 1988.

Catalogue records for this title are available from the British Library and the Library of Congress

ISBN 0-632-05866-8 (this book)
    0-632-05567-7 (set)

Commissioning Editors: Mike Stein and
    Rachel Robson
Project Manager (RCP): Filipa Maia
Editorial Assistant (RCP): Katherine Bowker
Production: Charlie Hamlyn and Jonathan
    Rowley
Layout and Cover Design: Chris Stone

DISTRIBUTORS

Marston Book Services Ltd
PO Box 269
Abingdon, Oxon OX14 4YN
(*Orders*: Tel: 01235 465500
        Fax: 01235 465555)

USA
Blackwell Science, Inc.
Commerce Place
350 Main Street
Malden, MA 02148-5018
(*Orders*: Tel: 800 759 6102
        781 388 8250
        Fax: 781 388 8255)

Canada
Login Brothers Book Company
324 Saulteaux Crescent
Winnipeg, Manitoba R3J 3T2
(*Orders*: Tel: 204 837 2987)

Australia
Blackwell Science Pty Ltd
54 University Street
Carlton, Victoria 3053
(*Orders*: Tel: 3 9347 0300
        Fax: 3 9347 5001)

For further information on Blackwell Science, visit our website:
www.blackwell-science.com

Contents

Respiratory Medicine

List of contributors

Praveen Bhatia MBBS MRCP
Staff Physician
Blackpool Victoria Hospital
Blackpool

Peter E. Glennon MB ChB Hons MD MRCP
BHF Clinical Lecturer
University of Cambridge
Addenbrooke's Hospital
Cambridge

Catherine E.G. Head MA MRCP
MRC Clinical Training Fellow and Specialist Registrar
University of Cambridge
Cambridge

Michael I. Polkey MRCP PhD
Consultant Physician
Royal Brompton Hospital
London

Paul R. Roberts MB ChB MRCP MD
Specialist Registrar, Cardiology
Southampton General Hospital
Southampton

Hamish A. Walker BA Hons MB BS MRCP
Clinical Research Fellow
Specialist Registrar Cardiology
Hammersmith Hospital
London

Veronica L.C. White BSc MSc MBBS MRCP
Research Fellow
Department of Respiratory Medicine
St. Bartholomew's Hospital
London

Foreword

Medical Masterclass is the most innovative and important educational development from the Royal College of Physicians in the last 100 years. Throughout our 480-year history we have pioneered and supported high-quality medicine, and while *Medical Masterclass* continues that tradition, it also represents a quantum leap for the College as it moves into the 21st century.

The effort that the College has put in to improve the Membership Examination, which started 150 years ago and is now run by all three UK Royal Colleges of Physicians, will now be matched by its attention to basic learning in general medicine—the grounding and preparation for the exam.

Teaching and learning for the exam have changed little over the past 50 years, relying on local courses, word-based teaching and commercial courses. *Medical Masterclass* is a completely new approach for those wishing to practise high-quality medicine. It is an imaginative multimedia programme with paper and CD modules covering the major areas of medicine, supported by a website which will provide summaries and links to the latest articles and guidelines, and self-assessment questionnaires with feedback. Its focus is on self-learning, self-assessment and dealing with realistic clinical problems—not just force-feeding facts. The series of interactive case studies on which the modules are based entail making diagnostic and treatment decisions, closely mimicking the situations found in the admission suite or outpatient clinic.

Medical Masterclass has been produced by the RCP's Education Department together with Blackwell Science. It represents a formidable amount of work by Dr John Firth and his team of authors and editors and is set to be the jewel in our crown. It also signals very clearly our intention to lead in the field of learning and to be supportive to our future members. I anticipate the package will also be invaluable for continued learning by our specialist registrars and consultants as part of continuing professional development.

I congratulate our colleagues for this superb product and commend it to you without reservation.

Professor Sir George Alberti
President of the Royal College of Physicians, London

Preface

Medical Masterclass comprises twelve paper-based modules, two CD-ROMs and a companion website. Its aim is to help doctors in their first few years of training to improve their medical skills and knowledge.

The twelve paper-based modules are divided as follows: two cover the scientific background to medicine, one is devoted to general clinical issues, one to emergency medicine and practical procedures, and eight cover the range of medical specialities. Medicine is often fairly straightforward when the diagnosis is clear, but patients rarely come to their doctor and say 'I've got Hodgkin's disease': they have lumps. The core material of each of the clinical specialities is defined by case presentations in the first part of each module: how do you approach the man who has lumps? Structured concise notes on specific diseases follow later. All practising doctors know that medicine is much more than knowing lots of facts about diseases: how do you tell someone they've got cancer? How do you decide when to stop treatment? Most medical texts say little about these issues: *Medical Masterclass* does not avoid them, nor does it talk in vague and abstract terms.

The two CD-ROMs each contain 30 interactive cases requiring diagnosis and treatment. The format is remarkably close to real life: you see the patient and are told the story; you have to decide how to investigate and treat; but you can't see all the results before you start to make decisions!

The companion website, which will be regularly updated, includes literature and guideline updates and review, and self-assessment questions. How much do you know, and are you improving? You will see how your score compares with your previous attempts, and also how your performance compares with others who have logged on to the site.

The *Medical Masterclass* is produced by the Education Department of the Royal College of Physicians of London and published by Blackwell Science. It is not a crammer for the MRCP exam and not written by those who set the exam. However, I have no doubt that someone putting effort into learning through the *Medical Masterclass* would be in a strong position to impress the examiners, although I am afraid that success—like much else in medicine and in life—cannot be guaranteed.

John Firth
Editor-in-Chief

Acknowledgements

Medical Masterclass has been produced by a team. The names of those who have written and edited material are clearly indicated elsewhere, but without the efforts of many other people *Medical Masterclass* would not exist at all. These include Professor Lesley Rees and Mrs Winnie Wade from the Education Department of the Royal College of Physicians of London, who initiated the project; Dr Mike Stein and Dr Andy Robinson from Medschool.com and Blackwell Science respectively, who have enthusiastically supported it from the beginning; and Ms Filipa Maia and Ms Katherine Bowker, who have run the office with splendid efficiency and induced authors and editors to perform to a schedule rarely achieved. I and the whole of the team of editors and authors are immensely grateful to all of these people for the energy that they have poured into *Medical Masterclass* in various ways.

John Firth
Editor-in-Chief

Key features

We have created a range of icon boxes to help you identify key information and to make learning easier and more enjoyable. Here is a brief explanation:

Clinical pointer

This icon highlights important information to be noted.

Further information

This icon indicates the source of further information and reference.

Hints

This icon highlights useful hints, tips and mnemonics.

Key points

This icon is used to highlight points of particular importance.

Quote

This icon indicates useful or interesting citations from notable individuals, including well-known physicians.

Think about

This icon indicates what the reader should reflect on after having read a passage from the text.

Warning/Hazard

This icon is used to indicate common or important drug interactions, pitfalls of practical procedures, or when to take symptoms or signs particularly seriously.

Cardiology

AUTHORS:
**P.E. Glennon, C.E.G. Head,
P.R. Roberts and H.A. Walker**

EDITOR:
P.R. Roberts

EDITOR-IN-CHIEF:
J.D. Firth

1 Clinical presentations

1.1 Paroxysmal palpitations

Case history

A 28-year-old teacher is referred to you in outpatients with a 5-year history of intermittent palpitations. Other than the sensation of palpitations she has no other symptoms. In her family, two relatives have died following a sudden collapse.

Clinical approach

The symptom of palpitations (abnormal awareness of the heart beat) can be caused by a range of clinical conditions from the very benign to the potentially life threatening; approach the patient with this in mind. It is unusual to see someone during a symptomatic episode, so as much information as possible should be gained from the history, with a main aim being to assess the patient's potential risk from life-threatening ventricular arrhythmias. You should always have in the back of your mind a list of the possible causes of palpitations (Table 1). In most situations it will be essential to have investigations during a symptomatic episode. Remember that the severity of symptoms does not always reflect the seriousness of the underlying problem: some patients in sinus rhythm may experience severe palpitations, whereas others may be asymptomatic when in ventricular tachycardia.

Table 1 Potential causes of palpitations.

Type of palpitation	Cause
No arrhythmia	Anxiety
	Panic attacks
	Depression
Extrasystoles	Atrial
	Ventricular
Bradyarrhythmia	Atrioventricular block
	Sinus node disease
Tachyarrhythmia	Ventricular tachycardia
	Atrial fibrillation/flutter
	AVNRT
	AVRT
	Sinus tachycardia

AVNRT, atrioventricular nodal re-entry tachycardia; AVRT, atrioventricular re-entry tachycardia.

In this case the family history should make you particularly keen to exclude significant inherited conditions that may predispose to arrhythmias, e.g. hypertrophic obstructive cardiomyopathy.

History of the presenting problem

Which came first—the anxiety or the palpitation, the chicken or the egg?
• Palpitations secondary to anxiety-induced sinus tachycardia are common
• Patients with cardiac arrhythmias are frequently anxious about their future.

What are the palpitations like?

The characteristics of the palpitations can provide valuable clues in making the diagnosis. Ask the following:
• 'Tap out' the rhythm—note how fast this is, and whether it is regular or irregular. Irregular means that atrial fibrillation is most likely. A 'missed beat' is typically caused by an extrasystole—after the compensatory pause the next sinus beat is felt with extra force. These missed beats are almost always of no pathological significance. However, they can cause worry that is likely to be reinforced because anxiety is the most common cause of awareness of extrasystoles, which are likely to have been long standing and previously asymptomatic.
• Do you feel the palpitations in your neck? These are suggestive of cannon waves, indicating atrioventricular (AV) block.
• How do they start, what brings them on and how do they stop? Do you get any warning at all? Do they come on gradually or suddenly? Palpitations that come on and go away gradually are most likely to be due to sinus tachycardia.
• Are there accompanying symptoms? Do you feel faint or dizzy with them? Have you ever collapsed? Arrhythmias causing these symptoms are more likely to be of a serious (potentially life-threatening) cause and clearly mandate thorough investigation. Some patients with supraventricular tachycardia (SVT) develop polyuria as a result of atrial stretch causing release of atrial natriuretic peptide.
• How frequent are the palpitations? Palpitations that occur infrequently are likely to be difficult to catch on tape.
• What treatments have been tried already? An SVT may be terminated by a Valsalva manoeuvre.

Other aspects

Ask about the following:
- General health: is there anything to suggest thyrotoxicosis? (See *Endocrinology*, Section 1.13.)
- Smoking, alcohol, tea and coffee consumption—acute excess of these can trigger arrhythmia in those predisposed.
- Drugs, prescribed and non-prescribed: a range of these can cause arrhythmia. Always consult the drug datasheet or *British National Formulary* (BNF).
- Is the patient prone to anxiety? Does he or she ever have anxiety attacks?
- Find out whether he or she has a history of recurrent presentation to doctors with medically unexplained symptoms.
- Family history: this is clearly an important element in this case, but always ask directly about it. A patient is much more likely to be concerned about palpitations, even if of benign cause, if a relative has died at a young age of heart disease.

Examination

Examination of the patient with palpitations:
- A normal examination does not rule out a significant arrhythmia
- Do not focus entirely on the cardiovascular system
- Patients with significant cardiovascular pathology may initially present with palpitations
- Take note of the patient's mental state.

General

As the patient is unlikely to be symptomatic at the time, the purpose of examination is to assess the patient's general well-being, including mental state, and to establish whether there is a cardiovascular or systemic cause for the symptoms. Is there any evidence of thyrotoxicosis, which might predispose to paroxysms of atrial fibrillation? In most patients with an SVT, examination will be entirely normal.

Cardiovascular

Take careful note of the following:
- Pulse rate, rhythm and character
- Blood pressure
- Jugular venous pressure (JVP)
- Heart sounds and murmurs
- Lung bases.

Cardiovascular examination is aimed at evaluating whether there is a structural abnormality that may make the patient susceptible to arrhythmias. Pay particular attention to auscultation of the heart:

- The findings of a diastolic murmur, opening snap and loud first heart sound may indicate mitral stenosis, which predisposes to atrial fibrillation as the size of the atria enlarges.
- The harsh systolic murmur found in patients with hypertrophic obstructive cardiomyopathy may suggest ventricular arrhythmias.
- Signs of congestive heart failure raise the possibility of ventricular arrhythmias and atrial fibrillation.

Approach to investigations and management

This should be guided by facts established from the history and examination. Auscultation may suggest a structural cardiac abnormality, such as valvular disease, and in such patients echocardiography may be warranted.

Investigations

ECG

In most situations only a 12-lead ECG in sinus rhythm is available. However, if an ECG has been recorded during symptoms and documents an arrhythmia, it may not be necessary to investigate further because this alone may enable a precise diagnosis to be made (see Section 3.1, p. 120).

Assessing the 12-lead ECG of a patient with palpitations:
- Look for sinus bradycardia/tachycardia.
- Are there any features suggestive of cardiac structural. abnormality, e.g. P mitrale, left ventricular hypertrophy (LVH) (Fig. 1)?
- Measure the PR interval.
- Look for evidence of AV block.
- Are there δ waves (Fig. 2)?
- Has the patient had a previous myocardial infarction (MI)?
- Measure the QT interval and calculate the QTc (QT adjusted for rate).
- Are there any ventricular/atrial ectopic beats?

Ambulatory monitoring

See Section 3.3 (p. 127). An example of an arrhythmia captured on an ambulatory monitor record is shown in Fig. 3.

Management

In many cases when an arrhythmia has been found to be associated with symptoms, the management will be straightforward.

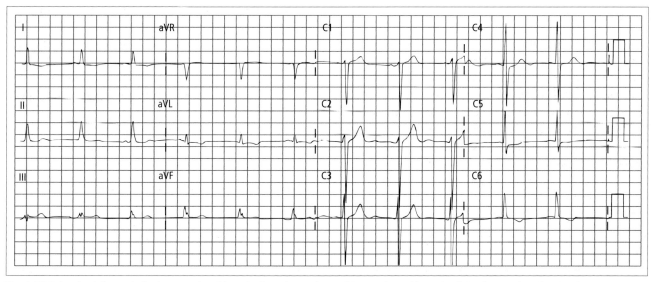

Fig. 1 ECG showing left ventricular hypertrophy with strain (lateral ST/T changes) in a patient with previously undiagnosed aortic stenosis.

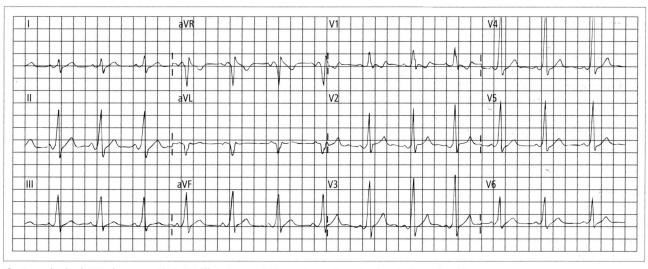

Fig. 2 Twelve-lead ECG of patient with the Wolff–Parkinson–White syndrome. Note the short PR interval and δ waves.

Fig. 3 Ambulatory monitor of a patient with supraventricular tachycardia (SVT). Sinus tachycardia is followed by ventricular bigeminy before the sudden onset of SVT.

Supraventricular arrhythmias

Most SVTs are amenable to pharmacological therapy with class 1, 2, 3 or 4 agents or suitable for radiofrequency ablation. (See Section 2.2.2, p. 59.)

Paroxysmal atrial fibrillation/flutter: initial therapy should be the maintenance of sinus rhythm pharmacologically. Drugs with a class 3 action are most efficacious in this instance, e.g. sotalol, amiodarone. Specific attention should be focused towards the need for anticoagulation. (See Section 2.14.1, p. 108.)

Bradyarrhythmias

See Section 2.2.1, p. 58.

Ventricular arrhythmias

Ventricular arrhythmias may be suitable for ablation or for implantation of an implantable cardioverter defibrillator (ICD). (See Section 3.4, p. 130.)

Others

In many cases a benign arrhythmia is detected, such as ventricular or atrial ectopy, and occasionally symptoms are clearly associated with sinus rhythm. In most cases explanation and positive reassurance to the patient are all that is required. Only in rare instances, where the patient is very debilitated, should a β blocker be prescribed.

Significant symptoms can occasionally be associated with sinus tachycardia; in these circumstances it is important to exclude causes of sinus tachycardia, the most common being anxiety, before attributing the arrhythmia to inappropriate sinus node function.

Brugada P, Gursoy S, Brugada J, Andries E. Investigation of palpitations. *Lancet* 1993; 341: 1254–1258.
Vohra JK. Palpitations: reassurance or more? *Med J Aust* 1999; 170: 442–448.
Zimetbaum P, Josephson ME. Evaluation of patients with palpitations. *N Engl J Med* 1998; 338: 1369–1373.

1.2 Palpitations with dizziness

Case history

A 57-year-old retired policeman presents with a 2-month history of rapid palpitations. Initially he was well during the episodes, but more recently he has noticed that he is dizzy when they go on for a longer time. He made an appointment to see his GP, who referred him directly to the medical admissions unit where you are asked to assess him.

Clinical approach

Your main concern is that this patient gives a history of presyncope, which places him in a higher risk category for life-threatening arrhythmia (see Section 1.1, p. 3). The main objective with this patient is to exclude a significant ventricular arrhythmia. With the little information available, it is apparent that the palpitations are directly related to the presyncope, which would be consistent with the diagnosis of ventricular tachycardia (VT).

It is vital to ensure that the patient is safe while a diagnosis has to be established; he should therefore be admitted for investigation and monitoring. It is essential to document the heart rhythm during an episode. Some patients with VT are asymptomatic, whereas others are extremely symptomatic of only short runs of VT. Both groups are at risk of cardiac arrest as a result of VT or from the VT degenerating into ventricular fibrillation.

 Broad complex tachycardia: do not attribute a broad complex tachyarrhythmia to SVT with aberration unless you are absolutely certain of the diagnosis.

History of the presenting problem

What is the relationship of the presyncope and palpitations?

It is important to determine the order of symptoms; many patients with presyncope or syncope will have a reactive sinus tachycardia after the event that might cause a feeling of palpitation. In this case it is clear that the presyncope is occurring with more prolonged episodes of palpitation.

Aside from ventricular arrhythmia, consider other causes of palpitations and syncope:
• Bradyarrhythmias
• Atrial flutter with 1 : 1 conduction
• Atrial fibrillation and Wolff–Parkinson–White syndrome
• Aortic stenosis.
  And do not forget the following:
• Vasovagal syncope: the most common cause of presyncope and syncope
• Acute blood loss: this will usually be obvious, but it is a mistake to miss the fact that the patient has had melaena!

Relevant past history

Ischaemic heart disease

This is a common cause of VT. Find out the following:

- Is there a previous history of angina/MI?
- Does the patient have symptoms consistent with angina?
- Does the patient have risk factors for ischaemic heart disease (IHD)?

Cardiomyopathy

Most forms of cardiomyopathy can cause VT. Ask the patient the following:
- Is there a history of breathlessness/lethargy?
- Have you had a recent viral illness?
- How much alcohol do you drink? Have you ever drunk heavily in the past?

Drug history

Drug toxicity can provoke VT, e.g. digoxin, quinidine, catecholamines. Check the datasheet or BNF for details of any drug that the patient is taking. Is arrhythmia reported as a side effect?

Family history

Particularly in young patients presenting with arrhythmias, always enquire if anyone in the family has had a similar problem.

Other

Ventricular tachycardia may be part of a primary electrophysiological disturbance or secondary to any pathology that produces structural changes in the ventricles. Any 'cardiac history' could therefore be relevant, e.g. valvular heart disease, congenital heart disease, right ventricular dysplasia, previous cardiac surgery.

Examination

The priorities are to establish the following:
- Is the patient unwell/hypotensive/sweating?
- Is the patient in VT or another arrhythmia at the moment? If the patient is having a symptomatic episode, specific signs may provide clues to the diagnosis.
- Are there any obvious cardiovascular causes for VT?
- Are there any other signs suggesting systemic upset?

General

In most cases the examination will be normal, but it is important to examine all systems thoroughly because many diseases can have an impact on the electrophysiological status of the heart, e.g. renal disease leading to

hyperkalaemia or respiratory disease causing hypoxaemia will both predispose to arrhythmia.

Cardiovascular

The main aim of the cardiovascular examination will be to elicit whether there are any structural abnormalities that may make the patient liable to ventricular arrhythmias. Pay specific attention to:
- pulse rate, rhythm and character
- JVP
- apex beat
- thrills or heaves
- heart sounds and murmurs
- lung bases.

Approach to investigations and management

 A broad complex tachycardia should always be treated as ventricular tachycardia until proven otherwise.

Investigations

12-lead ECG

Obtaining an ECG during an episode is a key objective in establishing a diagnosis (Fig. 4). Beware of confusing VT and SVT with aberrant conduction. (See Section 3.1, p. 120.)

Ambulatory monitoring

If the diagnosis is not apparent, monitoring for longer periods may be necessary. (See Section 3.3, p. 127.)

Electrophysiological study

If symptoms are infrequent or doubt exists as to the diagnosis, then provocation of the rhythm during an electrophysiological study will provide definitive evidence. (See Section 3.2, p. 125.)

Other

If VT is suspected, investigations to identify possible causes should be considered:
- Chest radiograph (cardiomegaly, heart shape, pulmonary oedema) (Fig. 5)
- Check electrolytes: abnormalities of potassium or magnesium can be associated with arrhythmia
- Echocardiogram (cardiac function, valve structure/ function, intracardiac masses) (Fig. 6)

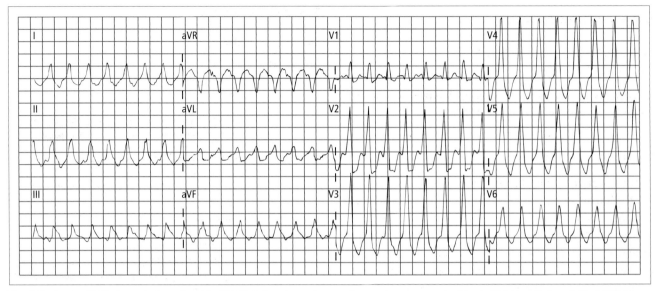

Fig. 4 Twelve-lead ECG of ventricular tachycardia (VT). Note broad complexes and concordance across chest leads. Right bundle-branch block (RBBB) morphology suggests left ventricular origin.

Fig. 5 Chest radiograph of patient with dilated cardiomyopathy. The cardiothoracic ratio is increased. There is a pleural effusion at the right base.

Fig. 6 Echocardiogram demonstrating dilated cardiomyopathy. This is a 'four-chamber' view with both ventricles dilated, particularly the left ventricle (seen in the centre at the top).

- Exercise ECG (ischaemia, exercise-induced arrhythmias)
- Cardiac catheterization (coronary atherosclerosis, valvular function)
- Computed tomography/magnetic resonance imaging (CT/MRI) (mediastinal pathology, pericardial/myocardial disease).

Management

The patient is likely to be having presyncope associated with VT and should be admitted for monitoring and observation. Management will consist of the following:
- Immediate cessation of arrhythmia if in VT (DC shock/pharmacological cardioversion)
- Identification of cause

- Correction of cause
- Antiarrhythmic therapy
- Assessment for ICD.

Immediate management

The priorities are as follows:
- If the patient does not have an output, start emergency resuscitation. (See *Emergency medicine*, Section 1.1.)
- If the patient is haemodynamically compromised, consider DC cardioversion (under general anaesthesia or sedation). (See Section 2.2.2, p. 59.)
- If the patient is not compromised, consider pharmacological intervention (lidocaine, amiodarone).
    Correct electrolyte (K^+/Mg^{2+}) imbalances.

Long-term management

IMPLANTABLE CARDIOVERTER DEFIBRILLATOR

All patients with VT should be considered for assessment for an ICD. (See Section 3.4, p. 130.)

ANTIARRHYTHMICS

In those patients who do not have an indication for an ICD, pharmacological therapy should be considered; in many circumstances either sotalol or amiodarone will be the drug of choice. It is essential to monitor the patient to ensure suppression of the arrhythmia; symptomatology is not always adequate because the drugs may slow but not prevent the VT, making it better tolerated or unnoticed. Monitoring will usually be in the form of ambulatory ECG recording, but exercise testing if the arrhythmia is exercise induced or by provocation at electrophysiological study may be appropriate in some cases.

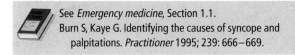
See *Emergency medicine*, Section 1.1.
Burn S, Kaye G. Identifying the causes of syncope and palpitations. *Practitioner* 1995; 239: 666–669.

1.3 Syncope

Case history

A 75-year-old woman presents to you in the accident and emergency (A&E) department with a history of sudden collapse. This occurred unexpectedly while she was shopping and there have been no previous similar episodes. When the paramedic team arrived at the scene she was alert and orientated, and all observations were normal.

Clinical approach

This is a very common clinical problem and accounts for up to 3% of attendances at A&E departments and 1% of hospital admissions. Your aim will be to determine the cause of the syncope, remembering that untreated cardiac related syncope has a 1-year mortality rate of 20–30%. A difficult aspect of managing patients such as this is that there are so many causes of syncope, both cardiac and non-cardiac (Table 2). A carefully taken history may exclude a large proportion of these, and a meticulous examination may elicit the cause. A history from a witness should be obtained if at all possible—it might be invaluable.

Table 2 Causes of syncope.

Type	Cause
Non-cardiac	Seizures
	Postural hypertension
	Cerebrovascular
	Drug induced
	Situational (micturition, defaecation, cough, swallow)
	Psychogenic (anxiety, panic, somatization, depression)
Cardiac	Bradyarrhythmias (including vasovagal)
	Tachyarrhythmias
	Left ventricular outflow obstruction (aortic stenosis, HOCM)
	Myxoma
	Mitral stenosis
	Cardiac ischaemia (MI, angina)
	Pulmonary obstruction (pulmonary stenosis, pulmonary hypertension, pulmonary embolism, Fallot's tetralogy, myxoma)
	Cardiac tamponade
	Aortic dissection

HOCM, hypertrophic obstructive cardiomyopathy; MI, myocardial infarction.

History of the presenting problem

Did the woman really have a syncopal episode, or did she just trip up? If syncope is likely, direct questions should be targeted at excluding all of the causes listed in Table 2. One of the most important of these is seizures.

Seizures or cardiac syncope?

Seizures are associated with the following:
- Blue face (not pale)
- Convulsive movements (usually, but not always)
- Tongue biting
- Incontinence
- Unconsciousness >5min
- Drowsiness and disorientation for a variable length of time on recovery.

A detailed description of the events leading up to the syncopal episode, and a description of the syncopal episode itself and of the recovery phase may provide information to establish the cause. Be very particular: 'Can you remember exactly what you were doing before you collapsed?' Do not accept: 'I was out shopping.' 'Were you sitting down . . . standing up . . . had you just turned your head?' This history should be obtained from the patient, from any witness and preferably from both. You may need to ask specific questions:
- Did you feel sweaty or nauseous before the episodes?
- Did you get palpitations beforehand?
- Did you get chest pain beforehand?
- Did you feel breathless beforehand?

All of these would suggest a cardiac cause, as opposed to seizures. And if someone has had more than one episode:

- How long have you had the symptoms?
- Are the episodes becoming more frequent?
- Have you had fits of any sort before?

Take particular care to consider those conditions that make the patient at high risk of recurrent syncope or death and for which specific treatments are available. These include the following:

- Aortic dissection: was syncope associated with chest pain? Is there a history of hypertension? Has the patient had any previous vascular conditions? (See Section 1.5, p. 15.)
- Pulmonary embolism: has the patient had a period of immobility? Any recent operations? Has there been a previous history of thromboembolism? (See Section 1.9, p. 28.)
- Aortic stenosis: has a murmur been noticed in previous examinations? Is there a history of dyspnoea? Is there a history of exertional presyncope?

Relevant past history

Identification of any underlying cardiac disease places the patient in a high-risk group. Establish whether there are other symptoms suggestive of cardiac abnormality:

- Is there a history of angina/MI?
- Is there any cardiac family history?
- Is there a history of rheumatic fever?
- Are there any risk factors for IHD?
- What medications is she taking? Are there any that might predispose to syncope, e.g. diuretics that could cause postural hypotension, or agents that might predispose to arrhythmia. (See Section 1.2, p. 6.)

Examination

Look for evidence of injury caused by the syncope, and concentrate specifically on cardiovascular and neurological assessment.

Cardiovascular

Take careful note of the following:
- Peripheral perfusion
- Pulse rate and rhythm
- Peripheral pulses, including left radial and femorals
- Pulse character: is it slow rising?
- Blood pressure: is there a postural drop? Is it the same in both arms?
- JVP
- Cardiac apex
- Are there carotid bruits (or bruits elsewhere)?
- Heart sounds and murmurs
- Lung bases
- Liver edge
- Peripheral oedema.

Any abnormal cardiac signs increase the chances of a cardiac cause of syncope.

Ask the patient to move her neck through its full range of movement: does this provoke feelings of presyncope or dizziness, which would suggest vertebrobasilar ischaemia as a likely cause for her syncope?

Consider carotid sinus massage to investigate carotid sinus sensitivity, but be extremely cautious in those patients at risk of atheromatous carotid disease.

Neurological

The presence of any focal neurological signs would raise the possibility that syncope was caused by a cerebrovascular event, but does not prove that this is the case. A cardiac cause of syncope could have led to cerebrovascular ischaemia.

Approach to investigations and management

 Remember that patients with syncope are likely to be in a high state of anxiety and that it is essential that all other explanations are carefully considered before attributing the problem to psychogenic causes.

This woman will need to be admitted to hospital for monitoring and assessment. The history and examination provide the basis for direct investigation and management. If it is felt that syncope is most likely to be neurological in origin then investigation should be pursued as described in *Neurology*, Section 1.20. However, a cardiac cause can never be totally excluded without thorough investigation.

Investigations

Immediate investigations

The immediate investigations of a patient with probable cardiac syncope are discussed below.

ECG

Of patients with a cardiac syncope, 10% will have an identifiable abnormality on the ECG to suggest a cause. Therefore, look for the following:
- Sinus rate
- PR interval
- QRS axis
- QRS width
- Left ventricular hypertrophy
- Right ventricular hypertrophy
- P-wave morphology

Fig. 7 Complete heart block demonstrated on a Holter monitor.

• Evidence of pre-excitation (Wolff–Parkinson–White syndrome)
• Evidence of acute MI/infarction.

CHEST RADIOGRAPH

Look for the following:
• Cardiac size and shape
• Prominent pulmonary vasculature
• Pulmonary oedema
• Aortic outline: is the mediastinum of normal width?

BLOOD TESTS

These are rarely helpful in establishing a diagnosis, but cardiac enzymes, full blood count (FBC), electrolytes, renal and liver function tests and inflammatory markers will usually be requested as a 'screen'. Electrolyte disturbance (particularly hypokalaemia) might predispose to arrhythmia and syncope (see Section 1.2, p. 6). Raised inflammatory markers may indicate a systemic problem.

Further investigations

DURING HOSPITAL ADMISSION

It is more than likely that the ECG, chest radiograph and screening blood tests will not demonstrate any clear cause of syncope, in which case consider the following:
• Ambulatory monitoring: 24-h Holter monitoring and patient-activated devices may be useful to exclude tachy-/bradyarrhythmias (Fig. 7). (See Section 3.3, p. 127.)
• Echocardiography: this may indicate structural or functional cardiac abnormality—transthoracic echocardiography (Fig. 8) is usually adequate, but in some instances, e.g. when aortic dissection is being considered, trans-oesophageal echocardiography (TOE) may be required.
• If pulmonary embolism is plausible, check blood gases and organize lung ventilation–perfusion scanning or CT angiography. (See Section 1.9, p. 28 and *Respiratory medicine*, Section 1.5.)

Fig. 8 Transthoracic echocardiogram of atrial myxoma. The myxoma (MYX) is seen to occupy most of the left atrium and is almost prolapsing through the mitral valve (MV) into the left ventricle (LV). The aorta (AO) is seen above the left atrium.

• If aortic dissection is plausible, organize a CT scan of the chest.

FOR THOSE WITH RECURRENT UNEXPLAINED SYNCOPE

Consider the following for patients with recurrent unexplained syncope.

Tilt-table test
A tilt-table test can be helpful in identifying vasovagal syncope, with continuous blood pressure and heart rate monitoring showing abnormal bradycardia and/or hypotension in response to upright tilt. However, the findings on tilt-table testing can be difficult to interpret, particularly in elderly patients, and it is important to adopt a strict protocol and use clear endpoints to define a positive result.

Electrophysiological studies
Abnormalities of sinus and AV node function may be

identified, suggesting a bradycardic cause of syncope. Similarly, provocation of atrial/ventricular arrhythmias may establish the diagnosis. (See Section 3.2, p. 125.)

Management

If a cardiac cause of syncope is established, then management is as indicated:
• Bradyarrhythmias: consider permanent pacemaker. (See Section 3.5, p. 132.)
• Tachyarrhythmias: pharmacological therapy, ablation or an ICD. (See Sections 2.2.2, p. 59 and 3.4, p. 130.)
• Valvular disease: consider surgical intervention. (See Section 2.5, p. 71.)
• Pulmonary embolism: will need anticoagulation. (See Sections 1.9, p. 28, 2.18, p. 115, and *Haematology*, Section 3.6.)
• Hypertrophic obstructive cardiomyopathy: advice on lifestyle changes and pharmacological therapy. (See Section 2.4.1, p. 66.)

If no cause for syncope is established and the patient is agitating to go home ('there's nothing wrong with me, doctor—I just had a faint'), then what should you do? If, after 24–48 h, there has been no recurrence of presyncope or syncope, the patient has 'mobilized' satisfactorily on the ward and serial 12-lead ECGs show no change, most physicians would be willing for the patient to be discharged home with the following:
• Reassurance that nothing terrible has been found, but also a clear statement that no firm diagnosis has been made—meaning that patient and doctors must remain alert.
• A letter for the patient's general practitioner.
• Instructions to report recurrence of presyncope or syncope immediately.
• Arrangements for a 24-h ambulatory monitoring (and perhaps echocardiography) if it has not been possible to obtain this during the patient's inpatient stay (which is preferable, but not always possible).

Most patients will be aware of the serious nature of most cardiac causes of syncope. It is essential to be aware of the psychological needs of such patients. Reassurance and appropriate information at an early stage may prevent problems at a later stage in their management.

See *Medicine for the elderly*, Section 1.1.
See *Emergency medicine*, Sections 1.1, 1.4 and 1.6.
See *Neurology*, Section 1.20.
Kapoor WN. Syncope and hypotension. In: Braunwald E (ed.) *Heart Disease: A textbook of cardiovascular medicine*, 5th edn. Philadelphia, PA: WB Saunders Co., 1997: 863–876.

1.4 Stroke and a murmur

Case history

A 58-year-old woman presents with a left-sided hemiparesis of sudden onset. She had previously been fit and well. However, a murmur had been noted, but not investigated, when she was 45 and undergoing a minor gynaecological procedure.

Clinical approach

A stroke can be a devastating condition with high morbidity and mortality. It is not possible to predict accurately the degree of recovery that this woman will make. It is important to identify whether or not she is at high risk of further events, and in particular whether she is at risk of cardiac embolic stroke. The majority of strokes are related to cerebrovascular atheromatous disease and not to cardiac disease, but most cardiac causes of embolic stroke are treatable, so further events are potentially preventable in this group. In most cases where there is a cardiac cause this will be elicited from the history or examination.

Consider the causes of cardiac embolic strokes when taking a history and examining a patient who has had a stroke:
• 'Non-valvular' atrial fibrillation
• Acute MI with mural thrombus
• Mechanical prosthetic valves
• Rheumatic heart disease
• Dilated cardiomyopathy
• Infective endocarditis
• Paradoxical embolism
• Left atrial myxoma
• Calcific aortic stenosis.

History of the presenting problem

The first priority will be to establish the diagnosis of stroke and then to focus on possible causes.

Identification of cardiac cause of stroke:
• Establish whether there have been any previous thromboembolic events
• Is the patient known to have any cardiac conditions?
• Does the patient have any cardiac symptoms? Specifically, is there a history of palpitations suggestive of atrial fibrillation?

Relevant past history

In most cases, it will be obvious if there is any pre-existing cardiac condition, but ask the patient the following:
- Are you known to have an irregular pulse?
- Have you had angina or a heart attack?
- Have you had rheumatic fever?
- Have you had any heart operations?
- Has a murmur ever been heard?
- Did you have a 'hole in the heart' as a child?

Examination

In the absence of previous cardiac conditions and with an entirely normal clinical examination, the likelihood of the stroke being cardiac in origin is small. It is therefore vital that the examination of the cardiovascular system is thorough. A patient with a recent stroke may have difficulty in co-operating with you during the examination, e.g. rolling the patient on to the side to listen for mitral stenosis may be difficult if he or she has a hemiparesis. However, it is important not to compromise the quality of your examination—seek help in moving the patient if necessary.

General

It is unlikely that there will be many signs from general examination that will help in establishing whether or not the cause was cardiac:
- The patient with a previous MI or dilated cardiomyopathy might be dyspnoeic as a result of cardiac failure, but there are many other causes of breathlessness, including aspiration pneumonia in someone who has just suffered a stroke.
- The patient with infective endocarditis may have fever and peripheral stigmata. (See Section 1.13, p. 38.)
- Look carefully for any signs of previous cardiac surgery, particularly if the patient is unable to give a history.

Do not forget to examine the back and the breast crease where there may be scars from previous mitral surgery (valvuloplasty).

Cardiovascular

Take careful note of the following:
- Peripheral perfusion.
- Peripheral pulses: is it possible that this woman has had an aortic dissection?
- Pulse rhythm and character: in particular, is there atrial fibrillation? Is there aortic stenosis or incompetence?
- Blood pressure: often elevated in someone who has just had a stroke.
- Cardiac apex.
- Heart sounds and murmurs: this woman is said to have a murmur—listen carefully for both mitral stenosis and

aortic incompetence, which are the easy murmurs to miss. You are most unlikely ever to hear the 'tumour plop' of an atrial myxoma, but it is absolutely certain that you will not if you never listen!
- Lung bases.
- Liver edge.
- Peripheral oedema.

 Consider non-thromboembolic cardiovascular causes for stroke:
- Aortic dissection involving the carotid arteries
- Vasculitis of the cerebral vessels (very rare).

Approach to investigations and management

In most cases, simple non-invasive investigations will provide the information needed to establish a cardiac cause of stroke.

Investigations

ECG and chest radiograph

Every patient who has a stroke should have a 12-lead ECG and chest radiograph. The ECG may provide valuable clues to the aetiology of thrombus (Fig. 9).

Echocardiogram

Echocardiography should be performed only if there is a clinical, ECG or chest radiographic indication of cardiac abnormality (Fig. 10). (See Section 3.11, p. 141.) CT or MRI of the chest may rarely be required to define a structural abnormality.

Blood tests

Check the FBC (?polycythaemia, ?thrombocytosis), electrolytes, renal and liver function tests, inflammatory markers (if raised, consider endocarditis, myxoma and vasculitis, and perform appropriate specialist blood tests), and blood cultures (if any suspicion of endocarditis).

CT scan of the brain

In any case where anticoagulation is to be considered, a CT brain scan is required to exclude haemorrhage.

Management

The patient will require care appropriate to the disability produced by their stroke. (See *Medicine for the elderly*, Section 1.4, *Emergency medicine*, Section 1.25 and *Neurology*, Sections 1.21 and 2.8.1.)

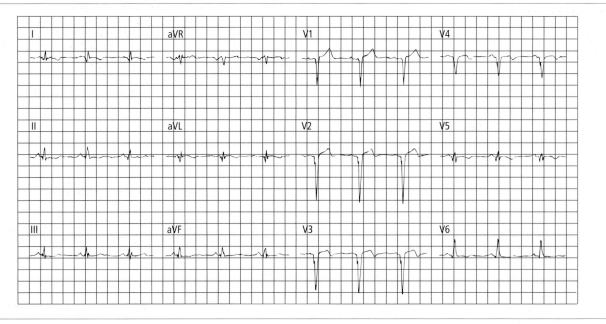

Fig. 9 ECG demonstrating anterior Q waves and poor R-wave progression across the chest leads. This is most probably secondary to a previous large anterior myocardial infarction. Left ventricular mural thrombus is possible in this scenario.

Fig. 10 Transoesophageal echocardiogram of cardiac thrombus. The left ventricle is seen in cross-section with a large mural thrombus.

Particular attention to anticoagulation, restoration of sinus rhythm (in some cases) and surgical correction of cardiac lesions (in rare cases) will be required in patients with a cardiac cause for stroke.

Anticoagulation

If a cardiac cause of stroke has been identified—meaning almost certainly that there is further substantial thromboembolic risk—then, if the stroke is confirmed as ischaemic on CT brain scan, consideration of anticoagulation is required. However, leaving the patient without anticoagulation keeps him or her at risk of further thrombo-

embolism; anticoagulation puts him or her at increased risk of haemorrhagic transformation of a cerebral infarct. There are no good data to determine when anticoagulation should be started. Assuming that the patient is recovering from the stroke, most physicians would begin with heparin (intravenous or low molecular weight) at some time between 7 and 14 days, with a view to longer-term warfarin therapy if the thromboembolic risk persists, and with very careful monitoring of the level of anticoagulation. (See *Haematology*, Section 3.6.)

 Strokes may be haemorrhagic, even in those at risk of thromboembolism.
Some features are more likely with cerebral haemorrhages:
- Nausea/vomiting
- Cerebral irritation
- Depressed conscious level.

But ischaemic and haemorrhagic strokes cannot be distinguished with certainty on clinical grounds and a CT brain scan should always be performed before commencing anticoagulation.

Antiarrhythmics

After anticoagulation, restoration of sinus rhythm should be the primary target in those with atrial fibrillation. Pharmacological cardioversion is preferable to DC cardioversion in the short term, because of the risks of a general anaesthetic in the context of a recent stroke. Sotalol or amiodarone are the drugs of choice. (See Section 2.2.2, p. 59.)

Table 3 Differential diagnosis of central chest pain.

Common cardiac	Myocardial infarction
	Unstable angina
Common non-cardiac	Oesophagitis
	Musculoskeletal
Must consider	Thoracic aortic dissection
Less common	Pericarditis
	Coronary vasospasm

Surgical correction of cause

Repair of an aortic dissection, replacement of an infected valve or removal of an atrial myxoma may be necessary immediately. There is increased risk of further cerebral insult when the patient goes on cardiac bypass, but this has to be balanced against the potential risk of not treating the underlying condition. In those with valvular pathology, it is usual to allow time for the patient to make as complete a recovery as possible from the stroke before considering surgery.

See *Medicine for the elderly*, Section 1.4.
See *Emergency medicine*, Section 1.25.
See *Neurology*, Sections 1.21 and 2.8.1.
See *Haematology*, Section 3.6.
Barnett HJM, Eliasziw M, Meldrum HE. Prevention of ischaemic stroke. *Br Med J* 1999; 318: 1539–1543.
Zipes DP. Specific arrhythmias: diagnosis and treatment. In: Braunwald E (ed.) *Heart Disease: A textbook of cardiovascular medicine*, 5th edn. Philadelphia, PA: WB Saunders Co., 1997: 654–656.

1.5 Acute central chest pain

Case history

A 52-year-old lorry driver presents with a tight, aching, central chest pain. This came on while loading his lorry with heavy boxes.

Clinical approach

If the patient is still in pain then your first concern is to decide whether or not he is having an MI. Your initial history must be brief and should be combined with an ECG because timely treatment with aspirin and thrombolytic therapy may be life saving (see Section 2.1.3, p. 55). Dissection of the thoracic aorta is much less common, but should be considered at an early stage because it can be fatal and is potentially remediable, and also because thrombolysis is contraindicated!

The differential diagnosis of central chest pain is set out in Table 3. The brief history given suggests that the pain is not pleuritic, but it is important to confirm this because the differential diagnosis of pleuritic pain is different. (See Section 1.9, p. 28.)

If a firm diagnosis cannot be established on the basis of history, examination and immediately available tests, you should assume that the patient has cardiac ischaemia. The emphasis then switches to assessing the patient's risk of death or MI in the ensuing hours or days.

History of the presenting problem

If the patient is still in pain, you must record an ECG as soon as practicable, not after you have finished the history and examination.

Is the pain the result of cardiac ischaemia?

When, where and how?

This man's pain came on when he was loading heavy boxes on to his lorry, but enquire about the following details if they do not emerge spontaneously in the account of any patient presenting with central chest pain:
- When did it come on?
- What were you doing at the time?
- Where did the pain start? (Ask the patient to indicate where in the chest)
- How did it start? Suddenly (in an instant) or gradually?
- Did it go anywhere else?
  Ischaemic cardiac pain:
- is typically brought on by exercise or emotion, but unstable angina and MI may start at rest or even during sleep
- tends to be felt in the middle of the chest
- does not come on suddenly, but usually builds up over a few minutes
- characteristically radiates to the neck, jaw or left arm.

What?

Ask for a specific description of the character of the pain. Patients sometimes have difficulty finding appropriate adjectives; you may have to make a few suggestions, e.g. aching, burning, stabbing, crushing, sharp, squeezing, tearing, throbbing, tight—but be careful to give enough options so as not to make your suggestions obviously leading. How bad was the pain? Ask the patient to rank it on a scale of 1–10, 10 being the worst pain that they could imagine. In patients with a clear previous history of stable angina, always ask whether the current pain at rest resembles their usual exertional pain.

Ischaemic cardiac pain is typically crushing, squeezing or tight.

Did you notice anything else with the pain?

Are there features that are commonly associated with MI?:
- Did you sweat?
- Were you nauseous? And did you vomit ?
- Did you think you were going to die?

How long did the pain last?

Ischaemic cardiac pain is not fleeting in nature (i.e. a few seconds only), nor does it persist constantly for several days.

Can you make an alternative diagnosis?

Make sure that you consider the options discussed below.

Could the pain be the result of aortic dissection?

If it came on suddenly, is described as 'tearing' or radiates to the back, you must look particularly carefully for evidence of aortic dissection.

Could the pain be caused by oesophagitis, which can be precipitated by bending and lifting?

Ask about belching and reflux, history of indigestion, use of remedies for indigestion or a history of previous investigation for indigestion ('You've never had a barium meal or an endoscopy, have you?'). (See *Gastroenterology*, Section 1.2.)

Could the pain be musculoskeletal?

Unaccustomed physical activity can provoke both ischaemic cardiac pain and musculoskeletal pain. Musculoskeletal pain tends to be less severe and of different character, and can usually be made better or worse by change in position; this is not a feature of ischaemic cardiac pain.

Could the pain result from pericarditis?

Most unlikely in this case—usually a concern in younger patients at low risk of coronary disease, when the most common cause is viral: 'Have you had 'flu or anything like that recently?' The pain often has a superficial quality and may be affected by position, typically improving when the patient leans forward. (See Section 1.14, p. 42.)

Could the chest pain result from anxiety?

Tingling fingers in association with chest pain suggests hyperventilation, but never jump immediately to the diagnosis of 'anxiety'—severe pain (e.g. cardiac ischaemia) may have produced the hyperventilation.

Relevant past history

This provides essential information to judge whether the patient's chest pain is likely to be caused by IHD or, in the jargon, 'to risk stratify the patient'. To put it simply, a young woman with no cardiac risk factors is exceedingly unlikely to have IHD, even if she gives a 'classic' history of angina, whereas it is almost inconceivable that a middle-aged or elderly man who smokes and gives the same history does not have IHD. Focus on the points discussed below.

Previous cardiac events

Ask the patient specifically about the following:
- Angina (stable or unstable)
- MI
- Cardiac catheterization
- Revascularization procedures (percutaneous transluminal coronary angioplasty [PTCA] or coronary arterial bypass grafting [CABG]).

Previous vascular events (non-cardiac)

Ask the patient about a history of the following:
- Stroke/transient ischaemic attack (TIA)
- Peripheral vascular disease.

Risk factors

It is essential to elicit a history of the following:
- Family history
- Smoking
- Hypertension
- Hypercholesterolaemia
- Diabetes.

 Oesophageal pain is often indistinguishable from ischaemic cardiac pain. Both may occur at rest, both may be severe and both are common. Cardiac pain may be associated with, and even relieved by, belching. Beware of discharging a high-risk patient with a clinical diagnosis of oesophageal pain.

Examination

Is the patient well, ill, very ill or nearly dead? Patients having an MI rarely look well; if they look nearly dead, call for intensive care unit (ICU) help immediately! All patients complaining of chest pain need prompt, rapid assessment.

Cardiovascular

Cardiovascular examination in patients presenting with acute central chest pain is frequently normal, which is probably why it is often performed in a cursory manner. Check: peripheral perfusion; pulse rate, rhythm and character; blood pressure; JVP; apex beat; for palpable heaves or thrills; heart sounds and murmurs; lung bases; peripheral pulses; and for ankle swelling. Do not forget key signs that are often missed, including the following:
• Unequal radial pulses and unequal blood pressures in the two arms (?aortic dissection)
• Early diastolic murmur of aortic regurgitation (?aortic dissection)
• Harsh ejection systolic murmur of aortic stenosis
• Pericardial rub.

Abdominal

Do not forget to palpate the epigastrium: is this tender? Is there guarding? Patients with an intra-abdominal catastrophe, e.g. perforated peptic ulcer or pancreatitis, can present with pain in the lower chest and signs of circulatory collapse, making it look very much as though they are having an MI.

Musculoskeletal

If the pain is worse on moving and reproduced by chest wall compression, a musculoskeletal cause is likely.

Approach to investigations and management

 A patient with previously stable angina who presents with increasing frequency and severity of chest pains over a few days ('crescendo angina') is very likely to have an unstable coronary plaque and should be admitted for treatment and further assessment, even if pain free at the time of consultation.

If the patient is hypotensive with poor peripheral perfusion, then proceed as described in *Emergency medicine*, Section 1.2; if not, then proceed to establish a diagnosis as follows.

Investigations

The key investigations are those that will indicate whether or not the patient is suffering from an acute coronary syndrome, i.e. the ECG and biochemical markers of heart muscle damage.

ECG

Look for specific abnormalities:
• ST-segment elevation/left bundle-branch block (LBBB) (MI) (Fig. 11)
• ST-segment depression (unstable angina) (Fig. 12)
• T-wave inversion (may be MI/unstable angina)
• ST-segment elevation concave upwards (pericarditis).

 An entirely normal ECG is associated with relatively low risk but does not rule out serious coronary disease or the presence of unstable angina.

 A patient presenting with a normal ECG, who has had normal coronary angiography within the preceding 5 years, is unlikely to be suffering from an acute coronary syndrome, but this cannot be completely excluded.

Biochemical markers of heart muscle damage

Creatine kinase (CK) and its more specific cardiac isoform, CK-MB, have been used to diagnose MI retrospectively in those with a 'non-diagnostic' ECG. Troponins are more specific and sensitive markers of heart muscle damage and are superseding CK. (See Section 3.7, p. 135.)

Fig. 11 Acute inferior myocardial infarction. The ECG shows ST segment deviation in the inferior leads (II, III and AVF). ST segment depression in leads V2 and V3 may indicate posterior extension.

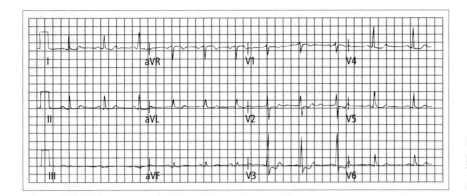

Fig. 12 ECG showing ST depression in a patient presenting with acute chest pain. Thrombolysis is not beneficial, and may be harmful in these circumstances.

Other blood tests

Check FBC, cholesterol, electrolytes, renal and liver function tests. In some cases where there is diagnostic doubt, it will be appropriate to measure the serum amylase.

Chest radiograph

Look for cardiomegaly, pulmonary oedema and mediastinal widening (aortic dissection).

Consider thoracic aortic dissection (see Section 2.11.1, p. 99) if there is the following:
- History of sudden onset, 'tearing' central chest pain, radiating to the back
- History of hypertension
- Patient looks 'marfanoid'
- Inferior infarction on ECG (dissection extended to right coronary artery)
- Mediastinal widening on chest radiograph.

Management

Give oxygen, analgesia (opiate if necessary) and aspirin 300 mg while the diagnosis is being established. Further treatment depends on the underlying cause:
- MI: see Section 2.1.3, p. 55
- Unstable angina: see Section 2.1.2, p. 53
- Oesophagitis: see *Gastroenterology*, Section 2.2
- Suspected aortic dissection: see Section 2.11.1, p. 99
- Pericarditis: see Section 2.6.1, p. 78
- Coronary vasospasm: treat with high doses of calcium antagonist; avoid β blockers which may exacerbate vasospasm.

Persisting pain of uncertain cause

Reassure the patient that there is no evidence for heart attack at present, but admit for overnight observation and repeat ECG/cardiac markers at 12–24 h.

Pain gone, diagnosis uncertain

Most patients require overnight admission. However, a negative troponin test in conjunction with favourable clinical and ECG criteria is increasingly being used to identify low-risk patients who may be discharged early without the need for overnight stay. However, it is important to realize that a negative troponin test does not rule out coronary disease. Patients discharged early in these circumstances must have more detailed risk assessment within the next few weeks, which should include an exercise test (see Section 3.1.1, p. 124). Patients should be invited to seek medical help again if their symptoms return.

In difficult cases, consider coronary vasospasm:
- Multiple admissions
- Negative coronary angiogram ('minor irregularities')
- Paroxysms of crushing central chest pain at rest
- Relieved by glyceryl trinitrate (GTN)
- No limitation of exercise
- Pain often associated with profuse sweating, occasionally with syncope
- Usually benign, but patients with significant ECG changes or ventricular arrhythmia during pain must be admitted for urgent treatment and investigation (Fig. 13).

See *Emergency medicine*, Sections 1.1, 1.2 and 1.3.
See *Gastroenterology*, Section 1.2.
Braunwald E. The history. In: Braunwald E (ed.) *Heart Disease*. Philadelphia, PA: WB Saunders Co., 1996: 3–7.
Crea F, Kaski JC, Maseri A. Key references on coronary artery spasm. *Circulation* 1994; 89: 2442–2446.
Goldman L, Cook EF, Johnson PA *et al*. Prediction of the need for intensive care in patients coming to the emergency department with acute chest pain. *N Engl J Med* 1996; 334: 1498–1504.
Hamm CW, Goldman BU, Heeschen C *et al*. Emergency room triage of patients with acute chest pain by means of rapid testing for cardiac troponin T or troponin I. *N Engl J Med* 1997; 337: 1648–1653.
Hillis SG, Fox KAA. Cardiac troponins in chest pain. *BMJ* 1999; 319: 1451–1452.

(a)   (b)

Fig. 13 Left coronary angiogram demonstrating coronary vasospasm. This 34-year-old woman presented with chest pain and anterior ST segment elevation on the ECG. Shortly afterwards, she had a VF arrest. After resuscitation, the ECG returned to normal. (a) Initial angiography showed a normal left coronary artery. (b) Intracoronary ergometrine induced localized spasm of the proximal left anterior descending coronary artery, and reproduced the chest pain with ECG changes.

1.6 Breathlessness and ankle swelling

Case history

A 48-year-old professor of mathematics presents with a 6-week history of progressive breathlessness and bilateral ankle swelling.

Clinical approach

These symptoms are most commonly caused by cardiac or pulmonary disease. The cause usually becomes apparent early in the history, and subsequent questions, examination and investigation should be directed to providing confirmatory details. The common differential diagnoses are given in Table 4.

History of the presenting problem

If the following do not emerge spontaneously, make specific enquiry about them:
• Chest pain: if present, does this sound like ischaemic cardiac pain or like pleurisy?
• Cough/sputum, and has there been haemoptysis?
• Wheeze, but note that this is not synonymous with

Table 4 Differential diagnosis of ankle swelling and breathlessness.

Cardiac	Left ventricular dysfunction*
	Valvular heart disease*
	Pericardial effusion/constriction
	Cyanotic congenital heart disease
	High-output cardiac failure secondary to anaemia
Pulmonary	Chronic airway or parenchymal lung disease*
	Chronic, repeated pulmonary embolism
	Primary pulmonary hypertension
Gastrointestinal	Liver failure
	Protein-losing enteropathy
Renal	Nephrotic syndrome
	Chronic renal failure
Endocrine	Hypothyroidism

*Most common causes.

airway disease—it may occur in pulmonary oedema when it is known as 'cardiac asthma'.

Cardiac

Progressive breathlessness associated with orthopnoea, paroxysmal nocturnal dyspnoea and cough productive of clear, frothy sputum would suggest a cardiac cause. The ankle swelling in cardiac failure is usually bilateral and symmetrical, but it is not uncommon for one ankle to swell initially. A preceding episode of severe central chest pain at rest, particularly if occurring against a background of stable angina, would suggest a precipitating MI—the 'really bad episode of indigestion' may have been something different.

Pulmonary

The development of increasing breathlessness and ankle swelling may indicate the development of cor pulmonale in a man with long-standing respiratory disorder. His symptoms are said to have started only 6 weeks ago, but what was he like before then? What is the most vigorous exercise he ever took? Three months ago was his breathing more laboured than that of his wife, family or friends?

Pulmonary embolism

Stepwise progression (sudden deterioration followed by periods of stability) should raise the suspicion of multiple recurrent pulmonary emboli, even in the absence of pleuritic chest pain or haemoptysis.

Relevant past history

Ask about the following:
• Is there anything at all to suggest IHD: heart attack, angina, chest tightness on exercise that may not have been recognized as significant?
• Rheumatic fever or cardiac murmur
• Recurrent asthma/bronchitis or any other respiratory problem
• Smoking, which is obviously a substantial risk factor for both chronic airway disease and IHD
• Alcohol intake
• Thromboembolism.

Examination

A full examination is required, but pay particular attention to the cardiac and respiratory systems. Do not finish your examination until you are absolutely sure where the JVP is.

General

Look for cyanosis, anaemia or stigmata of chronic liver disease.

Cardiac

Look for signs of cardiac dysfunction, check:
• Pulse rate, rhythm, volume and character: a sinus tachycardia may be caused by anxiety or cardiac failure;

consider specifically 'is this man in atrial fibrillation?'. A low-volume pulse might indicate cardiac failure, but is there anything about the character to suggest either aortic stenosis or incompetence?
• Blood pressure, including pulsus paradoxus, which suggests pericardial effusion/tamponade (see Section 2.6.2, p. 80).
• JVP—is this raised?
• Apex beat—is this displaced?
• Is there an S3 gallop?
• Are there murmurs (especially diastolic)?
• Are there basal crepitations? But remember that these are not specific for pulmonary oedema and cardiac failure.

Look for signs of pulmonary hypertension, which is indicated by the following:
• Raised JVP
• Left parasternal heave (palpable right ventricle)
• Loud pulmonary component of the second heart sound.

Also note whether one leg is much more swollen than the other, which might indicate deep venous thrombosis.

Respiratory

Check the shape and expansion of the chest: does this suggest chronic airways disease? Are there any abnormal chest signs (other than basal crepitations)? If there are, a respiratory cause of breathlessness and oedema is likely. Check the peak flow. (See *Respiratory medicine*, Section 1.1.)

 Oedema of the hands and face is a feature of hypoalbuminaemia, and is very rarely the result of congestive cardiac failure (Fig. 14).

Approach to investigations and management

Investigations

These will focus on the heart and lungs. Initial investigations should include an ECG, chest radiograph, urine stick tests for protein and 'screening' blood tests.

Fig. 14 Hand oedema in a patient with hypoalbuminaemia.

Fig. 15 ECG showing left atrial strain (inverted P wave in V1) and partial left bundle-branch block in a patient with severe congestive cardiac failure secondary to alcoholic cardiomyopathy.

ECG

Look for the following:
• Previous MI, LBBB or poor R-wave progression indicating left ventricular disease.
• A dominantly negative P wave in lead V1, reflecting left atrial hypertrophy—an indirect sign of left heart dysfunction (Fig. 15).
• Right ventricular hypertrophy (right bundle-branch block [RBBB] with dominant R waves in V1) secondary to any cause of pulmonary hypertension.
• Low voltages and electrical alternans, which occur with a large pericardial effusion.
• Atrial arrhythmias: common in both cardiac and pulmonary disease.

Chest radiograph

In the context of an elevated JVP:
• A large heart should prompt echocardiography (Fig. 16).
• Are there signs of pulmonary oedema?
• If the heart size is normal, inspect the lung fields closely for evidence of chronic obstructive airway disease or parenchymal lung disease.
• If the heart size and lung fields are both normal, consider pulmonary embolism or pericardial constriction.

Blood tests

Check the FBC, electrolytes, and renal, liver and thyroid function tests.

Urinalysis

Do not forget this simple test. If there is significant

Fig. 16 Chest radiograph showing cardiomegaly and pulmonary oedema in a patient with congestive cardiac failure caused by severe mitral regurgitation. Note cardiomegaly and enlarged left atrium.

proteinuria on dipstick testing (≥2+), the nephrotic syndrome is possible. Check serum albumin and 24-h urinary protein excretion. Remember that proteinuria of up to 1 g/day can be caused by severe cardiac failure.

If the history, examination and tests described above suggest a cardiac cause for breathlessness and oedema, the following cardiac investigations may be needed to make a precise diagnosis.

Echocardiogram

Echocardiography is most useful for ruling out significant valvular or left ventricular disease. Pericardial effusion is commonly found, but careful clinical and echocardiographic assessment is required to judge whether this is contributing to symptoms (see Section 2.6.2, p. 80). Assessment of right heart function is largely subjective, but reasonably accurate indirect measurements of pulmonary artery systolic pressure can be obtained. Echocardiography may suggest pericardial constriction or restrictive cardiomyopathy, which requires cardiac catheterization for confirmation. (See Sections 2.4.3, p. 70 and 2.6.3, p. 82.)

Cardiac catheterization

Right heart catheterization is the most accurate way to measure pulmonary artery pressures. It is useful for detection and quantification of an intracardiac shunt, e.g. atrial septal defect (ASD). It can confirm pericardial constriction and help distinguish it from restrictive cardiomyopathy (see Section 2.4.3, p. 70). It also allows pulmonary angiography if pulmonary embolism is suspected.

Left heart catheterization allows coronary angiography and assessment of valvular dysfunction.

CT of the chest

Spiral CT has a high sensitivity for the detection of pulmonary embolism. It is preferred to ventilation–perfusion scanning if the lung fields are abnormal on a chest radiograph (see Section 2.18, p. 115). It may be helpful in suspected pericardial constriction. (See Section 2.6.3, p. 82.)

- The presence of bilateral basal crackles on auscultation of the chest has a very poor positive predictive value for the presence of pulmonary oedema—a chest radiograph is much more accurate.
- Beware that marked abnormality of renal and liver function tests commonly occurs in congestive cardiac failure, and does not necessarily indicate primary disease in these organs.
- The severity of left ventricular dysfunction on echocardiography correlates poorly with severity of the clinical syndrome of heart failure. However, normal systolic left ventricular function on echocardiography should prompt review of a diagnosis of heart failure.

When the cause of breathlessness is not obvious, consider chronic repeated pulmonary thromboembolism.

This is a commonly missed diagnosis. Multiple small pulmonary emboli lead to progressive occlusion of the pulmonary arteriolar bed, classically presenting with breathlessness that becomes more severe in a stepwise manner. Pulmonary hypertension eventually leads to right ventricular failure and ankle swelling. Prominent pulmonary arteries may be the only finding on a chest radiograph. Diagnosis is made by ventilation–perfusion scan or spiral CT.

Consider primary pulmonary hypertension, particularly in young women with unexplained breathlessness.

This is a rare condition that predominantly affects young women. Although usually idiopathic, there is a link with appetite-suppressant drugs. It presents with progressive breathlessness and fatigue, and is commonly misdiagnosed as asthma. Exertional chest pain ('right ventricular angina') is sometimes a feature. In the later stages, the condition is complicated by peripheral oedema resulting from right heart failure. Diagnosis is by exclusion of recognized causes of pulmonary hypertension, and requires cardiac catheterization. (See Sections 1.10, p. 30, and 2.12.1, p. 101.)

Management

Where breathlessness and oedema are caused by cardiac dysfunction, loop diuretics are central to the relief of symptoms in most cases. Give intravenously if symptoms are severe, but be aware that aggressive diuresis may precipitate circulatory collapse in those who require a high filling pressure, e.g. chronic pulmonary thromboembolism, cor pulmonale, pericardial disease, cyanotic congenital heart disease.

Further management depends on the underlying cause:
- Left ventricular dysfunction: see Section 2.3, p. 63
- Valvular heart disease: see Section 2.5, p. 71
- Pericardial effusion/constriction: see Section 2.6, p. 78
- Cyanotic congenital heart disease: see Section 2.7, p. 84
- Chronic lung disease: see *Respiratory medicine*, Sections 2.3 and 2.11
- Chronic, repeated pulmonary embolism: see Section 2.18, p. 115
- Primary pulmonary hypertension: see Section 2.12.1, p. 101
- Chronic liver disease: see *Gastroenterology*, Section 2.10
- Nephrotic syndrome: see *Nephrology*, Section 2.1.4
- Chronic renal failure: see *Nephrology*, Section 2.1.2.

It is always worth checking that patients with oedema are aware of the need to avoid adding salt to their food. If salt is essential then modest amounts of 'Lo-Salt' (KCl) are better than NaCl. Also check what food they are eating—you would be surprised how many people with oedema insist that they 'do not add any salt to their food', but eat crisps, salted peanuts or tinned soup containing large amounts of it.

See *Emergency medicine*, Section 1.5.

Cohn JN. Drug therapy: the management of chronic heart failure. *N Engl J Med* 1996; 335: 490–498. Review article.

Gaine SP, Rubin LJ. Primary pulmonary hypertension. *Lancet* 1998; 352: 719–725. Review article.

Goldhaber SZ. Pulmonary embolism. *N Engl J Med* 1998; 339: 93–104. Review article.

Watson RDS, Gibbs CR, Lip GYH. ABC of heart failure: clinical features and complications. *BMJ* 2000; 320: 236–239. Review article.

1.7 Hypotension following myocardial infarction

Case history

A 59-year-old man was admitted with an inferior MI for which he was treated with aspirin and thrombolysis. Three hours after admission his condition was judged stable enough to give atenolol. The following morning he was reviewed by a consultant cardiologist on the post-take round, and was felt to have had an uncomplicated course. A CK of 3651 IU/mL was noted, and an ACE inhibitor was recommended. Before this drug could be given, the senior house officer (SHO) was asked to see the patient urgently because he had become drowsy with a systolic blood pressure of 60 mmHg.

Clinical approach

The cause of profound hypotension after MI can usually be established by examining the patient, obtaining an ECG and chest radiograph, and scrutinizing the drug chart. Consider the diagnoses listed in Table 5.

History of presenting problem

Pay particular attention to the following:
• Chest pain: recurrent pain may indicate reinfarction or cardiac rupture.
• Onset: a period of stability followed by an abrupt drop in blood pressure indicates a catastrophic event, but

Table 5 Differential diagnosis of hypotension after myocardial infarction.

Drug induced	Streptokinase infusion
	Intravenous nitrate
	β Blocker
	Angiotensin-converting enzyme inhibitor
Cardiac	Bradyarrhythmia
	Tachyarrhythmia
	Acute left ventricular dysfunction (including reinfarction)
	Acute right ventricular dysfunction (right ventricular infarct)
	Acute mitral regurgitation
	Ventricular septal defect (VSD secondary to septal rupture)
	Cardiac rupture with tamponade
	Aortic dissection
Other (less likely)	Dehydration
	Haemorrhage
	Pulmonary embolus
	Sepsis

hypotension resulting from left ventricular pump failure tends to be more insidious.
• Drugs: look for a temporal relationship of hypotension to administration of drugs—hypotension during infusion of streptokinase is common and usually occurs during the first 20 min.
• Breathlessness: acute breathlessness associated with hypotension may indicate pulmonary oedema.
• Volume depletion: may rarely be caused after MI by vomiting without adequate fluid replacement. This is unlikely to be the explanation, but examine the fluid balance charts.

Examination

General

Assess the general clinical condition of the patient:
• If the patient looks as though he or she is about to arrest, call for resuscitation team help immediately. Do not wait until you are sure that the heart has stopped.
• Conscious level: check the Glasgow Coma Score.
• Pain level.

Cardiovascular

Pay specific attention to the following:
• Peripheral circulation: it is a poor prognostic sign if the patient is shut down—how far up the arms and legs are they cold?
• Heart rate and rhythm
• Blood pressure: measure this yourself. Can you feel the pulse and measure the blood pressure in the left arm? Could the patient have had a dissection, presenting with inferior MI and now progressing?
• JVP: if markedly elevated consider right ventricular infarction, ventricular septal defect (VSD), tamponade or pulmonary embolism.
• S3 gallop.
• New pansystolic murmur: which would suggest VSD or mitral regurgitation, perhaps as a result of chordal or papillary muscle rupture.

Approach to investigations and management

Investigations

The diagnosis should become apparent with the following basic investigations:
• ECG: arrhythmia or reinfarction?
• Chest radiograph: do not assume there is no pulmonary oedema unless you have seen a recent chest radiograph.

- Arterial blood gases: will document hypoxia, which is likely to be the result of pulmonary oedema, but in the presence of a normal chest radiograph would suggest pulmonary embolus.
- Echocardiogram: provides rapid information about left (and to a lesser extent right) ventricular function. Also useful in detection of tamponade, acute mitral regurgitation and VSD.
- Urea and electrolytes to establish renal function.
- Cardiac enzymes: has there been reinfarction?

Differential diagnosis

Consider the diagnoses listed in Table 5—look particularly for evidence of the following:

Acute mitral regurgitation

- Inferior infarction
- Severe pulmonary oedema
- Murmur may not be present as a result of rapid equalization of left ventricular and left atrial pressures
- Echocardiography is diagnostic (Fig. 17).

Acquired ventricular septal defect

- Very high JVP
- Less severe pulmonary oedema than acute mitral regurgitation
- New systolic murmur
- Usually picked up by echocardiography
- Consider a Swan–Ganz pulmonary artery catheter—this will demonstrate a 'step up' in oxygen saturation at the level of the right ventricle, indicating left-to-right shunting.

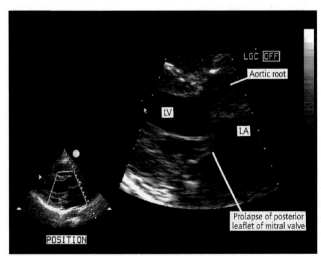

Fig. 17 Transoesophageal echocardiogram showing prolapse of the posterior mitral valve leaflet (indicated) into the left atrium (LA) after papillary muscle rupture. LV, left ventricle.

Ischaemic left ventricular dysfunction

- Severe coronary disease (especially critical left main-stem stenosis)
- Recurrent chest pain accompanied by transient hypotension, pulmonary oedema and widespread ischaemia/acute infarction on the ECG
- Patients are at high risk of death: refer for cardiac catheterization and appropriate revascularization.

Right ventricular infarction

- Inferior infarction
- Hypotensive patient with high JVP
- Clear lung fields on chest radiograph.

Management

Hypotension after an MI should always be taken seriously and treated quickly, even if the patient appears not to be *in extremis*. Monitor heart rhythm, blood pressure, pulse oximetry, hourly urine output, fluid balance, daily electrolytes and renal function. Then:

- Stop drugs that may contribute to hypotension
- Give high-flow oxygen
- If possible, identify and treat the underlying cause: acute mitral regurgitation and VSD are indications for urgent referral to a cardiothoracic surgeon.

Does the patient require fluid or inotropes? It is often difficult to know. The obvious risk is that fluid could precipitate pulmonary oedema, and monitoring of the pulmonary capillary wedge pressure (PCWP) with a Swan–Ganz catheter is very helpful in this context. As a general rule:

- If the lungs are reasonably clear, the patient is not profoundly hypoxic, and hypotension is the main problem, then give intravenously 250 mL 0.9% saline and reasses, repeating if necessary. This will help those with right ventricular infarction because increasing the preload will increase right ventricular output (See *Physiology*, Section 1.2). Consider inotropes, e.g. dobutamine, epinephrine (adrenaline).
- If there are lots of crackles in the lungs and the patient is hypoxic as well as hypotensive, a bolus of saline will not help and could be fatal. Start inotropes, e.g. dobutamine, epinephrine (adrenaline). Call for ICU help—the patient is likely to die soon if not ventilated electively.

 In a patient who has become breathless and hypotensive with pulmonary oedema on the chest radiograph, inotropic agents may be started without the insertion of a Swan–Ganz catheter because the left atrial filling pressure is almost certainly high. PCWP measurement becomes useful if the clinical situation has not become satisfactory over the next 12–24 h.

Communication

The prognosis of profound hypotension after MI is very poor. You, or one of your colleagues, may have talked to the patient's next of kin when he or she was first admitted and warned of the gravity of the diagnosis. They certainly need to be spoken to now. If they are not present, phone them as soon as management is under way to see if they wish to come up to the hospital. Take your time, speak slowly and do not be afraid of silence or tears:
- 'This is Dr Brown from the hospital . . .'
- 'We promised that we would call if there was any change in the situation . . .' (warning that you are about to give bad news)
- 'I'm calling to say that I'm afraid that your husband has taken a turn for the worse . . .'
- 'His blood pressure has fallen . . .'
- 'We're doing some tests to find out why, and have started to give him some treatment to help the heart, but the situation is serious . . .' (The wife may say 'is he going to die?')
- 'His heart is under a lot of strain; we're doing everything we can; but I don't know whether he is going to pull through . . .' (The wife may say 'how long?')
- 'We have to take things as they come, an hour at a time.'

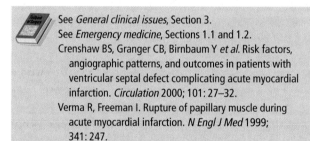

See *General clinical issues*, Section 3.
See *Emergency medicine*, Sections 1.1 and 1.2.
Crenshaw BS, Granger CB, Birnbaum Y *et al.* Risk factors, angiographic patterns, and outcomes in patients with ventricular septal defect complicating acute myocardial infarction. *Circulation* 2000; 101: 27–32.
Verma R, Freeman I. Rupture of papillary muscle during acute myocardial infarction. *N Engl J Med* 1999; 341: 247.

1.8 Breathlessness and haemodynamic collapse

Case history

You are bleeped urgently by A&E to see a 55-year-old woman brought in by ambulance. Her husband called 999 this morning when he found her acutely breathless at home. She had a brief syncopal episode on being moved into the ambulance, but is now conscious, although extremely dyspnoeic, and her blood pressure is only 80 mmHg systolic.

Clinical approach

The following are the priorities:
- Resuscitate (**a**irway, **b**reathing, **c**irculation) and secure venous access while taking the history
- Give high-flow oxygen
- Examine with a clear idea of possible causes of breathlessness and haemodynamic collapse in mind (Table 6)
- Exclude tension pneumothorax—insert a large bore cannula into the silent side of the chest (second intercostal space, midclavicular line) if this is the clinical diagnosis
- Exclude other diagnoses that can be established quickly: arrhythmia, acute MI with definitive ECG changes.

History of presenting problem

If you can obtain a history from the patient and/or her husband, ask particularly about the following:
- Sudden or gradual onset: sudden onset suggests pneumothorax, massive pulmonary embolus (PE), acute valve dysfunction, dissection or arrhythmia
- Central chest or interscapular pain: suggesting MI or aortic dissection
- Pleuritic chest pain or haemoptysis: suggesting smaller PEs preceding a larger one

Table 6 Differential diagnosis of acute dyspnoea and haemodynamic collapse. Note that, although tension pneumothorax is uncommon, this diagnosis should be considered before all others.

General cause	Comment	Specific cause
Cardiac	Common	Myocardial infarction/complications (acute mitral regurgitation, VSD, acute left ventricular failure)
		Arrhythmia (VT)
	Less common	Aortic dissection
		Cardiac tamponade
		Acute aortic regurgitation
Cardiorespiratory	Common	Massive PE (occluding >50% pulmonary vasculature)
Respiratory	Common	Acute life-threatening asthma
	Less common	Tension pneumothorax
Other	Common	Sepsis
	Less common	Intra-abdominal catastrophe
		Severe haemorrhage ('air hunger')
		Anaphylaxis

PE, pulmonary embolism; VSD, ventricular septal defect; VT, ventricular tachycardia.

- Symptoms suggestive of pulmonary oedema: orthopnoea, paroxysmal nocturnal dyspnoea (PND), pink frothy sputum
- Worsening asthma
- Abdominal pain, vomiting, haematemesis, melaena: could there have been an intra-abdominal catastrophe?
- Symptoms suggestive of sepsis: the most common infective cause of hypotension and breathlessness would be septicaemia and acute respiratory distress syndrome (ARDS), but with 'flu-like illness also consider pericardial effusion with sudden decompensation
- Exposure to a known allergen.

Relevant past history

There is not time for a lengthy history, but ask about the following:
- Pulmonary embolism or deep venous thrombosis and relevant risk factors (see Section 2.18, p. 115)
- Cardiac: MI, angina, previously undiagnosed anginal pain, valve disease, rheumatic fever, 'heart murmur' (and if so any recent dental work or surgery—could she have acute valve dysfunction caused by infective endocarditis); hypertension (risk factor for IHD and aortic dissection)
- Respiratory: asthma, chronic airflow obstruction, pneumothorax
- Abdominal: peptic ulcers, pancreatitis, gallstones
- Anaphylaxis: allergy to anything?
- Drugs: a useful rapid marker for past medical history in this context!

 If no history is available, check bags and pockets for inhalers, GTN, etc.

Examination

 This woman will look very ill or nearly dead; if nearly dead, call for ICU help or the cardiac resuscitation team immediately. Do not wait until she has a cardiac arrest if she looks as though she is deteriorating.

Immediate assessment

- Vital signs: pulse (rate and rhythm), blood pressure, respiratory rate, temperature.
- Is there cyanosis? Check pulse oximetry (but do not remove the high-flow oxygen to 'check value on air' in someone who is desperately ill!).
- Conscious level: the Glasgow Coma Score.
- Is there swelling of the lips and tongue (anaphylaxis)?

Is this a tension pneumothorax?

- Chest looks asymmetrical, with side under tension 'blown up'.

- Tracheal deviation away from the side under tension.
- Mediastinal shift: apex beat not in the normal place; cardiac dullness moved to left or right away from the side under tension.
- Side of chest under tension is silent.

Cardiovascular

- Is there paradox? If the pulse becomes impalpable on inspiration, this could be severe asthma or cardiac tamponade.
- Can you feel the left radial pulse? Is the blood pressure the same in the left arm as the right? Could this be an aortic dissection?
- Where is the JVP? This is a critical piece of information: if high, this suggests that the cause of hypotension and breathlessness is cardiac or respiratory; if low, then go for bleeding, intra-abdominal catastrophe or sepsis.
- Are there features to suggest massive pulmonary embolism? High JVP, right ventricular heave, tricuspid regurgitation.
- Could there be acute mitral regurgitation or an acute VSD? Listen for a pansystolic murmur (see Section 1.7, p. 23 for further information). Note that acute aortic regurgitation might not produce an audible early diastolic murmur.
- Can you hear the heart sounds and is there a pericardial rub? Quiet sounds might indicate pericardial fluid and a rub would suggest pericarditis—both making tamponade a likely diagnosis in this context.

Respiratory

- A silent chest would suggest life-threatening asthma.
- Are there any other dramatic signs? A chest full of crackles is likely to indicate severe pulmonary oedema or aspiration. An area of bronchial breathing may indicate that pneumonia is the primary diagnosis.

Abdominal

- Is there tenderness, guarding or an abdominal aortic aneurysm?
- Is there melaena on rectal examination?

Legs

- Signs of a deep venous thrombosis are not necessary for a diagnosis of PE, but would strongly support the diagnosis.

Skin and nails

- Could those spots be meningococcal?
- Are those splinters endocarditic?

Approach to investigations and management

 Always remember that the history, examination, investigation and management should be in parallel, not in series, when dealing with patients who are severely ill.

Investigations

The following investigations are required immediately in all patients who present with severe hypotension and breathlessness.

Blood tests

Check BM stix immediately in anyone who is severely ill. Check arterial gases. Take samples for FBC, electrolytes, renal and liver function tests, cardiac enzymes and blood cultures.

ECG

Perform a 12-lead ECG immediately, and repeat after 1 h (sooner if clinically indicated), looking for the following:
• Arrhythmia (see Section 2.2, p. 58).
• Localized ST segment elevation of acute MI (see Section 2.1.3, p. 55).
• ECG changes compatible with acute PE, the most common being sinus tachycardia and T-wave inversion in leads V1–V4. The 'typical' right axis deviation and 'S1Q3T3' are actually quite unusual (see Section 2.18, p. 115).
• Generalized ST-segment elevation of pericarditis (much less common in this context) or low voltages/voltages of pericardial effusion (see Section 2.6, p. 78).

Chest radiograph

Look for pneumothorax, pulmonary oligaemia (PE), pulmonary oedema, consolidation, effusions, heart size, mediastinal shift and the widened mediastinum of aortic dissection.

 A normal mediastinal width on the chest radiograph does not exclude aortic dissection.

Further investigations may be indicated depending on clinical findings and the results of immediate tests.

Echocardiogram

An echocardiogram is the examination of choice to look for effusion, valve regurgitation and VSD, and to assess ventricular function. Remember that right ventricular dysfunction in the context of acute severe dyspnoea and hypoxia is highly suspicious of a massive PE.

Other investigations

Discuss with a senior colleague whether further imaging is required to establish the diagnosis: tests that may be indicated for suspected PE include ventilation–perfusion ($\dot{V}/\dot{Q}$) scanning, contrast CT of the chest, pulmonary angiography and ultrasound of the leg veins. Check CT abdomen if your assessment suggests an abdominal cause.

Management

'General supportive measures' will be required by all patients:
• First priority is always airway, breathing, circulation
• High-flow oxygen, with monitoring of arterial blood gases
• Rapid restoration of intravascular volume in those who are volume deplete (low JVP, postural hypotension—lying and sitting, as standing will clearly not be possible).
    Specific management will depend on the diagnosis:
• Tension pneumothorax: immediate insertion of a wide-bore cannula into the pneumothorax will decompress it and relieve the life-threatening mediastinal shift. (See *Emergency medicine*, Section 1.1; *Respiratory medicine*, Sections 3.2 and 3.4.)
• PE: the two major treatment options for massive PE with haemodynamic collapse are thrombolysis and surgical embolectomy. (See Section 2.18, p. 115.)
• Arrhythmia: see Sections 1.1, p. 3, 1.2, p. 6, 1.3, p. 9 and 2.2, p. 58.
• Complications of MI: see Section 1.7, p. 23.
• Tamponade: urgent pericardiocentesis. (See Section 2.6.2, p. 80.)
• Asthma: see *Emergency medicine*, Section 1.7; *Respiratory medicine*, Section 2.2.2.
• Intra-abdominal catastrophe: call for surgical help immediately; resuscitate while considering surgery and in the anaesthetic room; do not say you will resuscitate and then call the surgeons.
• Anaphylaxis: see *Emergency medicine*, Section 1.29; *Rheumatology and clinical immunology*, Section 1.7.
    And, if you do not know the diagnosis, give broad-spectrum antibiotics to cover sepsis. (See *Emergency medicine*, Section 1.28 and *Infectious diseases*, Section 1.2.)

Communication

After making your clinical assessment, performing immediate investigations and initiating management, you will need to speak to her husband to explain the situation. (See Section 1.7, p. 25, for guidance on how to do this.)

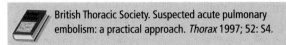

British Thoracic Society. Suspected acute pulmonary embolism: a practical approach. *Thorax* 1997; 52: S4.

1.9 Pleuritic pain

Case history

A 36-year-old male computer programmer presents with a 4-h history of moderately severe left-sided pleuritic chest pain. He was well until yesterday but became unusually breathless while cycling to work today.

Clinical approach

Pleuritic pain is the result of pleural irritation (e.g. by air) or inflammation, which may be caused by infarction (peripheral PE), infection (pneumonia) or as part of a systemic inflammatory disorder, e.g. autoimmune rheumatic disease.

The differential diagnosis of the patient presenting with pleuritic pain is shown in Table 7. The two most important acute diagnoses to consider in this case are pneumothorax and PE. Pneumothorax is easily confirmed or excluded on chest radiograph, but the diagnosis of PE may not be so straightforward.

• A low-grade fever (<38°C) does not necessarily indicate infection, it can be associated with inflammation of any cause, including pulmonary infarction
• Pneumonia may present in a variety of ways and sputum production is not generally an early feature
• Rib fracture tends to be associated with a clearly memorable episode of trauma and is therefore not usually a diagnostic difficulty, but remember the possibility of pathological fracture.

Table 7 Differential diagnosis of patient presenting with pleuritic chest pain.

Common causes	Pulmonary embolism
	Pneumothorax
	Pneumonia
	Musculoskeletal: rib fracture, costochondritis, Bornholm's myalgia (Coxsackie B virus, self-limiting), non-specific
Less common causes	Autoimmune rheumatic disease
	Pericarditis
	Neoplasia: primary or secondary
	Herpes zoster ('Shingles' difficult to diagnose before the rash)

History of presenting problem

Bear in mind the diagnoses listed in Table 7 when taking the history—which is most likely?

Description of the pain

Check the following:
• The pain is definitely pleuritic—sharp, localized and exacerbated by deep inspiration and coughing. If not you need to consider other causes of chest pain. (See Section 1.5, p. 15.) If it is exacerbated by movement and associated with tenderness, a musculoskeletal cause becomes more likely.
• Whether the onset of pain was sudden, associated with coughing or straining (pneumothorax, PE) or gradual. Did it follow a 'flu-like illness (pneumonia, Bornholm myalgia) or an incident of chest trauma (pneumothorax, rib fracture)?

Associated symptoms

Ask about the following:
• Dyspnoea: when did this occur in relation to the pain? How severe—'at rest'/'can't walk'/'can't hurry'?
• Cough: non-specific, but production of purulent sputum indicates likely infection and haemoptysis is a feature of PE, pneumonia and (exceedingly unlikely in this case) malignancy.
• Fever: sweats, rigors and temperature >38.5°C would suggest pneumonia.
• Unilateral leg pain, swelling or tenderness, all suggestive of venous thrombosis and strongly supporting the diagnosis of PE in this case.

Relevant risk factors

Pulmonary embolism

Ask about recent immobility/surgery/travel/dehydration, smoking and family history of PE, deep venous thrombosis or hypercoagulable states. In a woman, ask about pregnancy or use of the oral contraceptive/hormone replacement therapy (HRT).

Pneumothorax

Ask about respiratory disease, recent flights or diving.

Relevant past history

Ask specifically about the following:
• Have there been similar previous episodes? (Always a good question to ask—the patient may tell you the diagnosis!)

- Pneumothorax.
- PE or deep venous thrombosis.
- Autoimmune rheumatic disease.

Examination

The first priority is always to establish how unwell the patient is:
- Is he breathless at rest?
- Does he look cyanosed? Check pulse oximetry.
- Can he speak easily?
- Check peripheral perfusion, pulse, blood pressure, respiratory rate and temperature.

This man is not very ill; he noticed his breathlessness when cycling, immediate assessment does not cause concern, and so the examination can be completed before investigation and treatment are considered.

General

Note the following:
- Habitus: tall thin 'marfanoid' young men have an increased risk of spontaneous pneumothorax
- Labial herpes: often seen in pneumonia
- Signs of autoimmune rheumatic disease.

Cardiovascular

Note particularly the following:
- Cardiac rhythm: atrial fibrillation can occur secondary to PE or pneumonia.
- Signs of right ventricular dysfunction: elevated JVP, parasternal heave, loud P2 and pansystolic murmur of tricuspid regurgitation—any or all of these would support the diagnosis of a large PE, but a patient presenting with a small peripheral PE causing lung infarction and pleurisy (as perhaps in this case) would not be expected to have any of these findings.
- Pericardial rub, indicating pericarditis.
- Calf swelling and tenderness: measure both sides—a difference of >2 cm may indicate venous thrombosis and would strongly support the diagnosis of PE in this clinical context.

Respiratory

Note particularly the following:
- Thoracic tenderness or rib crepitus: exquisite local tenderness clearly suggests a musculoskeletal cause, but there can be local tenderness with pleurisy. Rib crepitus proves that a rib has been broken.
- Expansion, percussion and auscultation: is there a pleural rub? These can be very localized; ask the patient to put a finger on the place that hurts most and listen at this

point and just around it—you may miss a rub if you do not take care to do this. In pneumothorax, expansion may be reduced, percussion note may be hyperresonant, and breath sounds may be diminished on the affected side, but with a small pneumothorax examination may be normal.

Other

Examine the abdomen for masses and the breasts in a woman.

Approach to investigations and management

Investigations

 In the patient presenting with pleuritic pain, the key initial investigation is the chest radiograph.

Chest radiograph

Look specifically for the following:
- Pneumothorax: look very carefully at the lung apex—is there an area within the chest that does not have any lung markings? Can you see a line indicating the edge of the lung? Are you absolutely sure?
- Lobar oligaemia: a rare sign, but suggesting large PE.
- Pleural effusion: this may be visible only as blunting of the costophrenic angle and would be consistent with the diagnosis of PE or pneumonia.
- Wedge-shaped peripheral infarcts: typical of PE.
- Consolidation: typical of pneumonia.

ECG

Look for arrhythmia, RV strain and pericarditis (see Section 3.1, p. 120). Remember that the ECG is most likely to be normal in someone with PE, and also that pain and fear are the most common causes of sinus tachycardia in a patient presenting to hospital.

Arterial blood gases

If the patient is unwell or pulse oximetry indicates oxygen saturation <95%, check arterial blood gases. Some would recommend that this be performed for all patients presenting with pleuritic chest pain. Typical findings in PE presenting with pleurisy are normal PO_2 (but there may be hypoxia) and reduced PCO_2 as a result of hyperventilation.

 If the probable diagnosis is pulmonary embolism, give anticoagulation (low-molecular-weight heparin) immediately, while waiting for confirmatory investigations.

Further investigations may be indicated depending on clinical findings and the results of immediate tests.

Definitive investigation for pulmonary embolism

Ventilation–perfusion scanning (see Section 3.10, p. 140) is the most common readily available imaging test, but CT angiography is increasingly used.

Blood tests

Full blood count, electrolytes, renal and liver function tests, clotting screen, blood cultures, atypical respiratory serology screen, inflammatory markers and tests for autoimmune rheumatic disease may all be indicated in some patients. In a patient who has recovered from a PE, consider checking thrombophilia screen after the therapeutic course of anticoagulation has been stopped. (See *Haematology*, Section 1.20.)

Sputum

If present, sputum should be sent for microscopy, culture and sensitivity, and also for cytology and acid-fast bacilli (TB) if the clinical picture is appropriate.

Management

This depends on the specific diagnosis:
• PE: see Section 2.18, p. 115; see also *Emergency medicine*, Section 1.8 and *Haematology*, Sections 1.13, 1.20 and 3.6.
• Pneumothorax: see *Emergency medicine*, Section 3.3 and *Respiratory medicine*, Sections 3.2 and 3.4.
• Pneumonia: see *Emergency medicine*, Section 1.9; *Infectious diseases*, Section 1.4; *Respiratory medicine*, Section 1.10.
• Musculoskeletal pain: analgesia and reassurance. Particularly in the case of rib fracture adequate analgesia is essential to allow the patient to inspire fully and avoid hypostatic pneumonia. Local intercostal nerve blocks can be very effective.
• Pericarditis: see Sections 1.14, p. 42 and 2.6.1, p. 78.

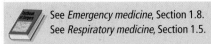
If you diagnose a PE for which there is no obvious cause (e.g. postoperative), perform rectal (and in a woman pelvic) examination and consider pelvic ultrasonography to exclude masses causing deep venous thrombosis by compression.

See *Emergency medicine*, Section 1.8.
See *Respiratory medicine*, Section 1.5.

1.10 Breathlessness and exertional presyncope

Case history

A 30-year-old woman is referred to outpatients because of gradually worsening fatigue and exertional dyspnoea. A year ago she was fit and active but is now unable to jog or attend her usual exercise classes. There has been no improvement with bronchodilator therapy. She is extremely anxious about an episode last week when she nearly fainted while hurrying for a train to a job interview.

Clinical approach

There are suggestions in this history that stress or anxiety may be contributing to this patient's symptoms, but your primary concern should be to exclude the significant organic conditions that can present insidiously like this, shown in Table 8.

Exertional syncope or presyncope is a symptom to be taken seriously. It usually indicates an inability to increase the cardiac output appropriately as a result of a fixed obstruction or ventricular dysfunction.

History of the presenting problem

Presenting symptoms

Ask the patient the following:
• Are you limited by fatigue (may indicate low cardiac output), breathlessness or by something else (what)?
• 'How far can you walk/run?' 'How many flights of stairs?' Be specific about this, and try to get a feeling for the pace of progression by asking: 'How does this compare with last Christmas/during your summer holidays?'
• Have there been any other instances of syncope/presyncope, and exactly what were the circumstances?

Associated symptoms

Ask specifically about the following:
• Chest pain: if present, is this pleuritic or anginal? This woman is young for IHD, but anginal pain can be associated with pulmonary hypertension. This is thought to originate from the hypertrophied (and therefore relatively hypoxic) right ventricle.
• Haemoptysis: a feature of pulmonary hypertension, but could also indicate pulmonary embolism.
• Cough/wheeze/sputum: features that would suggest chronic lung disease.

Table 8 Differential diagnosis of exertional dyspnoea and presyncope.

Pathophysiology	Specific conditions
Left ventricular outflow tract obstruction	Hypertrophic cardiomyopathy Aortic subvalvular/valvular/supravalvular stenosis
Pulmonary hypertension	Primary pulmonary hypertension Secondary, e.g. to respiratory disease, pulmonary thromboembolism or mitral valve disease (see Section 2.12.2, p. 103)
Right ventricular outflow tract obstruction	Infundibular/pulmonary stenosis
Left ventricular dysfunction	See Section 2.3, p. 63
Pericardial compromise of cardiac filling	Effusion Constriction
Anaemia	–
Sustained arrhythmia	Atrial fibrillation Complete heart block

- Orthopnoea/PND: suggests pulmonary oedema.
- Palpitations: see Section 1.2, p. 6.
- Ankle oedema/calf swelling or tenderness: unilateral problems raise the possibility of venous thromboembolism; bilateral swelling suggests RV failure.
- Raynaud's phenomenon: this may be present in autoimmune rheumatic disease and also in 10% of women with primary pulmonary hypertension.
- Any features that would suggest autoimmune rheumatic disease, e.g. joint pains, rashes.

Relevant past history

Enquire specifically about a history of the following:
- Venous thromboembolism
- Rheumatic fever or 'heart murmur'
- Chest trauma or TB—may lead to pericardial problems
- Respiratory disease.
  Also ask about the following:
- Smoking
- Alcohol
- Other risk factors for IHD (see Sections 1.5, p. 15 and 2.1, p. 51)
- Other risk factors for PE (see Sections 1.9, p. 28 and 2.18, p. 115)
- If a cause is not obvious, it may also be appropriate to enquire regarding risk factors for HIV infection (see *General clinical issues*, Section 2).

Drug history

Ask directly about the use of the following:
- Oral contraceptive: risk factor for thromboembolism
- Appetite suppressants: implicated in valve disease and pulmonary hypertension
- Cardiotoxic chemotherapy

- Cocaine: can cause LV dysfunction and pulmonary hypertension.

Family history

Ask about any family history of the following:
- IHD
- PE
- Hypertrophic cardiomyopathy
- Pulmonary hypertension.

 Ask broad questions such as 'has anyone in the family died suddenly?'

 Think about pregnancy

Many previously silent cardiorespiratory conditions manifest themselves in pregnancy because of the physiological changes (see Section 1.16, p. 48).

Examination

General

Is she well or ill? Is she breathless at rest or climbing on to the couch? Look for clinical anaemia, clubbing, cyanosis, malar flush, and signs of autoimmune rheumatic disease or endocarditis.

Cardiovascular and respiratory

Full assessment, noting particularly the following:
- Pulse volume, character, rate and rhythm: is the pulse slow rising (left ventricular outflow tract obstruction) or jerky (hypertrophic cardiomyopathy)? If arrhythmia, see Section 1.2, p. 6.

- Blood pressure: is there a narrow pulse pressure suggesting left ventricular outflow tract obstruction?
- JVP: look very carefully for this—you must decide where it is. It could be very high if the right ventricle is hypertrophied or failing or there is pericardial disease (effusion or constriction).
- Heart sounds and murmurs: added sounds suggest ventricular dysfunction; quiet sounds might be the result of chronic lung disease or pericardial effusion. Is that rather loud third sound a pericardial knock?
- Are the lung fields clear?
- Is there any oedema or hepatomegaly: if there is hepatomegaly, is this pulsatile? If it is, there is tricuspid regurgitation and the JVP must be elevated, even if you did not see it the first time around—look again!

Look for the following patterns:
- Pulmonary hypertension: loud P2 and associated RV hypertrophy (parasternal heave), dilatation (pansystolic murmur of tricuspid regurgitation) and dysfunction (raised JVP, oedema and hepatomegaly)
- LV dysfunction: tachycardia, gallop rhythm and fine basal crackles of pulmonary oedema
- PE: pleural rub, calf swelling and tenderness.

Approach to investigations and management

Investigations

The echocardiogram is the key investigation in the patient with dyspnoea and syncope on exertion.

Blood tests

Check pulse oximetry. Perform arterial blood gases if the oxygen saturation is <95% or the patient looks cyanosed. Check FBC, electrolytes, renal and liver function, glucose, cholesterol and inflammatory markers (CRP and ESR). Other tests for autoimmune rheumatic disease may be indicated. (See *Rheumatology and clinical immunology*, Section 3.2.)

Urinalysis

Look specifically for protein, blood and glucose. Could there be a multisystem inflammatory condition?

ECG

Note the rhythm, axis, and any atrial or ventricular hypertrophy (see Section 3.1, p. 120). LBBB is commonly associated with a dilated LV.

Chest radiograph

Note the heart size and shape, pulmonary arteries, lung fields and any valve calcification or pleural effusions.

Echocardiography

Echocardiography allows visualization of ventricular dimensions, hypertrophy and function, together with outflow tracts and valves (with gradients) and any intracardiac shunt or pericardial effusion. If there is significant pulmonary hypertension a dilated, hypertrophied RV, compressing the LV into a D shape (Fig. 18), can usually be seen and the presence of tricuspid regurgitation allows the measurement of pulmonary artery pressure.

Other

- If the echocardiogram suggests pulmonary hypertension but no cause is apparent, further investigations are needed (see Section 2.12.1, p. 101). These are initially directed towards excluding secondary causes of pulmonary hypertension. If a cause is not discovered and the diagnosis of primary pulmonary hypertension is made, other investigations, e.g. right heart catheterization, are used to determine prognosis and optimize treatment.
- Pulmonary function tests.

Management

Further management will depend on the specific diagnosis:

Fig. 18 Short axis echo view of a patient with primary pulmonary hypertension showing the high pressure, dilated right ventricle (RV) compressing the left ventricle (LV) into a characteristic D shape. (Courtesy of Dr LM Shapiro.)

- Pulmonary hypertension: see Section 2.12, p. 101
- Hypertrophic cardiomyopathy: see Section 2.4.1, p. 66
- Valve disease: see Section 2.5, p. 71
- LV dysfunction: see Section 2.3, p. 63
- Pericardial effusion/constriction: see Sections 2.6.2, p. 80 and 2.6.3, p. 82
- Sustained arrhythmia: see Sections 2.2, p. 58
- Anaemia: see *Haematology*, Section 2.1 for discussion.

Examination and investigations normal

Provide reassurance and encourage the patient to maintain activity, but retain an open mind and keep her under review.

 Peacock AJ. Primary pulmonary hypertension. *Thorax* 1999; 54: 1107–1118.

1.11 Dyspnoea, ankle oedema and cyanosis

Case history

A reclusive 45-year-old man is referred by his GP, having sought medical attention for the first time in his life because of ankle swelling that prevented him from putting on his shoes on. The GP was surprised to find that he was centrally cyanosed and moderately dyspnoeic.

Clinical approach

Cyanosis can be of cardiac (right-to-left shunting) or respiratory origin or, rarely, associated with abnormal haemoglobin. Chronically, cyanosis can be reasonably well tolerated, but complications develop (see Section 2.7, p. 84). The differential diagnosis in this man, previously unknown to the medical profession, is wide:
- Respiratory failure and cor pulmonale secondary to chronic obstructive pulmonary disease, but also bronchiectasis, pulmonary fibrosis or hypoventilation syndromes.
- Eisenmenger's syndrome: see Section 2.7.2, p. 86.
- Secondary pulmonary hypertension of another cause.
- Other congenital heart disease: patients with Ebstein's anomaly or mild cases of tetralogy of Fallot may survive to middle age.

You need to determine the cause of the patient's cyanosis by looking for evidence of respiratory disease, pulmonary hypertension and intracardiac shunts.

History of the presenting problem

Ask about the duration and severity of the patient's presenting symptoms:
- How long has his ankle been swelling up for?
- Has he noticed that he has become blue and, if so, when? Has he been a 'funny colour' for as long as he can remember? If this has been very long standing, it suggests a cardiac rather than a respiratory explanation.
- Is he limited by breathlessness? Quantify his functional status—how far can he go on the flat? Can he go up stairs? How many times does he have to stop?

Enquire specifically regarding the following:
- Has he had any symptoms of hyperviscosity? These would include dizziness, headache, visual disturbance or paraesthesiae, probably indicating secondary polycythaemia in this case.
- Has he had any episodes of syncope or presyncope? These are a poor prognostic sign in patients with pulmonary hypertension.
- Does he find it difficult to stay awake sometimes? Has he ever fallen asleep during the day when he was not trying to, e.g. when driving a car? Has anyone ever complained that he snores a lot when he goes to sleep? Does he wake up with headaches in the mornings? Any of these features would make you think that he might have obstructive sleep apnoea.
- Does he smoke, which would put him at risk of chronic lung disease? Does he have chronic cough, sputum or wheeze—all features suggesting that he has chronic lung disease? Is there any history of asbestos exposure?

Ask about features that suggest thromboembolic disease:
- Asymmetrical calf swelling or tenderness
- Pleuritic chest pain
- Haemoptysis.

Also ask about the following:
- Symptoms of liver disease or autoimmune rheumatic disease.
- Use of prescribed medications (unlikely in this man), other drugs and risk factors for HIV (see *General clinical issues*, Section 2).
- History of stroke or transient ischaemic attack: these would be uncommon in a patient aged 45 years, but may be attributable to paradoxical embolism from right-to-left shunting in this case.

Relevant past history

Ask specifically about the following:
- Was he a blue baby? Did he have a heart murmur? Did he have rheumatic fever (try St Vitus' dance)?
- TB and whooping cough: these would put him at risk of bronchiectasis.
- Did any siblings die young? If so, consider cystic fibrosis.

Examination

Concentrate on a full cardiovascular and respiratory examination, noting particularly the following:
- Cyanosis—and check pulse oximetry.
- Neck and oropharynx: is obstructive sleep apnoea likely?
- Clubbing: a feature of congenital cyanotic heart disease, bronchiectasis and fibrosing alveolitis, but not of other causes of secondary pulmonary hypertension or primary pulmonary hypertension.
- Pulse rate and rhythm.
- Blood pressure.
- JVP: this will almost certainly be grossly elevated.
- Is there a left parasternal heave? This would suggest RV hypertrophy (RVH).
- Heart sounds: listen specifically for the fixed split S2 of an ASD, the right ventricular S4 of pressure overload, the loud P2 of pulmonary hypertension or inaudible P2 of right ventricular outflow tract obstruction, e.g. in Fallot's tetralogy.
- Murmurs: listen for the pansystolic murmurs of tricuspid regurgitation and VSD and the ejection systolic murmur of right ventricular outflow tract obstruction, but remember that these may not be dramatic.
- Hepatomegaly: is the liver pulsatile, which would indicate tricuspid regurgitation?
- Oedema.
- Any signs of chronic lung disease, in particular airflow obstruction, fibrosis or bronchiectasis.

Approach to investigations and management

 Cardiac cyanosis will not improve with maximal inspired oxygen whereas respiratory cyanosis generally will.

Investigations

Blood tests

Check arterial blood gases for PO_2 and PCO_2 when the patient is breathing air and (monitoring patient continuously in case he or she is a CO_2 retainer dependent on hypoxic drive) after 10 min on high-flow oxygen (see *Respiratory medicine*, Section 3.6.1.).

Check FBC: is the patient polycythaemic? Check electrolytes, renal and liver function. Other tests, e.g. for autoimmune rheumatic disorders, may be indicated in some cases.

ECG

Look for evidence of RVH. (See Section 3.1, p. 120.)

Chest radiograph

Look for signs of pulmonary hypertension and chronic lung disease, in particular the hyperexpansion of chronic obstructive pulmonary disease and the interstitial shadowing of parenchymal lung disease.

Echocardiography

Echocardiography is a key investigation to assess RV function, RVH and pulmonary pressures, to examine the heart valves, and to look for septal defects and shunts.

Pulmonary function tests

Does the patient have severe obstructive or restrictive lung disease? Check spirometry, lung volumes and gas transfer.

Further investigations

Depending on the initial results consider the following:
- High-resolution CT scan of the chest.
- Transoesophageal echocardiography for ASD if there is pulmonary hypertension and a shunt is suspected but not seen on transthoracic echo.
- Ventilation–perfusion scan or spiral CT if pulmonary thromboembolism is considered possible.
- MRI of the heart to define anatomy more clearly.

Management

Depends on the underlying condition. Note that, in all patients with pulmonary hypertension, great care must be taken with the use of diuretics for oedema—the risk is that overzealous fluid removal can lead to reduction in right ventricular filling pressure and thereby cause circulatory collapse.

 Do not fluid deplete in right-to-left shunting because this increases the shunt.

- Secondary pulmonary hypertension: see Section 2.12.2, p. 103
- Eisenmenger's syndrome and other congenital heart disease: see Section 2.7, p. 84
- Chronic respiratory failure and cor pulmonale: see *Respiratory medicine*, Section 2.11
- Pulmonary thromboembolism: see Sections 1.9, p. 28, and 2.18, p. 115.

 See *Respiratory medicine*, Sections 1.6 and 1.8.

1.12 Chest pain and recurrent syncope

Case history

A 63-year-old retired accountant presents with a 4-month history of syncopal episodes and chest pain on exertion.

Clinical approach

The combination of chest pain and syncope is very suggestive of a cardiac problem. The causes of recurrent syncope are given in Table 9 (see also Table 2, p. 9)—the main differential in this case is between left ventricular outflow tract obstruction from aortic stenosis or hypertrophic obstructive cardiomyopathy, and arrhythmias, which may be supraventricular or ventricular. Complete heart block only rarely causes chest pain, although coexistent IHD may cause angina. Orthostatic hypotension is common in patients treated with antianginal medication, and can lead to syncope. Also remember that pain from any cause, including angina, can cause vasovagal syncope.

History of the presenting problem

Get a good description of the syncopal episodes

Although a patient's recall of the events surrounding a collapse may be limited, try to ascertain as much information as possible from the patient or any witnesses. (See Section 1.3, p. 9 and *Neurology*, Section 1.20.)

When does it happen?

Classically, syncope caused by outflow tract obstruction occurs only on exertion as a result of reflex bradycardia

and vasodilatation. Arrhythmias can occur at any time, but they may happen only on exercise or stress if they are sensitive to increased sympathetic outflow or ischaemia. Syncope from orthostatic hypotension occurs on standing, but may be more prominent after exertion.

Chest pain

The obvious assumption is that this man's pain is the result of angina. This needs to be confirmed—ask specifically: 'Show me where you feel the pain. When do you get the pain? What is it like? Does it go anywhere else? How long does the pain last and what makes it go away?, etc.' (See Sections 1.5, p. 15 and 2.1, p. 51.) Angina with associated dyspnoea on exertion is found in outflow tract obstruction, although not in association with syncope.

Relevant past history

It is obviously important to establish a past history of heart disease. Ask specifically about a history of IHD, valvular disease and arrhythmias:
• Any heart trouble in the past?
• Ever had a heart attack or been told that you have angina?
• Any palpitations or fluttering sensations before?
  Try also to ascertain whether there is a history of rheumatic fever. Patients may remember a period of illness as a child with joint pains, or a long period off school or away from sport. Patients with a bicuspid aortic valve may have been told that they have a murmur.

Risk factors

Ask about risk factors for IHD such as hypertension, smoking and family history. A family history of sudden death may reflect hereditary hypertrophic obstructive cardiomyopathy or long QT syndrome with underlying ventricular arrhythmias.

Examination

Examination of a patient with exertional chest pain and syncope:
• General impression: is the patient well or unwell?
• Full cardiovascular examination
• Is the carotid pulse slow rising, suggesting aortic stenosis?
• Is there any arrhythmia?

General

As always, assess whether the patient looks unwell. A patient with critical aortic stenosis or hypertrophic

Table 9 Causes of syncope.

Symptom—syncope with:	Diagnosis to consider
Angina and dyspnoea occurring on exertion	Aortic stenosis or hypertrophic obstructive cardiomyopathy
Associated palpitations	Arrhythmia
Preceded by a definite prodrome with progressive nausea and sweating	Vasovagal syncope
A history of severe dizziness, blurring of vision, weakness or syncope on standing or after exertion in a patient treated with antianginal medication	Orthostatic hypotension
Prolonged episode with involuntary limb movements or tongue biting	Epilepsy

obstructive cardiomyopathy may be dyspnoeic simply on getting undressed.

As you examine the patient with syncopal episodes, consider the following diagnoses:
• Aortic stenosis: slow rising carotid upstroke, undisplaced thrusting apex, ejection systolic murmur radiating to carotids, perhaps with a palpable thrill
• Hypertrophic obstructive cardiomyopathy: jerky carotid pulse, diffuse 'rolling' or double apical pulsation, ejection systolic murmur
• Arrhythmia: look for abnormal rhythm, and for evidence of sinus node disease or ischaemia on the ECG
• Orthostatic hypotension: look for a postural drop in blood pressure.

Cardiovascular

Take careful note of the following:
• Pulse rate and rhythm
• Pulse character
• Blood pressure supine and on standing
• JVP
• Apex
• Heart sounds and murmurs
• Lung bases
• Peripheral oedema.

Approach to investigations and management

Investigations

Investigation of a patient with exertional syncope and chest pain:
• ECG: is there arrhythmia or left ventricular hypertrophy?
• Echocardiography: investigation of choice to exclude severe outflow tract obstruction.

ECG

Look for evidence of left ventricular hypertrophy and ischaemia, also arrhythmias or evidence in support of a rhythm disturbance, e.g. δ waves, long QT interval, bi- or trifascicular block (Fig. 19).

Chest radiograph

Cardiomegaly may suggest severe left ventricular hypertrophy with or without dilatation. Is the aortic valve calcified?

Echocardiography

Assess for evidence of aortic stenosis or hypertrophic obstructive cardiomyopathy and degree of severity. Remember that symptoms are unlikely unless obstruction

(a)

Fig. 19 Twelve-lead ECGs: (a) left ventricular hypertrophy, (b) old anterior myocardial infarction, (c) long QT.

(b)

(c)

Fig. 19 *Continued*

is severe. The presence of an old infarct may predispose to ventricular arrhythmia. (See Section 2.1.1, p. 51.)

Twenty-four-hour ambulatory monitor

This may uncover evidence of arrhythmias such as ventricular tachycardia (Fig. 20).

Tilt-table testing

Hypotension with or without bradycardia may be precipitated in a vasovagal syndrome.

For further discussion of the investigation of syncope, see Section 1.3, p. 9.

Fig. 20 Twelve-lead ECG showing ventricular tachycardia.

Management

There should be a low threshold for admitting patients with syncope caused by arrhythmia or left ventricular outflow tract obstruction. Remember that it may happen while crossing a road.
- Aortic stenosis: see Section 2.5.1, p. 71
- Arrhythmias: see Sections 1.1, p. 3, 1.2, p. 6, 1.3, p. 9 and 2.2, p. 58
- Hypertrophic obstructive cardiomyopathy: see Section 2.4.1, p. 66
- Orthostatic hypotension: changing antianginal medications to those with less antihypertensive action may reduce the incidence of problems
- Epilepsy and other neurogenic syncope: see *Neurology*, Sections 1.20 and 2.7.

See *Medicine for the elderly*, Section 1.1.
See *Neurology*, Section 1.20.
Abboud FM. Neurocardiogenic syncope. *N Engl J Med* 1993; 328: 1117.
Bradenburg RO. Syncope and sudden death in hypertrophic cardiomyopathy. *J Am Coll Cardiol* 1990; 15: 962.
Grech ED, Ramsdale DR. Exertional syncope in aortic stenosis. *Am Heart J* 1991; 127: 603.
Leitch JW, klein GJ, Yee R *et al.* Syncope associated with supraventricular tachycardia: An expression of tachycardia rate or vasomotor response? *Circulation* 1992; 85: 1064.
Lipsitz L. Orthostatic hypotension in the elderly. *N Engl J Med* 1989; 321: 952.

1.13 Fever, weight loss and new murmur

Case history

A 68-year-old, previously well man with a 6-week history of fever and weight loss is referred to the A&E department by his GP, who has also noticed a heart murmur.

Clinical approach

The list of diagnoses associated with the constitutional symptoms of fever and weight loss that have persisted for more than a few weeks is large—the most common causes are shown in Table 10. However, in the presence of a murmur, whether new or not, the diagnosis of infective endocarditis must go to the top of the list and should initially dominate your approach, even in the absence of any other stigmata. A careful history and examination are essential; other chronic infection, occult malignancy or autoimmune rheumatic disease may be uncovered.

History of the presenting problem

Given the non-specific nature of the symptoms, a careful and thorough history is essential—only scant information is available thus far. The history and examination are

Table 10 Differential diagnosis of 6 weeks' fever and weight loss.

Category	Common example	In presence of a murmur
Infective	Infective endocarditis TB Liver abscess	Infective endocarditis is the number one consideration
Autoimmune rheumatic disorder/vasculitis	SLE Rheumatoid arthritis Polymyalgia rheumatica	SLE (also some other rheumatic disorders) can affect the heart valves and cause substantial diagnostic difficulty
Malignancy	Lymphoma Hypernephroma	Consider atrial myxoma—is this the only case that you will ever diagnose? 'Marantic' endocarditis is possible

SLE, systemic lupus erythematosus; TB, tuberculosis.

dominated by consideration of the most likely diagnosis, infective endocarditis, but clues may emerge that take you off on another tack. Bear the diagnoses listed in Table 10 in mind as you take the history and go on to examine the patient.

General

Gauge the severity of the debilitation. In acute infective endocarditis, the fever is high with rigors and prostration: 'Have you had attacks of really bad shivering and shaking?' 'Have you sweated so much that you had to change your clothes or the sheets on the bed?' The current history is more suggestive of a subacute presentation, which is associated with a low-grade fever, malaise and weight loss.

Cardiac and respiratory symptoms

Ask about symptoms of heart failure:
• Have you been getting breathless going about your business or in bed at night?
• Have your ankles become swollen?

These may be insidious; if present they raise the possibility of haemodynamic compromise from aortic or mitral regurgitation. Sudden episodes of pulmonary oedema can be found in atrial myxoma.

Ask about chest pain, and—if present—get a good description:
• MI is rare in endocarditis, but can arise from coronary artery embolus.
• Pleuritic chest pain and/or haemoptysis may suggest pulmonary abscess or infarction from tricuspid valve endocarditis, as well as TB or other lung pathology. Haemoptysis is also a feature of left atrial myxoma.

Extracardiac manifestations

These may dominate the clinical picture in endocarditis if the patient presents, for example, with an arterial embolus leading to a stroke, or limb or splanchnic infarc-

tion, or more rarely as a result of some other systemic manifestation of endocarditis. This is not so in this case, but enquire about the following:
• Any skin rashes?
• Any changes in your nails recently?
• Have you noticed any blood in your urine?
• Have you had any back or abdominal pain?
• Any changes in your vision?
• Have you had any sudden periods of arm or leg weakness, or episodes of difficulty speaking?

Vasculitic rashes can occur with infective endocarditis, although uncommon, but are not specific and may occur with several of the differential diagnoses. Also rare, but much more suggestive, are transient changes in the hands and feet, which may be painful in the finger or toe pulps (Osler's nodes), or painless in the palms or soles (Janeway's spots or lesions).

Usually causing microscopic haematuria and unnoticed, the glomerulonephritis that may accompany infective endocarditis can cause gross haematuria, as may renal infarction; however, macroscopic haematuria would clearly lead you towards hypernephroma as the diagnosis. Back pain may simply result from myalgia, but severe loin pain suggests renal infarction and could be caused by a renal abscess or tumour. Pain in the left hypochondrium radiating to the left shoulder may result from splenic infarction or an abscess.

Relevant past history

Ask the following:
• Has anyone ever told you that you have a heart murmur, or that they've heard a 'sound' or 'hole' in your heart?
• Have you had rheumatic fever?
• Any recent trips to the dentist for surgery or invasive investigations?
• It may also be appropriate to ask regarding any history of intravenous drug abuse. (See *General clinical issues*, Section 2.)

(a)

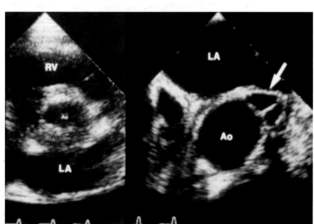

(b)

Fig. 22 (a) Aortic vegetation and (b) para-aortic abscess (arrow).
(Courtesy of Dr J Chambers.)

 See *Infectious diseases*, Sections 1.8 and 1.10.
See Section 2.8.1, p. 92.
Arnow PM. Flaherty JP. Fever of unknown origin. *Lancet* 1997;
   350: 575–580.
Chien JW. Making the most of blood cultures. Tips for optimal
   use of this time-honored test. *Postgrad Med* 1998; 104:
   119–124; 127.
Krivokapich J, Child JS. Role of transthoracic and transesophageal
   echocardiography in diagnosis and management of
   infective endocarditis. *Cardiol Clin* 1996; 14: 363–382.
Saccente M, Cobbs CG. Clinical approach to infective
   endocarditis. *Cardiol Clin* 1996; 14: 351–362.

1.14 Chest pain following a 'flu-like illness

Case history

A 25-year-old woman presents to A&E complaining of a 4-day history of chest pain. She has been unwell with 'flu for the last week. You are referred the patient by the A&E officer who thinks the pain may be pericarditic.

Clinical approach

The history immediately suggests an acute pericarditis of viral aetiology. The risk arises not from this diagnosis, which is usually mild and self-limiting, but from the failure to recognize more serious pathology that presents in a similar manner (Table 11). You must initially decide whether or not the pain is caused by pericarditis, excluding the other causes of chest pain along the way and, if so, whether there is a more serious underlying aetiology. Only then should you assume the diagnosis of viral pericarditis.

As there is some overlap between the symptoms of pericardial and pleural inflammation, you will need to consider pulmonary pathologies, in particular pneumonia and PE. Remember that serositis is also a feature of some autoimmune rheumatic diseases, such as systemic lupus erythematosus (SLE) and rheumatoid arthritis.

In this patient, both MI and aortic dissection would be extremely unlikely, but because of their potentially fatal consequences they should always be borne in mind in any patient presenting with chest pain.

History of the presenting problem

What and where?

Get as much information as possible:
• Show me where you feel the pain?
• What is the pain like?
• Does it go anywhere else?

If a clear description of the pain is not forthcoming, offer suggestions—'like a knife', 'raw'—both of which

Table 11 Differential diagnosis of pericarditic chest pain.

Comment	Diagnosis
Common	Acute pericarditis
	Musculoskeletal
	Oesophagitis
Must consider	Pneumonia
	Pulmonary embolism
	Autoimmune rheumatic disease
Do not completely forget	Myocardial ischaemia
	Aortic dissection

may suggest pericarditic pain, or 'like a heavy weight' or 'squeezing', which do not. The pain of pericarditis is usually located retrosternally, and like angina it may radiate to the neck or shoulders.

How and when?

Ask specifically about the pattern:
- Did the pain start suddenly?
- Do you have pain all the time? If not, when do you get it?
- Does it hurt when you breathe in?
- When you sit forward, does the pain get less?
- Is the pain worse lying in bed?

Pericarditic pain is usually continuous, but does not typically have a sudden onset, unlike PE. It is exacerbated by inspiration, movement and lying supine, and is typically eased by sitting forward. Aside from movement itself, there is no relationship with exertion, unlike angina.

Any other symptoms?

This woman has had 'flu-like symptoms recently, but ask any patient presenting with chest pain the following:
- Have you been feeling 'under the weather' or feverish recently?
- Do you feel breathless?
- Have you coughed up any phlegm? What colour was it? Any blood?
- Any joint pains?
- Do you ever get an acid taste at the back of your mouth?

Acute pericarditis often presents with a story of a recent 'flu-like infection. Although painful breathing may cause dyspnoea in pericarditis, prominent respiratory symptoms are clearly more in keeping with pulmonary pathology. Haemoptysis would suggest pulmonary embolism. The presence of arthralgia may simply reflect the associated viraemia, but could also suggest connective tissue disease. Acid reflux may suggest oesophagitis, as would a history of indigestion.

When taking a history in a young patient, at low risk of IHD, presenting with chest pain—look for the following patterns:
- Pericarditis: sharp or raw retrosternal continuous discomfort, worse on lying down, and relieved by sitting forwards, often with a history of a 'flu-like illness
- Musculoskeletal pain: history of unaccustomed activity with chest wall tenderness
- Oesophagitis: suggested by dyspeptic symptoms, particularly belching and reflux, worse at night
- Pneumonia: fever (sometimes rigors), breathlessness, malaise and (sometimes) pleuritic pain; dry painful cough initially, later productive of sputum
- PE: sudden onset of pleuritic pain with breathlessness and haemoptysis
- MI or aortic dissection: however unlikely you consider these may be in a young patient, think of them if the symptoms are 'ischaemic' or 'tearing' in nature.

Relevant past history

You will obviously ask whether there have been any similar episodes in the past and, if so, what diagnosis (if any) was made.

Although the most likely cause of pericarditis in this case is viral infection and, assuming that the woman is unlikely to have sustained an MI or undergone cardiac surgery, ask about other conditions that are associated with pericarditis:
- Rheumatoid arthritis and other autoimmune rheumatic disease
- Renal failure
- Hypothyroidism
- Rheumatic fever
- Contact with TB
- Malignancy, e.g. breast
- Chest radiotherapy.

Examination

As always, get an overall impression first. A patient with uncomplicated pericarditis is unlikely to look very unwell—he or she will be in pain, which may be severe, and is likely to be sitting forward rather than lying supine. If the patient is unwell, this should prompt a rapid assessment for evidence of tamponade, pulmonary embolism or pneumonia, which may be life threatening.

General

- Check the temperature: pyrexia indicates an inflammatory cause of pain
- Examine the sputum pot: haemoptysis suggests PE
- Does it hurt when I press you on the chest where the pain is? This would clearly suggest a local musculoskeletal cause, but remember that there can be tenderness in pleurisy.

Cardiovascular

Perform a full cardiovascular assessment, taking particular note of the following:
- Peripheral perfusion: is this impaired? It should not be in uncomplicated pericarditis.
- Pulse rate, rhythm and character.
- Blood pressure: does it fall on inspiration?
- JVP: is this elevated?
- Auscultation: is there a pericardial rub?

Respiratory and other systems

- Look for chest signs suggestive of pneumonia or PE.
- Is the patient euthyroid?
- Are there any signs of malignancy, e.g. breast?
- Is there evidence of autoimmune rheumatic disorder, e.g. joint inflammation or deformity, rash?

When examining a young patient, at low risk of IHD, presenting with chest pain, look specifically for the following:
- Pericarditis: is there a pericardial rub? Look for an underlying aetiology.
- Is there evidence of cardiac tamponade? Look for poor peripheral perfusion, elevated venous pressure and tachycardia with a small volume pulse exhibiting pulsus paradoxus (blood pressure falls significantly on inspiration). This is an emergency and requires pericardiocentesis.

- Musculoskeletal pain: pain that is well localized and reproduced by local pressure on the chest wall.
- Pneumonia: fever with signs of focal lung consolidation. Listen for a pleural rub.
- Pulmonary embolism: is there haemoptysis in the sputum pot? Listen for a pleural rub. Are there signs of pulmonary hypertension? (See Sections 1.9, p. 28 and 1.10, p. 30.)
- Aortic dissection: a rank outsider—but does the woman look as though she may have Marfan's syndrome? Can you feel the left radial pulse? Is the blood pressure the same in both arms? (See Section 1.5, p. 15.)

(a)

(b)

Fig. 23 ECGs: (a) anterior myocardial infarction and (b) acute pericarditis, where widespread ST segment elevation, concave upwards, is seen.

Approach to investigations and management

Investigations

ECG

Along with chest pain and pericardial rub, the ECG changes encountered in acute pericarditis form a triad of characteristic findings that can establish the diagnosis (Fig. 23).

Blood tests

Check FBC, electrolytes, renal and liver function, thyroid function, inflammatory markers (ESR and CRP) and cardiac enzymes. If clinically indicated, check blood cultures and serology for evidence of autoimmune rheumatic disorders. (See *Rheumatology and clinical immunology*, Section 3.2.) Checking 'viral titres' is not generally useful.

Chest radiograph

Look for cardiomegaly, suggesting an effusion, and for any areas of consolidation or pleural effusion (Fig. 24).

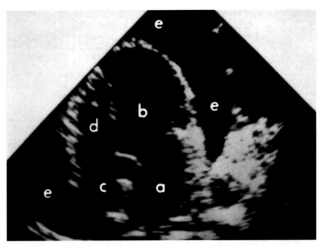

Fig. 25 Large pericardial effusion: the heart is surrounded by an echo-free space (e) formed by the effusion. a, left atrium; b, left ventricle; c, right atrium; d, right ventricle. (Courtesy of Dr J Chambers.)

Echocardiography

An echocardiogram that reveals a small amount of pericardial fluid can be very helpful in making the diagnosis of pericarditis. This is mandatory and urgent if the cardiac shadow is enlarged and you suspect cardiac tamponade (Fig. 25).

Other tests

Other tests, e.g. ventilation–perfusion scanning, should be performed if clinically indicated.

Management

This depends on the specific diagnosis:
• Acute pericarditis: see Section 2.6.1, p. 78
• Cardiac tamponade: see Section 2.6.2, p. 80
• Pneumonia: see *Infectious diseases*, Sections 1.2 and 1.4
• Pulmonary embolism: see Section 2.18, p. 115
• Connective tissue disease: see *Rheumatology and clinical immunology*, Sections 2.3.3 and 2.4.1
• Reflux oesophagitis: see *Gastroenterology*, Section 1.2.

In uncomplicated acute viral or idiopathic pericarditis, the illness is self-limiting. The patient should be reassured that they have not had a heart attack, and can be allowed home with simple analgesia, non-steroidal anti-inflammatory drugs (NSAIDs) often being particularly effective. Follow-up in a few weeks' time should be organized to ensure that the symptoms have settled. Admission will be warranted if the pain is severe, there is evidence of a large pericardial effusion or tamponade (which is a medical emergency), or if treatment of an underlying aetiology is indicated.

Fig. 24 Cardiomegaly. Note the increased cardiothoracic ratio in this posteroanterior film.

See *Infectious diseases*, Section 1.9.

Fowler NO. Cardiac tamponade. A clinical or an echocardiographic diagnosis? *Circulation* 1993; 87: 1738.

Shabetai R. Acute pericarditis. *Cardiol Clin* 1990; 8: 639–644.

Spodick DH. ECG in acute pericarditis. *Am J Cardiol* 1974; 40: 470.

Spodick DH. Pericarditis in systemic diseases. *Cardiol Clin* 1990; 8: 709–716.

1.15 Elevated blood pressure at routine screening

Case history

An obese 55-year-old publican is referred to your outpatient clinic for management of his blood pressure. He had attended his GP with pains in his legs and was found to have a blood pressure of 170/115 mmHg during the consultation. His father died of an MI at the age of 61. He takes no medication but smokes 20 cigarettes and drinks 4 pints of beer a day.

Clinical approach

This is an extremely common problem. The benefits of good control of elevated blood pressure are unassailable —this man already has several risk factors for vascular disease and failure to recognize and treat hypertension will add yet another. Your approach should be directed towards confirming an elevated blood pressure. By far the most likely diagnosis is essential hypertension, but do not fail to consider secondary causes (Table 12). Treatment

Table 12 Differential diagnosis of hypertension.

Comment	Diagnosis
Common	Essential hypertension False elevation as a result of inadequate blood pressure cuff size Isolated clinic ('white coat') hypertension
Must consider	Renal hypertension Renovascular hypertension Primary hyperaldosteronism (Conn's syndrome) Phaeochromocytoma Coarctation of the aorta
Other causes	Cushing's syndrome Acromegaly

offered must aim to reduce all modifiable cardiovascular risk factors.

History of the presenting problem

Hypertension is usually asymptomatic until organ damage intervenes. Some patients, on being given a diagnosis of hypertension, will ascribe many different and varied complaints to it. A multitude of symptoms, e.g. headache, epistaxis, tinnitus, dizziness, fainting, are often blamed on an elevated blood pressure, but probably occur with similar frequency in those whose blood pressure is normal.

Review of organ systems

Patients with chronic hypertension may present in cardiac failure, with breathlessnes and orthopnoea. Nocturia may suggest renal failure, which can be both a cause and a consequence of hypertension. In accelerated (malignant) phase hypertension (exceedingly unlikely in this case given the level of blood pressure) visual changes may result from retinal changes.

Could there be a secondary cause of hypertension?

A history of IHD, cerebrovascular disease or peripheral vascular disease would increase the likelihood of hypertension secondary to atheromatous renovascular disease. Are there any symptoms to support these diagnoses? His leg pains could be the result of intermittent claudication.

Is there any history of renal problems? Has he had medicals for work or insurance purposes? Have these been OK, or has he ever been told that he had protein in his urine? These questions might give a lead to the diagnosis of renal hypertension.

Episodes of palpitations, sweating or headaches might indicate a phaeochromocytoma, but would be much more likely to have a less exotic explanation (e.g. alcohol withdrawal).

Note that a strong family history of hypertension would support the diagnosis of essential hypertension.

Risk factors

In any patient presenting with hypertension it is very important to assess other cardiovascular risk factors, including the following:
- Smoking
- Diabetes
- Hyperlipidaemia
- Family history of cardiovascular events
- Alcohol consumption.

Examination

Examination and investigation of the patient with hypertension

Measurement of blood pressure—make sure that you take the time to do this properly:
- The patient should be recumbent for at least 3 min
- Use an adequate sized blood pressure cuff—a large cuff if the arm is large
- Measure blood pressure three times (at first visit it is recommended that the pressure is taken in both arms and the one with the higher value used thereafter)
- Record all readings, with the average of the second and third taken as the patient's value for consideration of treatment.

Unless the blood pressure is very high (diastolic BP >110 mmHg) measurements should be repeated on more than one occasion before deciding on whether or not to treat. A method similar to this has been used to measure blood pressure in most of the trials of treatment of hypertension, and to condemn someone to perhaps life-long drug treatment on the basis of a single reading taken casually is not good medicine.

The main objectives are to:
- assess for evidence of target organ damage
- uncover a secondary cause of hypertension.

General and cardiovascular

Perform a full examination, but take particular note of signs strongly suggesting secondary cause:
- Abdominal bruits
- Radiofemoral delay.

Look for signs indicating that there might be secondary cause. Is there peripheral vascular disease? Check for carotid or femoral bruits, abdominal aortic aneurysm and absent peripheral pulses.

Search for evidence of end-organ damage by hypertension:
- Cardiac: is there left ventricular hypertrophy or cardiac failure?
- Fundoscopy: are there hypertensive changes? (See Section 2.17, p. 110.)

When examining the patient with hypertension, consider the following:
- Essential hypertension: if elevated blood pressure, evidence of left ventricular hypertrophy or hypertensive retinopathy in the absence of a suspicion of a secondary cause.
- Isolated clinic hypertension: look for anxiety, e.g. tachycardia. Is the blood pressure lower when measured by the clinic nurse or the GP, or at place of work or at home? There must be no evidence of target organ damage.
- Renovascular disease: are there abdominal bruits, abdominal aortic aneurysm or other evidence of atherosclerosis?
- Coarctation: look for absent femoral pulses and radiofemoral delay, collaterals in the back muscles and a widespread systolic murmur heard best over the back.

Approach to investigations and management

Routine investigations

Urine

The way to detect renal disease causing hypertension is to test the urine with dipstix for proteinuria and haematuria. If this is positive for protein, quantification with a 24-h collection is required; if positive for blood, microscopy (to look particularly for red cells and casts) and culture are needed.

Blood tests

Check the FBC, electrolytes, renal and liver function, uric acid, fasting glucose and lipid profile. The most common cause of hypokalaemia is diuretic treatment, but low values are often found in untreated accelerated phase hypertension and in primary hyperaldosteronism. Is renal function normal? Is there glucose intolerance or frank diabetes? Is the cholesterol elevated?

ECG

Look particularly for evidence of left ventricular hypertrophy.

Chest radiograph

Assess heart size and look for pulmonary oedema and coarctation (Fig. 26).

Fig. 26 Coarctation of aorta: in this angiogram the tapering of the aorta can be seen shortly after the arch on a plain radiograph the feature to look for is rib notching produced by collateral vessels (see Fig. 67, p. 92).

Fig. 27 Left ventricular hypertrophy: compare with the normal parasternal M-mode (see Fig. 112, p. 141). The interventricular septum is grossly thickened in this patient. (Courtesy of Dr J Chambers.)

Other investigations required in some cases

Echocardiography

This is more sensitive than the ECG at detecting left ventricular hypertrophy, especially if patients are of Afro-Caribbean descent (Fig. 27).

Twenty-four-hour ambulatory blood pressure monitoring

This may be needed to confirm a suspicion of 'white coat hypertension'.

Other tests

Specific tests to diagnose primary renal disease (serological tests, renal biopsy), renovascular disease (captopril renography, renal angiography), Conn's syndrome (plasma renin and aldosterone levels) or phaeochromocytoma (urinary catecholamines) will be required in some cases, but only where there is substantial clinical suspicion.

A number of other conditions, e.g. Cushing's syndrome or acromegaly, can be complicated by hypertension, but it is rare for hypertension to be the presenting feature.

Management

Management depends on the precise diagnosis:
• Essential hypertension: see Section 2.17, p. 110
• Isolated clinic hypertension: reassurance and avoidance of poisons (drugs)!
• Renal and renovascular disease: see *Nephrology*, Sections 1.11, 2.1.3 and 2.5.1

• Coarctation of the aorta: surgery to be considered
• Phaeochromocytoma: see *Endocrinology*, Section 2.2.5
• Primary hyperaldosteronism: see *Endocrinology*, Section 2.2.3
• Accelerated (malignant) hypertension: see Section 2.17.1, p. 113.

Do not forget to offer advice and treatment (where possible) to reduce other cardiovascular risk factors. Decisions regarding the treatment of hypertension (or hypercholesterolaemia) should never be taken in isolation. It would be better for this man to stop smoking with some reduction in his blood pressure than to have 'perfect blood pressure' and a pack of cigarettes a day.

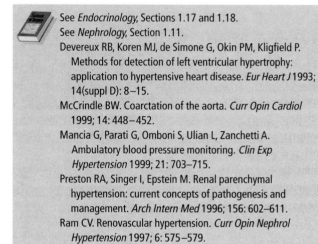

See *Endocrinology*, Sections 1.17 and 1.18.
See *Nephrology*, Section 1.11.
Devereux RB, Koren MJ, de Simone G, Okin PM, Kligfield P. Methods for detection of left ventricular hypertrophy: application to hypertensive heart disease. *Eur Heart J* 1993; 14(suppl D): 8–15.
McCrindle BW. Coarctation of the aorta. *Curr Opin Cardiol* 1999; 14: 448–452.
Mancia G, Parati G, Omboni S, Ulian L, Zanchetti A. Ambulatory blood pressure monitoring. *Clin Exp Hypertension* 1999; 21: 703–715.
Preston RA, Singer I, Epstein M. Renal parenchymal hypertension: current concepts of pathogenesis and management. *Arch Intern Med* 1996; 156: 602–611.
Ram CV. Renovascular hypertension. *Curr Opin Nephrol Hypertension* 1997; 6: 575–579.

1.16 Murmur in pregnancy

Case history

A 23-year-old woman is referred by her GP to the cardiology clinic after the discovery of a systolic murmur picked up during a routine antenatal visit. She is 29 weeks' pregnant with her first child.

Clinical approach

Your major concern will be to differentiate an innocent murmur from one that suggests underlying pathology (Table 13). Can you reassure the patient or, if there is a structural cardiac lesion, can you predict and prevent problems that might arise during the pregnancy? The most common diagnosis will be an innocent systolic murmur due to the hyperdynamic circulation, requiring no further intervention. Mitral or aortic valve disease, hypertrophic obstructive cardiomyopathy and congenital abnormalities, such as VSD, may require careful monitoring; at the very least they require antibiotic prophylaxis during vaginal delivery. Occasionally, rare and severe conditions such as cardiomyopathy of pregnancy can present in the third trimester.

Table 13 Differential diagnosis of a systolic murmur during pregnancy.

Comment	Diagnosis
Common	Innocent systolic murmur
	Venous hum
	Mammary soufflé
	Mitral valve prolapse
Must consider	Mitral valve disease (regurgitation/mixed/stenosis with tricuspid regurgitation)
	Aortic valve disease (stenosis/mixed/regurgitation with flow murmur)
	Hypertrophic cardiomyopathy
	Atrial or ventricular septal defect
Other causes	Peripartum cardiomyopathy

History of presenting problem

Most patients who present in this way will be asymptomatic. The presence of symptoms should raise the suspicion of significant pathology, but bear in mind that a degree of weakness, exertional dyspnoea, dizziness and peripheral oedema are quite common during pregnancy and are a result of physiological adaptation rather than intrinsic cardiac disease. Be sure to gauge the precise severity of the symptoms and relate it to the stage of the pregnancy.

Ask some general questions:

- Have you been getting out of breath more easily?
- How far can you walk?
- Have you woken up breathless at night?
- Any chest pains?
- Any palpitations? When do you get them?
- Any blackouts? What were you doing at the time?
- Do you ever feel as if you are going to pass out?

Relevant past history

Enquire about any previous cardiac history. Occasionally, a minor abnormality will have been documented in infancy or childhood and the patient may have been told that she has a murmur, 'hole' or 'sound' in her heart. Ask about any difficulties before the pregnancy that might also suggest a congenital abnormality; also ask about any heart problems in other family members. A history of sudden death at a young age might raise the possibility of a hereditary cardiomyopathy or Marfan's syndrome.

Examination

Examination of the pregnant patient with a systolic murmur:
- Do you think the patient looks unwell?
- Does the patient look Marfanoid?
- Is the carotid pulse slow rising or collapsing, suggesting severe aortic valve disease? Or is it jerky, suggesting hypertrophic cardiomyopathy (can be difficult to distinguish from the hyperdynamic circulation of pregnancy)?
- Does the murmur suggest valvular or structural abnormality or does it sound innocent?
- Is there any evidence of cardiac failure?
The bottom line is:
- Do you think that the heart is normal?

General

Be vigilant for evidence of systemic disease, which can present with valvular abnormalities. A complete examination is necessary. Most patients presenting with a murmur in pregnancy will look well: remember that if they do not, they are much more likely to have serious pathology.

Check temperature, and look carefully for any stigmata of endocarditis. (See Section 1.13, p. 38.)

Cardiovascular

A careful and thorough examination for signs of cardiac disease will form the main part of your assessment. Thinking all the time about the potential diagnoses, as listed in Table 13, take note of the following:

- Peripheral perfusion
- Pulse rate, rhythm and character
- Blood pressure
- JVP
- Apex
- Heart sounds
- Murmurs and radiation
- Lung bases
- Liver edge
- Peripheral oedema.

Approach to investigations and management

Investigations

ECG

Minor flattening of the T waves or axis shift are common in normal pregnancy, as are sinus tachycardia and ectopic beats. Look for evidence of atrial enlargement, left or right ventricular hypertrophy, or conduction abnormalities (Fig. 28).

Chest radiograph

This test is best avoided unless there are clear clinical indications.

Fig. 28 ECG: axis shift in pregnant woman.

(a)

(b)

Echocardiography

This is the investigation of choice to confirm or rule out cardiac pathology (Fig. 29).

Management

- Innocent murmur, venous hum, mammary soufflé: no treatment required; reassure
- Aortic or mitral valve disease: see Section 2.5, p. 71
- ASD or VSD: see Section 2.7, p. 84
- Hypertrophic cardiomyopathy: see Section 2.4.1, p. 66
- Peripartum cardiomyopathy: see Section 2.15, p. 109.

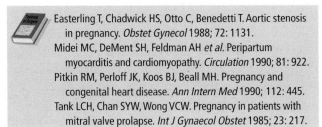

Easterling T, Chadwick HS, Otto C, Benedetti T. Aortic stenosis in pregnancy. *Obstet Gynecol* 1988; 72: 1131.
Midei MC, DeMent SH, Feldman AH *et al.* Peripartum myocarditis and cardiomyopathy. *Circulation* 1990; 81: 922.
Pitkin RM, Perloff JK, Koos BJ, Beall MH. Pregnancy and congenital heart disease. *Ann Intern Med* 1990; 112: 445.
Tank LCH, Chan SYW, Wong VCW. Pregnancy in patients with mitral valve prolapse. *Int J Gynaecol Obstet* 1985; 23: 217.

Fig. 29 (a) Mitral valve prolapse (MVP) and (b) ventricular septal defect (VSD). MVP: in the two-dimensional image on the left, the anterior mitral valve leaflet is seen to bow into the left atrium (arrow). The effect of this can be seen in the colour flow mapping on the right—a broad regurgitant jet can be seen. VSD: in these parasternal long and short axis views, a small jet of orange colour represents the abnormal blood flow across the septum from the left to right ventricle. LA, left atrium; LV, left ventricular; RV, right ventricle; Ao, aorta. (Courtesy of Dr J Chambers.)

2 Diseases and treatments

2.1 Coronary artery disease

2.1.1 STABLE ANGINA

Aetiology/pathophysiology/pathology

Chronic atheromatous plaques reduce coronary blood flow. Increased myocardial oxygen demand on exercise cannot be met, resulting in myocardial ischaemia and chest pain (angina pectoris).

Epidemiology

The estimated prevalence of this condition is 3–4% of the population.

Clinical presentation

Common

Common features include the following:
• Heavy central chest pain on exertion, relieved by rest
• Typically worse in cold weather, after meals
• Lower jaw or left arm pain.

Uncommon

• Exertional breathlessness ('angina equivalent').

Physical signs

Usually there are no physical signs in uncomplicated stable angina. Look for hypertension and signs of peripheral or cerebrovascular disease.

Investigations

An algorithm for investigation of the patient presenting with suspected angina is set out in Fig. 30:
• Resting ECG: often normal, but this does not rule out serious coronary disease.
• Exercise ECG: used to confirm the clinical diagnosis, assess exercise capacity objectively and determine prognosis. (See Section 3.1.1, p. 124.)
• Myocardial perfusion imaging (see Section 3.12.1, p. 143) or dobutamine stress echocardiography (see Section 3.11,

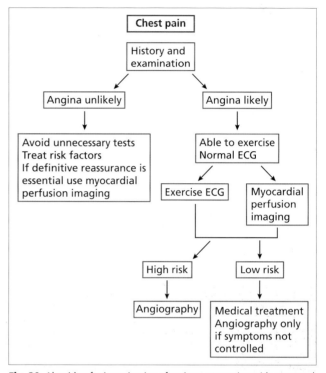

Fig. 30 Algorithm for investigation of patients presenting with suspected stable angina.

p. 141) may be used instead of exercise ECG in those unable to exercise or who have bundle-branch block.
• Lipid profile.
• FBC.
• Cardiac catheterization (see Section 3.8.1, p. 136).

Consider other causes of exertional chest pain:
• Syndrome X: typical exertional angina, positive exercise test and normal coronary angiogram. Usually in middle-aged women, possibly as an abnormality of coronary microvascular function; the treatment is medical
• Hypertrophic cardiomyopathy
• Severe anaemia
• Aortic stenosis.

Treatment

Short term

Aspirin, GTN and a β blocker are the first-line drugs.

Long term

Medical: other antianginal drugs (calcium antagonist, long-acting nitrate or nicorandil) may be added according to symptoms.

Percutaneous transluminal coronary angioplasty (PTCA) (see Section 3.8.2, p. 138) is generally indicated if there is symptomatic angina with suitable lesions in one or two coronary arteries. An improved life expectancy has not been demonstrated.

Coronary artery bypass grafting (CABG) improves life expectancy in patients with the following:
• Left main-stem stenosis
• Severe, proximal, three-vessel coronary disease, especially with impaired LV function (Fig. 31)
• Possibly proximal LAD lesion with one other vessel involved.

It is also indicated for symptomatic patients with less severe disease, in whom PTCA is not feasible or has failed.

Fig. 31 Left coronary angiogram demonstrating proximal stenoses in two major vessels with retrograde filling of a blocked right coronary artery (arrow) via collaterals. This patient therefore has three-vessel coronary artery disease.

Non-medical (interventional) management of coronary artery disease is summarized in Fig. 32.

Complications

• Unstable angina
• MI
• Arrhythmia.

Prognosis

The prognosis is generally good; cardiac catheterization is the best means of risk stratification. The mortality rate ranges from 2% per year (single vessel disease) to 20% per year (left main-stem stenosis). Impairment of left ventricular function is an independent risk factor.

Prevention

Primary

• Stop smoking
• Treat hyperlipidaemia
• Treat hypertension
• Aggressive control of diabetes
• Hormone replacement therapy in women: controversial; observational studies suggest benefit but a large randomized trial did not confirm this
• Alcohol: observational studies suggest some benefit in moderation, but not proven to be effective.

Secondary

Continue with primary preventive measures (see above). Aspirin (plus a statin if indicated) reduces risk of MI. Clopidogrel is an alternative for those with aspirin allergy.

Disease associations

• Peripheral vascular disease
• Cerebrovascular disease.

Fig. 32 Interventional treatment of coronary artery disease. CABG, coronary artery bypass grafting; PTCA, percutaneous transluminal coronary angioplasty.

Important information for patients:
• Explain that there are significant coronary narrowings but that the situation is stable
• Exertion within limits of symptoms is not dangerous, but avoid heavy lifting
• GTN may be used before exercise
• Gentle exercise (e.g. 30-min walk per day) is beneficial for the heart.

Antiplatelet Trialists' Collaboration. Collaborative overview of randomised trials of antiplatelet therapy. I: Prevention of death, myocardial infarction and stroke by prolonged antiplatelet therapy in various categories of patients. *BMJ* 1994; 308: 81–106.

Hillis LD, Rutherford JD. Coronary angioplasty compared with bypass grafting. *N Engl J Med* 1994; 331: 1086–1087.

Jackson R. Guidelines on preventing cardiovascular disease in clinical practice. *BMJ* 2000; 320: 659–661.

Swanton RH. Coronary artery disease. In: Swanton RH (ed.) *Cardiology* (Pocket Consultant). Oxford: Blackwell Science, 1998: 137–218.

Myers WO, Schaff HV, Gersh BJ *et al.* Improved survival of surgically treated patients with triple vessel coronary artery disease and severe angina pectoris. A report from the Coronary Artery Surgery Study (CASS) registry. *J Thorac Cardiovasc Surg* 1989; 97: 487–495.

Fig. 34 Angiogram of right coronary artery in a patient with unstable angina. There is extensive thrombus present, seen as filling defects within the lumen (arrows).

2.1.2 UNSTABLE ANGINA

Aetiology/pathophysiology/pathology

An atheromatous coronary artery plaque erodes or splits, producing a thrombogenic surface that attracts platelets (Fig. 33). The resulting thrombus reduces (but does not completely block) coronary blood flow, producing acute ischaemia of the heart muscle (Fig. 34).

Epidemiology

There are over 230 000 admissions per year for this condition in the UK.

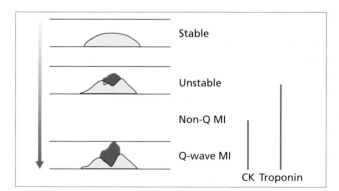

Fig. 33 Schematic diagram illustrating the sequence of events within a coronary artery during an acute coronary syndrome. Fissuring or erosion of an atherosclerotic plaque (yellow) leads to thrombosis (red), a rapid reduction in coronary blood flow and unstable angina. Transient complete occlusion leads to non-Q-wave (subendocardial) infarction, sustained occlusion to Q-wave (transmural) infarction. Highly sensitive troponin assays can detect microembolic heart muscle damage in unstable angina, allowing identification of those at higher risk of progression to infarction. CK, creatine kinase; MI, myocardial infarction.

Clinical presentation

Common

- Waxing and waning central chest pain at rest; partial relief from GTN
- Pain may be in the jaw or left arm
- Increasingly frequent and severe chest pain coming on with progressively less exertion (crescendo angina).

Uncommon

- Acute breathlessness (pulmonary oedema secondary to transient ischaemic LV dysfunction).

Physical signs

There are usually no specific signs in uncomplicated unstable angina.

Investigations

- ECG: may be normal; look for transient ST shift with pain; T-wave changes are less specific
- Cardiac biochemical markers: see Section 3.7, p. 136
- Stress testing may be useful if pain has settled but diagnosis in doubt, or to risk stratify once an unstable episode has settled
- Cardiac catheterization: see indications below.

Differential diagnosis

The differential diagnosis is as for MI (see Section 2.1.3, p. 55). Also consider coronary vasospasm.

Treatment

Myocardial infarction requiring thrombolysis must be excluded as soon as possible. The emphasis then switches to preventing progression to MI. Medical (antianginal and antithrombotic) treatment is the initial strategy, with cardiac catheterization reserved for persisting unstable symptoms or for certain high-risk subgroups.

Emergency

Emergency treatments include the following:
• Oxygen, analgesia, bedrest
• Aspirin, sublingual GTN, β blocker, low-molecular-weight heparin
• Consider heart-rate-lowering calcium antagonists (e.g. diltiazem) if a β blocker is contraindicated because of asthma, but avoid if there is significantly impaired LV function
• Glycoprotein IIb/IIIa inhibitors (e.g. tirofiban, eptifibatide, abciximab) are a new class of intravenous antiplatelet agents that improve outcome, particularly in patients undergoing urgent PTCA. Selective treatment of high-risk subgroups (e.g. troponin positive) may be the most effective way to use these expensive drugs (see recent NICE guidelines at www.nice.org.uk).

Short term

For continuing symptoms, use the following:
• Buccal nitrate or intravenous nitrate infusion
• Nicorandil.

If unstable symptoms do not resolve by 48 h, consider urgent cardiac catheterization with a view to revascularization (PTCA or CABG). This should also be considered in patients with the following:
• Post-infarct unstable angina
• Pulmonary oedema
• ST-segment shift with pain
• Recurrent unstable angina.

Long term

Once the acute episode has settled, the patient should be risk stratified in the same way as for stable angina (see Section 2.1.1, p. 51). This is done routinely in some hospitals before the patient is discharged.

Complications

Common

• Intractable or recurrent unstable angina
• MI.

Uncommon

• Pulmonary oedema
• Ventricular arrhythmias.

Prognosis

Morbidity

Fifteen per cent of patients with unstable angina progress to MI within 6 weeks.

Mortality

Ten per cent of patients die in the year after an episode of unstable angina.

Prevention

See Section 2.1.3, p. 55.

Important information for patients:
• Explain that the pain is a warning, not a heart attack
• Reassure that there is no significant heart muscle damage
• Explain that problems are best settled down with medication, if possible, but other treatments are available if they become necessary.

Braunwald E. Unstable angina: an aetiologic approach to management. *Circulation* 1998; 98: 2219–2222.
Heeschen C, Hamm CW, Goldmann B *et al.* Troponin concentrations for risk stratification of patients with acute coronary syndromes in relation to therapeutic efficacy of tirofiban. *Lancet* 1999; 354: 1757–1762.
Theroux P, Fuster V. Acute coronary syndromes. *Circulation* 1998; 97: 1195–1206.
Yeghiazarians Y, Braunstein JB, Askari A *et al.* Unstable angina pectoris. *N Engl J Med* 2000; 342: 101–114.

2.1.3 MYOCARDIAL INFARCTION

Aetiology/pathophysiology/pathology

Thrombus overlying an unstable plaque (see Fig. 33, p. 53) completely occludes the coronary artery, resulting in heart muscle necrosis. If the coronary occlusion is transient, only limited heart muscle death results (non-Q-wave infarction).

Epidemiology

• Each year there are 300 000 MIs in the UK.
• The mortality from coronary disease is in decline, but it remains the single most common cause of death in the UK (approximately 1 : 4 deaths).
• Death from an MI is almost three times higher in unskilled manual workers than in professional or managerial workers.

Clinical presentation

Common

• Acute onset with severe, crushing, central chest pain radiating to the jaw and/or left arm—unrelieved by nitrate
• Acute breathlessness (pulmonary oedema)
• Cardiac arrest (ventricular fibrillation).

Uncommon

• Pain in left arm alone, epigastrium or back
• Vomiting and sweating without pain
• Unexplained collapse
• Silent infarction (especially in people with diabetes and elderly people).

Physical signs

Common

There may be no abnormality on examination, but fre-quently the patient is pale, sweaty and obviously in pain. The patient may be hyper- or hypotensive. There may be pulmonary oedema.

Uncommon

The patient may present with only epigastric tenderness (inferior MI).

Investigations

Consider the following:
• ECG: ST-segment elevation and new bundle-branch block with an appropriate clinical history are both indications for thrombolysis (Fig. 35)
• Cardiac biochemical markers: see Section 3.7, p. 136
• Echocardiogram: indicated after an anterior MI or if there are haemodynamic complications (i.e. cardiogenic shock and/or pulmonary oedema)
• Serum cholesterol level is useful to guide initial statin therapy; sample <6 h after onset of pain because MI itself reduces cholesterol.

Differential diagnosis

The following may present in a similar way:
• Unstable angina
• Oesophagitis
• Musculoskeletal chest pain
• Thoracic aortic dissection.

Fig. 35 Anterior myocardial infarction.

Treatment

Emergency

Indications for thrombolysis
- Typical chest pain at rest for >20 min
- ST elevation in two contiguous leads (≥1 mm inferiorly, ≥2 mm anteriorly) OR new bundle branch block
- Within 12 h of onset, but consider thrombolysis if 12–24 h with continuing pain

Act quickly; delay in thrombolysis increases mortality. A 'door-to-needle' time of 20 min should be achievable in most cases.
- Take history while obtaining intravenous access.
- Simultaneous recording of baseline observations and ECG by nurse.
- Oxygen, opiate analgesia and antiemetic.
- Aspirin 300 mg if no contraindication.
- Once diagnosis confirmed, quickly examine patient while nurse draws up thrombolytic agent. Ensure no contraindications to thrombolysis (Table 14).
- Thrombolysis.
- Transfer to cardiac care unit (CCU) for monitoring. Emergency coronary angioplasty ('primary angioplasty') is an alternative to thrombolysis for MI. This may be a slightly better option if it can be performed by an experienced operator within 90 min of presentation, but most UK hospitals do not have these facilities.

Streptokinase (1.5 million units in 50 mL 0.9% saline over 1 h) is the first-line thrombolytic in the UK.
Consider recombinant tissue plasminogen activator (rTPA) if:
- Anterior MI; age <60 years; presenting within 6 h of onset
- Hypotension (streptokinase tends to lower blood pressure further)
- Streptokinase given ≥5 days before (neutralizing antibodies)
- Streptokinase allergy.

Table 14 Contraindications to thrombolysis.

Active internal bleeding
Active peptic ulcer
Bleeding tendency
Cerebrovascular accident in past 6 months (or at any time if haemorrhagic stroke)
Aortic dissection
Uncontrolled hypertension (>180/110 mmHg—bring down with nitrate infusion then thrombolyse)
Recent (<4 weeks) major trauma or surgery
Pregnancy

Note that anticoagulation in the therapeutic international normalized ratio (INR) range is a relative contraindication. Proliferative diabetic retinopathy is not a contraindication. Prior cardiopulmonary resuscitation is also not a contraindication unless prolonged or associated with obvious trauma.

Short term

The following have been shown to improve prognosis:
- β Blocker: orally within 24 h and continue indefinitely. Underused post-MI because of unfounded fears of side effects. Intravenous β blocker now controversial—may not confer added benefit. Oral diltiazem and verapamil are alternatives in patients with asthma, providing that LV function is not significantly impaired.
- ACE inhibitor: in patients with signs or echocardiographic evidence of LV dysfunction.
- Statin: year 2000 UK guidelines are to start if total cholesterol ≥5 mmol/L, which in practice is most patients post-MI.
- Warfarin: if there is persistent AF or large anterior MI with the risk of thromboembolism.
- Intensive insulin therapy (intravenous infusion for 24 h followed by insulin subcutaneously four times daily for 3 months) reduces mortality after MI in people with diabetes.
- Patients are usually kept in hospital for at least 5 days. Other antianginal drugs may be added to deal with residual stable angina (see Section 2.1.1, p. 51).

NEVER SMOKE AGAIN.

Long term

When appropriate, stress testing (see Section 3.1.1, p. 124) is usually undertaken 4–6 weeks after MI to identify high-risk patients who should undergo cardiac catheterization. Many of these will have severe coronary disease, the prognosis of which is improved by CABG.

Complications

Common

- Haemorrhage induced by thrombolysis: transfuse as required. For life-threatening bleeds, consider reversal of streptokinase with fresh frozen plasma or cryoprecipitate.
- Ventricular fibrillation/tachycardia: promptly cardiovert; antiarrhythmic drugs rarely necessary if it occurs in the first 24 h.
- Atrial fibrillation: see Section 2.2.2, p. 59.
- Complete heart block: see Sections 2.2.1, p. 58 and 3.5, p. 132.
- Pulmonary oedema: see Section 2.3, p. 63.
- Cardiogenic shock: inotropic support, monitor pulmonary artery wedge pressure, consider intra-aortic balloon pumping and ventilation in patients with surgically correctable cause, e.g. VSD, acute mitral regurgitation.

Fig. 36 Left ventriculogram showing apical mural thrombus (arrowed) after anterior myocardial infarction.

- Post-infarct unstable angina (16%).
- Reinfarction (3%).
- Pericarditis: usually benign; settles with NSAIDs.
- Stroke: consider reversing thrombolysis, request urgent CT scan of head.
- Arterial thromboembolism (AF or ventricular mural thrombus—Fig. 36).
- Deep venous thrombosis/pulmonary embolism.

Uncommon

- Left ventricular aneurysm
- Cardiac rupture: papillary muscle → acute mitral regurgitation (see Section 1.7, p. 23); septal → acquired VSD (see Section 1.7); free wall → tamponade (often sudden death).

Rare

- Dressler's syndrome: fever, pleuropericarditis, anaemia, raised ESR beginning 1–4 weeks after MI
- Frozen shoulder.

Prognosis

Morbidity

In the year after Q-wave MI:
- 25% develop unstable angina
- 10% have another infarction.
  The majority of patients admitted with an uncom-

plicated first MI will make a full recovery. Prognosis is determined by LV function at discharge and the results of stress tests (or cardiac catheterization if performed).

Non-Q-wave or subendocardial MI has a better prognosis than Q-wave MI over the first 6 weeks, but by 12 months the incidence of death is the same because of late reinfarction. Patients with non-Q-wave MI are therefore investigated more aggressively in the hope that prompt revascularization will prevent these late complications.

Mortality

- Of patients with a first MI, 30% do not reach hospital alive
- Of patients admitted to hospital, 10% die before discharge
- Of patients admitted to hospital, 10% die in the year after discharge.

Prevention

Primary

Prevention is via the control of the major risk factors for atherosclerosis (see Section 1.5, p. 15), usually managed in a primary care setting.

Secondary

- Aspirin, β blocker, ACE inhibitor
- Statin as indicated by cholesterol level.

Disease associations

Disease associations are cerebrovascular disease and peripheral vascular disease.

Important information for patients

On admission:
- Explain to the patient that he or she is having a heart attack, but that effective treatment is available
- The risk of haemorrhage following thrombolysis (3 per 1000) is outweighed by the benefits
- There is no net effect on stroke (increased haemorrhagic strokes offset by less ischaemic strokes).

On discharge:
- Good recovery is expected if there are no in-hospital complications
- Always carry GTN, even if free of angina
- Seek medical help if prolonged chest pain (>20 min) is not relieved by GTN
- You must give up smoking—reduces risk of reinfarction by 50%
- Gradually return to normal activities over the next 5 weeks. If available, a formal programme of cardiac rehabilitation is useful to reinforce these educational messages and restore patients' confidence.

pathway). If conduction is in an antegrade direction through the pathway, e.g. the Wolff–Parkinson–White syndrome, pre-excitation is seen on the surface ECG.

Ventricular tachycardias

Almost any pathological process affecting the ventricles may predispose to VT:
- MI (acute/chronic)
- Dilated cardiomyopathy
- Hypertrophic cardiomyopathy
- Valvular heart disease (especially aortic stenosis and mitral prolapse)
- Hypertension
- Congenital heart disease
- Long QT syndrome
- Cardiac tumours.

Pathophysiology/pathology

Tachyarrhythmias occur as a result of:
- Abnormal automaticity, e.g. VT after an MI
- Triggered activity, e.g. VT with long QT syndrome
- Re-entry, e.g. atrial fibrillation/flutter, AVRT/AVNRT, VT/ventricular fibrillation.

Clinical presentation

Common

- Palpitations
- Presyncope/syncope
- Breathlessness
- Chest pain.

Uncommon

Patients may complain only of lethargy.

Rare

Thromboembolism is unusual, except in AF.

Physical signs

Examination in sinus rhythm may be unremarkable. However, during tachycardia some physical signs may help to establish a diagnosis.

Atrial fibrillation/flutter

For the physical signs of AF, see Table 17.

Table 17 Clinical features distinguishing atrial fibrillation from atrial flutter.

	Atrial fibrillation	Atrial flutter
Pulse	Irregularly irregular	May be regular
JVP	Absence of 'a' waves	Rapid flutter waves
First heart sound	Variation in intensity	Constant intensity

JVP, jugular venous pressure.

AVNRT/AVRT

Physical signs are not especially helpful in making the diagnosis:
- Regular pulse
- JVP may be raised, but waveform is normal
- Constant intensity of first heart sound.

Ventricular tachycardias

Patients may or may not be significantly compromised:
- Hypotension
- Cannon waves.

Investigations

Investigations aim to exclude a structural thoracic/cardiac or metabolic cause: aside from an ECG, a chest radiograph, echocardiogram, thyroid function tests, renal function and electrolytes are appropriate in most cases.

Twelve-lead ECG

Documenting the arrhythmia with a 12-lead ECG will, in most cases, establish the diagnosis. In some cases where there is evidence of pre-excitation, the diagnosis can be relatively confidently made in sinus rhythm. Distinguishing some arrhythmias can be difficult:
- Atrial flutter versus atrial fibrillation: characteristic flutter waves (Figs 38 and 39)
- AVNRT versus AVRT: distinguishing these is rarely of clinical importance because, in most cases, the management is similar (Fig. 40)
- VT versus AVNRT/AVRT with aberrant conduction: see Section 3.1, p. 120.

Ambulatory monitoring

Documentation of an infrequent rhythm may be possible using 24-h Holter monitoring or patient-activated devices.

Fig. 38 ECG of atrial flutter: note the characteristic saw-tooth appearance of the baseline.

Fig. 39 ECG of atrial fibrillation. Notice the 'chaotic' baseline in comparison to Fig. 38 and the complete irregularity of QRS complexes.

Electrophysiological studies

See Section 3.2, p. 125.

Treatment

 There are many different classifications of antiarrhythmic agents. The Vaughan–Williams classification is the most commonly used and is based on the cellular action of the drug (Table 18).

Emergency

Atrial fibrillation/flutter

If the patient is compromised, consider DC cardioversion or intravenous amiodarone.

AVNRT/AVRT

Most will respond to intravenous adenosine. Verapamil may be used if you are confident that the rhythm is not VT.

Fig. 40 ECG of atrioventricular nodal re-entry tachycardia. Note the very rapid rate, regular rhythm and absence of discernible P waves.

Category	Action		Example
1	A	Prolong action potential	Quinidine, procainamide, disopyramide
	B	Shorten action potential	Lidocaine, mexiletine
	C	Slow conduction	Propafenone
2		Block β-adrenergic receptors	Propranolol, atenolol, metoprolol
3		K$^+$ channel blockers, prolong repolarization	Sotalol, amiodarone
4		Block slow calcium channels	Verapamil, diltiazem, nifedipine

Table 18 Vaughan–Williams classification of antiarrhythmic drugs.

Ventricular tachycardias

For resuscitation, see *Emergency medicine*, Section 1.1.

Short term

Atrial fibrillation/flutter

The main aim of treatment is the restoration of sinus rhythm. This may be achieved pharmacologically or electrically with DC cardioversion. In all cases, the risk of thromboembolism and the requirement to anticoagulate should be considered. Consider the following:
- Anticoagulation
- DC cardioversion
- Class III agent
- Digoxin (rate control only)
- Class I agent (if no coronary artery disease).

AVNRT/AVRT

- Class IA and IC agents
- Class II (β blockers)
- Class III (sotalol)
- Class IV (verapamil).

Ventricular tachycardias

- Class III agents
- Class I agents
- Class II agents
- Temporary pacing may prevent VT in patients with bradycardia-induced VT or long QT syndrome.

Long term

Most short-term drugs may be used long term, but more definitive therapies should be considered.

Atrial fibrillation/flutter

Consider the following:
- Anticoagulation
- Ablation for atrial flutter
- Ablation of AV node and permanent pacemaker for AF not controlled with drugs
- Implantable atrial defibrillator.

AVNRT/AVRT

Consider ablation (see Section 3.4.1, p. 130).

Ventricular tachycardias

Consider referral for ablation/ICD. (See Section 3.4, p. 130.)

 DC cardioversion does the following:
- It terminates most arrhythmias secondary to re-entry mechanisms
- Depolarizing all excitable myocardium interrupts the re-entry circuit.

Cardioversion of atrial fibrillation/flutter

The following can be used as guidelines for anticoagulation:
- Duration <48 h: proceed without anticoagulation
- Duration >48 h: anticoagulation for 4–6 weeks before and 4 weeks after cardioversion
- Duration >48 h and no evidence of intracardiac thrombus on TOE: proceed without anticoagulation.

Sinus rhythm is achieved in approximately 85% of cases of atrial fibrillation/flutter, but recurrence rates may be high (up to 75% at 12 months).

Complications

Atrial fibrillation/flutter

Thromboembolism is the most significant and devastating condition.

AVNRT/AVRT

Complications are uncommon but, with the Wolff–Parkinson–White syndrome, rapid conduction of AF down an accessory pathway may precipitate ventricular fibrillation.

Ventricular tachycardias

Haemodynamic collapse and death is a potential risk in most cases of VT.

Prevention

Primary and secondary prevention of stroke/TIA. (See Section 2.14.1, p. 108.)

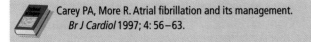 Carey PA, More R. Atrial fibrillation and its management. *Br J Cardiol* 1997; 4: 56–63.

2.3 Cardiac failure

Aetiology/pathophysiology/pathology

The common causes of heart failure are listed in Table 19.

After a single episode of cardiac damage, e.g. an MI, left ventricular dysfunction is often progressive even in the absence of further cardiac insults. This appears to result from the neurohumoral response to reduced cardiac output, which is initially compensatory but becomes detrimental in the long term (Fig. 41).

Epidemiology

The prevalence of heart failure is approximately 4 : 1000 (28 : 1000 at age >65). Heart failure is the primary diagnosis in about 4% of general medical admissions to hospital.

Increasing prevalence is the result of:
- an ageing population
- better survival after MI
- better survival with heart failure.

Clinical presentation

Heart failure commonly presents with the following:
- Exertional breathlessness
- Orthopnoea

Table 19 Causes of heart failure.

Cause	Relative frequency (%)
Ischaemic heart disease	40
Valve disease	9
Hypertension	6
Dilated cardiomyopathy/unknown	45

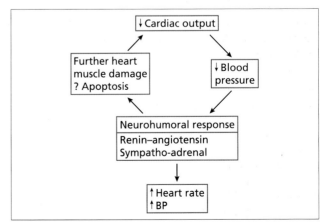

Fig. 41 The vicious cycle of progressive left ventricular damage.

- Paroxysmal nocturnal dyspnoea
- Cough productive of clear, frothy sputum
- Ankle swelling
- Fatigue.

 Severity of breathlessness in heart failure is graded according to the New York Heart Association (NYHA) class:
- NYHA I: impaired LV function but no symptoms
- NYHA II: breathless on vigorous exertion, e.g. walking briskly, walking uphill
- NYHA III: breathless during everyday activities, e.g. walking around the house
- NYHA IV: breathless at rest.

Physical signs

The physical signs include the following:
- Irregularly irregular pulse (AF)
- Elevated JVP (if up to angle of jaw suspect tricuspid regurgitation—check for systolic 'v' wave that coincides with contralateral carotid; check for pulsatile liver)
- Left parasternal heave (usually right ventricular hypertrophy, occasionally the result of greatly enlarged left atrium)
- Third heart sound (probably most sensitive and specific physical sign for LV dysfunction)
- Pansystolic murmur of functional mitral regurgitation
- Basal lung crackles
- Bilateral ankle oedema
- Ascites.

Investigations

Chest radiograph

Look for:
- heart size
- pulmonary oedema
- pleural effusions.

ECG

Look for:
- rhythm
- left atrial strain
- previous MI
- bundle-branch block.

Blood tests

- Urea and electrolytes: associated hyponatraemia, hypokalaemia (diuretic treatment), renal dysfunction
- Liver function tests: often mildly deranged in congestive cardiac failure.

Differential diagnosis

Consider the following:
- Cor pulmonale
- Nephrotic syndrome
- Liver failure.

Treatment

Emergency

In acute pulmonary oedema:
- sit up
- give oxygen (monitor blood gases)
- give intravenous diamorphine
- give intravenous furosemide (frusemide) 40–80 mg
- offload with intravenous infusion of nitrate titrated to maximum tolerated dose (but keep BP >90 mmHg systolic)
- check FBC, urea and electrolytes, cardiac enzymes
- consider pulmonary artery catheter, inotropic support or ventilation if these measures are unsuccessful.

Short term

Hospital treatment of congestive cardiac failure:
- Monitor fluid balance chart, daily weight (aim to lose 0.5–1 kg daily), and daily urea and electrolytes
- No-added-salt diet (but do not recommend a low-salt diet, which is extremely unpalatable)
- Intravenous loop diuretic, e.g. furosemide (frusemide) 80 mg once or twice daily
- ACE inhibitor (angiotensin II receptor blocker can be used if ACE inhibitor not tolerated)
- Consider anticoagulation (AF or grossly dilated left ventricle)
- Avoid calcium antagonists and NSAIDs.

If there is a good response, change to oral diuretics after 48 h. Aim to continue hospital treatment until the oedema is clearly improved, but in patients with impaired renal function it is better to accept some residual oedema than to precipitate acute-on-chronic renal failure. Do not use the JVP as the sole guide for treatment because this is often persistently elevated as a result of tricuspid regurgitation.

If weight loss is not satisfactory, add bendrofluazide 5 mg or metolazone 2.5–5 mg daily, but watch the renal function closely. If there is still no diuresis, consider higher doses of furosemide (frusemide) given by intravenous infusion over 2–6 h. Fluid restriction should be held in reserve for resistant cases. Rarely, inotropes (dopamine or dobutamine) are required for a few days to assist diuresis.

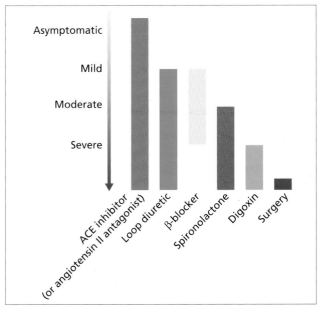

Fig. 42 Escalation of treatment for left ventricular dysfunction.

Long term

 You are a physician, doctor. You would promise life to a corpse if he could swallow pills. (Napolean Bonaparte)

Counselling the patient with heart failure can be very difficult as the prognosis is often poor. However, it is important to judge each case individually and not to give the patient unrealistic expectations.

Figure 42 shows long-term treatment options for those with heart failure. The following improve symptoms and life expectancy:
• ACE inhibitor in most patients.
• β Blocker, e.g. bisoprolol or carvedilol in patients with stable NYHA II or III symptoms. Start low, go slow. Hypotension should be dealt with by reducing the ACE inhibitor, fluid retention by increasing the loop diuretic. Try to continue the β blocker if at all possible, because these side effects are usually transient.
• Spironolactone in patients with NYHA III–IV and creatinine < 200 μmol/L, K$^+$ < 5.5 mmol/L. Check electrolytes weekly for 2 weeks and stop spironolactone if K$^+$ > 6.0 mmol/L.

Digoxin does not prolong life, but improves symptoms and reduces hospital admissions in more severe heart failure.

Cardiac transplantation is indicated for the following:
• Acute heart failure not responding to ventilation and inotropic support. A ventricular assist device (VAD—an artificial heart) may be used as a 'bridge to transplanta-

tion' if a suitable donor is not immediately available (Fig. 43). Heart function may improve (and transplantation be avoided) when 'rested' by one of these devices. However, use of a VAD is frequently complicated by thromboembolism and infection.
• Chronic progressive heart failure in patients with peak oxygen consumption (VO_{2max}) of <15 mL/kg/min during exercise (poor prognosis).

 … it is infinitely better to transplant a heart than to bury it so it can be devoured by worms. (Christiaan N. Barnard)

Complications

• AF
• VT
• Sudden death
• Progressive heart failure.

Prognosis

• Mortality related to ejection fraction and NYHA class
• Chronic stable heart failure: overall annual mortality rate = 10%
• Hospital series annual mortality rate = 30–50%
• Mortality rate of NYHA IV up to 60% in 1 year.

Prevention

Primary

• Prevention of MI (see Section 2.1, p. 51)
• Prompt reperfusion therapy for acute MI
• Avoid excess alcohol.

Secondary

ACE inhibitors, β blockers and spironolactone all reduce progression of heart failure and mortality.

 Important information for patients:
• Advice about no-added-salt diet
• Moderate alcohol intake
• Avoid heavy lifting (potentially arrhythmogenic)
• May feel worse for a few days after starting β blocker
• Weigh daily and report to GP or increase diuretic if weight gain (>1 kg in 3 days or >2.5 kg in 2 weeks).

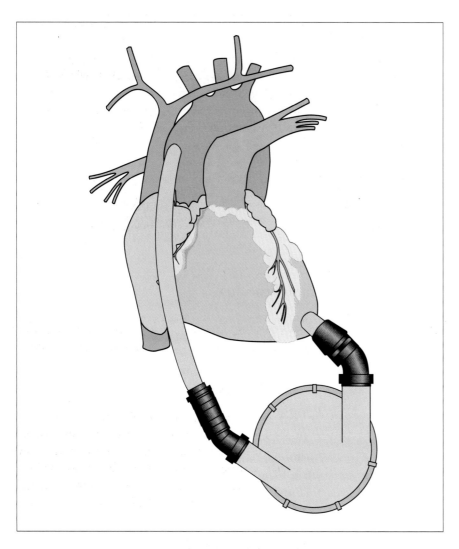

Fig. 43 Left ventricular assist device.

Houser SR, Lakatta EG. Function of the cardiac myocyte in the conundrum of end-stage, dilated human heart failure. *Circulation.* 1999; 99: 600–604.

Millane T, Jackson G, Gibbs CR *et al.* ABC of heart failure: acute and chronic management strategies. *BMJ* 2000; 320: 559–562.

Mann DL, Willerson JT. Left ventricular assist devices and the failing heart: a bridge to recovery, a permanent assist device, or a bridge too far? *Circulation* 1998; 98: 2367–2369.

Sharpe N. Benefit of beta-blockers for heart failure: proven in 1999. *Lancet* 1999; 353: 1988–1989.

2.4 Diseases of heart muscle

2.4.1 HYPERTROPHIC CARDIOMYOPATHY

Aetiology/pathophysiology/pathology

- Autosomal dominant
- Mutations found in at least eight genes (all encode contractile proteins, e.g. myosin β heavy chain, troponin T)
- Unexplained hypertrophy of the left (and occasionally the right) ventricle, which is usually focal, e.g. asymmetrical septal hypertrophy, apical hypertrophy
- Mechanism of hypertrophy unknown—possibly secondary to impaired function of contractile proteins (i.e. a compensatory phenomenon)
- Degree of hypertrophy variable even between individuals with the same mutation
- Left ventricular outflow tract obstruction may occur secondary to septal hypertrophy (Fig. 44)
- Mitral regurgitation may also be a feature, usually as a result of the Venturi effect in the presence of septal hypertrophy (Fig. 44).

Epidemiology

The prevalence of hypertrophic cardiomyopathy is 1 : 500 and it is the most common single-gene cardiac disorder.

Fig. 44 Effect of asymmetrical septal hypertrophy in hypertrophic cardiomyopathy. In late systole, the septum contracts down on the outflow tract, obstructing flow and generating a gradient. This generates a negative pressure (Venturi effect) just proximal to the obstruction, sucking the mitral valve anteriorly (systolic anterior motion) and producing mitral regurgitation. AO, aorta; LA, left atrium; LV, left ventricle; MV, mitral valve.

Clinical presentation

Common

- Exertional chest pain
- Palpitations
- Asymptomatic murmur
- Abnormal ECG on screening.

Uncommon

- Syncope.

Rare

- Sudden death.

Physical signs

There may be no abnormal findings.

Common

- Jerky pulse
- Prominent apical impulse
- Systolic murmur at left lower sternal edge/apex.

Uncommon

- Fourth heart sound: often easier to feel (as a double apical impulse) than hear.

Investigations

The ECG and echocardiogram must be interpreted together because they provide complementary information.

ECG

The ECG is sensitive but not very specific. It varies from T-wave inversion to overt left ventricular hypertrophy.

Echocardiography

Echocardiography is specific but less sensitive than the ECG. Classically, there is asymmetrical septal hypertrophy with systolic anterior motion of the mitral valve leaflet, left ventricular outflow tract obstruction and secondary mitral regurgitation. Alternative patterns include apical, free wall or concentric LVH.

Twenty-four-h ECG

This is used to identify the cause of palpitations or detect asymptomatic arrhythmia.

Exercise ECG

This is used to provoke arrhythmia and assess the blood pressure response (important for prognosis or for vocational driving licence).

Magnetic resonance imaging

MRI may confirm the diagnosis if echocardiographic images are not clear (Fig. 45).

> It is possible to have hypertrophic cardiomyopathy without any hypertrophy. The diagnosis may be made on the family history plus an abnormal ECG.

Differential diagnosis

- Hypertensive cardiac hypertrophy: a concentric pattern of hypertrophy with documented hypertension.

Fig. 45 Magnetic resonance imaging of the heart in the short axis, showing asymmetrical hypertrophy of the interventricular septum in hypertrophic cardiomyopathy (arrowed). LV, left ventricular cavity; RV, right ventricular cavity.

- Athlete's heart: differentiation may be difficult because some highly trained athletes, especially weight-lifters, rowers and cyclists, have an identical pattern of physiological hypertrophy. However, this will regress if training is discontinued. A septal thickness of >1.6 cm is likely to be pathological.

Treatment

No treatment is indicated in asymptomatic patients who do not have significant arrhythmia.

Antibiotic prophylaxis is generally recommended for dental and surgical procedures likely to produce a bacteraemia. Breathlessness and chest pain can be treated with β blockers or calcium antagonists, but often these only partially relieve symptoms. Severe breathlessness associated with an LV outflow tract gradient may be treated in a number of non-medical ways:

- Dual-chamber pacing: postulated to reduce gradient by activating the left ventricle from apex to base, so that the hypertrophied septum only contracts once most of the blood has been ejected from the left ventricle. Recent studies have been disappointing.
- Surgical myectomy: partial excision of the hypertrophied septum relieves gradient, but mortality rate is 1–2% at best.
- Percutaneous transluminal septal myocardial ablation is a promising new technique. A selected area of the obstructing septum is destroyed by alcohol injected into a carefully chosen septal artery (Fig. 46).

Complications

Common

- Atrial fibrillation: always anticoagulate because there is a high risk of thromboembolism. Often poorly tolerated, so consider cardioversion, with antiarrhythmic drugs to maintain sinus rhythm. Note that digoxin is contraindicated if there is significant LV outflow tract gradient (>50 mmHg), so use a β blocker or calcium antagonist for rate control.

Uncommon

- Ventricular tachycardia: give amiodarone—it may improve survival (although data from small retrospective studies). Consider ICD (see Section 3.4, p. 130).
- Progression to dilated cardiomyopathy: documented in up to 15% of early series, but certainly less common than this in modern practice.
- Sudden death.

Rare

- Endocarditis.

Prognosis

Risk of premature death associated with the following:
- Strong family history of sudden early death
- Diagnosis of hypertrophic cardiomyopathy in childhood
- Ventricular tachycardia on 24-h ECG monitoring
- Blood pressure drop on exercise
- Presence of certain high-risk mutations.

Disease associations

Friedreich's ataxia and the Wolff–Parkinson–White syndrome.

 Important information for patients

Explain the following:
- It is an inherited condition
- There is a 50% chance of transmission to children
- It is benign in most cases, hence reassure low risk if appropriate
- Continue as far as possible with a normal life, but avoid competitive physical sports
- Seek medical advice in the event of palpitations, dizziness or blackouts
- Careful discussion before screening—no treatment is indicated in the absence of symptoms, and knowledge of the diagnosis will adversely affect life insurance, mortgages, etc.

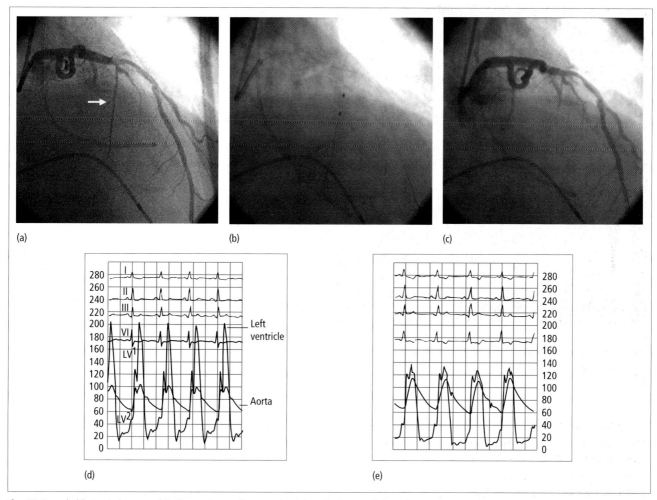

(a) (b) (c)

(d) (e)

Fig. 46 Septal ablation in hypertrophic obstructive cardiomyopathy. (a) A wire is passed through a coronary guide catheter into the target septal artery, indicated by arrow. A balloon catheter is passed, the wire is removed and the balloon inflated to occlude the artery. (b) Dye is injected down the lumen of the balloon catheter into the distal septal artery to confirm correct positioning. (c) Absolute alcohol is then injected to destroy selectively the septal artery, leaving a stump. Simultaneous pressure recordings reveal a left ventricular outflow tract gradient (peak ventricular minus peak aortic pressure) of approximately 100 mmHg (d) before the procedure, falling to (e) 15 mmHg afterwards.

Occupational aspects

Patients should not be professionals in sports requiring vigorous physical exertion. They may still hold vocational driving licences if they meet the DVLA criteria. (See Section 2.19, p. 118.)

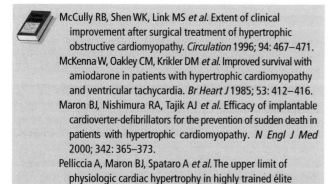

McCully RB, Shen WK, Link MS *et al.* Extent of clinical improvement after surgical treatment of hypertrophic obstructive cardiomyopathy. *Circulation* 1996; 94: 467–471.

McKenna W, Oakley CM, Krikler DM *et al.* Improved survival with amiodarone in patients with hypertrophic cardiomyopathy and ventricular tachycardia. *Br Heart J* 1985; 53: 412–416.

Maron BJ, Nishimura RA, Tajik AJ *et al.* Efficacy of implantable cardioverter-defibrillators for the prevention of sudden death in patients with hypertrophic cardiomyopathy. *N Engl J Med* 2000; 342: 365–373.

Pelliccia A, Maron BJ, Spataro A *et al.* The upper limit of physiologic cardiac hypertrophy in highly trained élite athletes. *N Engl J Med* 1991; 324: 295–301.

Spirito P, Seidman CE, McKenna WJ *et al.* The management of hypertrophic cardiomyopathy. *N Engl J Med* 1997; 336: 775–785.

2.4.2 DILATED CARDIOMYOPATHY

Aetiology/pathophysiology/pathology

This is a chronic progressive disorder, of unknown aetiology, characterized by dilatation and systolic dysfunction of the left (and sometimes the right) ventricle. Some cases are probably the result of unrecognized alcohol abuse, 'burn-out' hypertension, or acute myocarditis. Familial dilated cardiomyo-pathy caused by mutations in cyto-skeletal proteins has recently been described. Dilated cardiomyopathy also complicates muscular dystrophy.

Clinical presentation

This condition presents with congestive cardiac failure or arrhythmia (atrial or ventricular).

Investigations

The ECG often shows poor R-wave progression or LBBB. Echocardiography reveals a dilated left ventricle with globally impaired contraction. Focal areas of hypokinesia suggest ischaemic damage or prior myocarditis. Definitive diagnosis requires cardiac catheterization to ensure that there is no occult coronary disease.

Treatment/prognosis

See Section 2.3, p. 63.

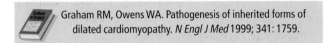
Graham RM, Owens WA. Pathogenesis of inherited forms of dilated cardiomyopathy. *N Engl J Med* 1999; 341: 1759.

2.4.3 RESTRICTIVE CARDIOMYOPATHY

Aetiology/pathophysiology/pathology

This is a chronic progressive condition characterized by excessively rigid ventricular walls that impair ventricular filling (diastolic dysfunction). Contractile (systolic) function is preserved. Causes are divided into the following:
• Myocardial, e.g. amyloid, sarcoid, storage diseases (often idiopathic)
• Endomyocardial, e.g. endomyocardial fibrosis, hypereosinophilic syndrome.

Epidemiology

This condition is rare in Western countries. Endomyocardial fibrosis is common in the tropics, particularly in Africa.

Clinical presentation

Symptoms

• Breathlessness, fatigue and ankle swelling.

Signs

• Elevated JVP, which rises on inspiration (Kussmaul's sign)
• Third and/or fourth heart sound

• Peripheral oedema
• Ascites.

Investigations

Chest radiograph

The heart size may be normal or increased. Pericardial calcification suggests constrictive pericarditis rather than restrictive cardiomyopathy. (See Section 2.6.3, p. 82.)

Echocardiography

Ventricular cavities are usually not dilated, but atrial cavities are often greatly enlarged. Rapid ventricular filling may be seen at the onset of diastole, which stops abruptly in early diastole.

Cardiac catheterization

Cardiac catheterization may be diagnostic in restrictive cardiomyopathy. Rapid ventricular filling in early diastole produces a 'square root sign' appearance of the LV diastolic pressure trace, which is also seen in pericardial constriction. However, other catheter data help differentiate the two conditions (Table 20).

Myocardial biopsy

This biopsy is sometimes useful to identify the cause of a restrictive cardiomyopathy.

Differential diagnosis

Restrictive cardiomyopathy must be distinguished from pericardial constriction, which is readily treated by surgery. Table 20 gives distinguishing features, but in up to 25% of patients it is not possible to tell and in these circumstances exploratory surgery may be justified.

Treatment

Response to medical treatment of heart failure is often poor. Successful combined heart and liver transplantation has been described in amyloid cardiomyopathy.

	Restrictive cardiomyopathy	Pericardial constriction
Third heart sound	Present	Absent
Pericardial calcification	Absent	In 50%
CT of the chest	Normal pericardium	Thickened pericardium
PA systolic pressure	Usually >50 mmHg	<50 mmHg
Diastolic pressure	LV > RV	LV = RV

Table 20 Differing features of restrictive cardiomyopathy and pericardial constriction.

LV, left ventricular; PA, pulmonary artery; RV, right ventricular.

Prognosis

The disease is generally relentlessly progressive with a high mortality.

Wynne J, Braunwald E. The cardiomyopathies and myocarditides. In: Braunwald E (ed.) *Heart Disease*. Philadelphia, PA: WB Saunders Co., 1996: 1426–1434.

2.4.4 ACUTE MYOCARDITIS

See *Infectious diseases*, Section 1.9.

2.5 Valvular heart disease

2.5.1 AORTIC STENOSIS

Aetiology/pathophysiology/pathology

Senile: calcific/degenerative

This is the most common form of aortic stenosis, especially in those aged >65 years. Diabetes, hypercholesterolaemia and chronic renal failure are risk factors. Coexistent coronary artery disease is common.

Congenital bicuspid valve

Symptoms usually appear at the age of 40–50 years.

Rheumatic heart disease

This is an unusual cause of aortic stenosis.

Stenosis results from a combination of fibrosis and calcification, with additional commissural fusion in the case of rheumatic fever. The increased LV pressure load results in compensatory LV hypertrophy and a prolonged ejection time, with diastolic dysfunction, myocardial ischaemia and an increased risk of ventricular arrhythmias.

Clinical presentation

Common

Common symptoms are exertional angina, dyspnoea and syncope, and occasionally palpitations. There are symptoms of LV failure if presentation is late.

Uncommon

Embolic phenomena from calcific emboli. Gastrointestinal bleeding (idiopathic/angiodysplasia) may occur. May present with infective endocarditis.

Physical signs

 The murmur is not a guide to severity. Look for clinical signs that reflect the haemodynamic significance.

In mild aortic stenosis, there may be few signs aside from the classic ejection systolic murmur at the base of the heart, radiating to the carotids. When haemodynamically significant, other features include the following:
- Slow rising carotid pulse ± thrill
- Prominent 'a' wave in the JVP
- Undisplaced thrusting apex beat with LV heave
- Soft first heart sound with single (calcified valve) or reversed splitting of the second heart sound
- Fourth heart sound
- Soft early diastolic murmur may be heard.

In late presentation, classic signs may lessen and LV failure and secondary pulmonary hypertension dominate.

Investigations

ECG

- Look for LVH and, rarely, conduction disturbance.

Chest radiograph

- May be normal but suspect aortic regurgitation, LV dilatation or severe hypertrophy if cardiomegaly present.

Echocardiography

Two-dimensional echocardiography shows bicuspid valves, thickening and reduced mobility of leaflets and calcification (Fig. 47). Continuous wave Doppler allows quantification of the pressure drop across the aortic valve and the aortic valve area (Table 21).

Coronary angiography

Coronary angiography will be required in most cases to assess the coronary arteries before surgery.

 Consider the following in your differential diagnosis:
- Innocent systolic murmur: pregnancy, fever, anaemia, thyrotoxicosis
- Aortic sclerosis
- Hypertrophic obstructive cardiomyopathy
- Atrial or ventricular septal defect.

(a)

(b)

Fig. 47 (a) Bicuspid aortic valve with arrow indicating abnormal fusion of cusps. (b) Calcific aortic stenosis. In this parasternal long axis view, the aortic valve cusps (arrowed) appear markedly thickened and calcified. (Courtesy of Dr J Chambers.)

Table 21 Grading of aortic stenosis by aortic valve area.

Aortic stenosis	Aortic valve area (cm^2)
Mild	>1.5
Moderate	1.1–1.5
Severe	≤0.8–1.0

Treatment

 Severe aortic stenosis is associated with a mean gradient of >70 mmHg. Note, however, that a lesser gradient can indicate critical stenosis if there is LV impairment.

Emergency

Admit the patient if there is heart failure and treat with diuretics. Exercise great caution with ACE inhibitors and other vasodilators, and never use them if the patient is hypotensive. Aim for early valve replacement as an emergency, if failure does not respond to treatment.

Long term

Follow moderate disease at yearly intervals with repeat echocardiography. Severe stenosis requires closer supervision to detect onset of symptoms. Antibiotic prophylaxis is required for dental procedures, etc. Valve replacement should be considered in all patients with severe aortic stenosis who become symptomatic. It is also indicated in asymptomatic patients who develop LV dysfunction.

Complications

The following are associated with aortic stenosis:
• Cardiac failure
• Sudden death
• Infective endocarditis
• Embolic disease
• Complete heart block.

Prognosis

Symptoms occur only after the stenosis has become severe. Mild aortic stenosis progresses to severe over 20 years in about 20% of cases, two-thirds remaining unchanged. Asymptomatic patients have an excellent prognosis. In symptomatic disease, the average survival with angina or syncope is 2–3 years, and with heart failure 1.5 years.

 Decena BF III, Tischler MD. Stress echocardiography in valvular heart disease. *Cardiol Clin* 1999; 17: 555–572.
Otto CM. Aortic stenosis: clinical evaluation and optimal timing of surgery. *Cardiol Clin* 1998; 16: 353–373.
Wierzbicki A, Shetty C. Aortic stenosis: an atherosclerotic disease? *J Heart Valve Dis* 1999; 8: 416–423.

2.5.2 AORTIC REGURGITATION

Aetiology/pathophysiology/pathology

Aortic regurgitation (AR) may result from primary disease of the valve leaflets, dilatation of the aortic root, loss of commissural support, failure of valve prosthesis, either alone or in combination. The result is the addition of a regurgitant volume to the normal inflow from the left atrium.

Aetiology of aortic regurgitation

Dilatation of the aortic root
- Degenerative (senile)
- Cystic medial necrosis: isolated/associated with Marfan's syndrome
- Aortic dissection
- Systemic hypertension
- Aortitis

Primary disease of valve leaflets
- Rheumatic heart disease
- Infective endocarditis
- Bicuspid valve
- Myxomatous degeneration
- Trauma

Loss of support of the aortic valve cusps
- High VSD
- Fallot's tetralogy

Failure of a prosthetic valve.

Clinical presentation

The patient may present with the following:
- Exertional dyspnoea
- Orthopnoea
- Paroxysmal nocturnal dyspnoea
- Palpitations and head pounding
- Angina.

Physical signs

Eponymous signs associated with aortic regurgitation:
- Quincke's: fingertip capillary bed pulsation
- de Musset's: head bobbing
- Corrigan's pulse: visible neck pulsations
- Müller's: uvular pulsations
- Duroziez's: systolic and diastolic murmurs heard over the femoral artery when compressed proximally or distally, respectively
- Traube's: pistol shot sounds over femoral arteries.

Examination in mild AR may be normal. More severe AR is associated with the following:
- Wide pulse pressure with a collapsing pulse
- Second heart sound single and loud; disappears in severe AR
- Displaced hyperdynamic apex beat ± systolic thrill
- Early diastolic murmur at left sternal edge: duration corresponds to severity
- Ejection systolic murmur ± third heart sound (increased flow)
- Austin Flint murmur: arising from mitral valve being struck by regurgitant blood.

Investigations

ECG

Look for the following:
- Normal/LVH
- Left atrial enlargement
- Prolongation of PR interval
- Non-specific ST segment and T-wave changes.

Chest radiograph

This is normal or shows cardiomegaly, which may be gross. There is pulmonary oedema in acute cases. Look out for evidence of aortic dissection.

Echocardiography

Two-dimensional echocardiography allows estimation of LV dimensions and ejection fraction, and determines the anatomy of the aortic valve and root. Dissection and endocarditis may be detected, but often require trans-oesophageal study. Continuous wave Doppler allows assessment of severity (Fig. 48).

Coronary angiography

Coronary angiography will be required before surgery to assess the coronary arteries in most cases.

Differential diagnosis

Consider pulmonary regurgitation and mitral stenosis with Graham Steell murmur.

Treatment

Emergency

In patients with acute severe AR or severe decompensated chronic AR, treat failure aggressively with diuretics

Fig. 48 Aortic regurgitation: in this parasternal long axis view, the broad regurgitant jet is seen mainly in blue. The diastolic timing can be seen from the lower velocity orange jet directly below, representing ventricular filling from the left atrium. (Courtesy of Dr J Chambers.)

± vasodilators ± inotropes. Look for the underlying cause and plan early or emergency valve replacement.

Short term

Treat heart failure with digitalis, diuretics and ACE inhibitors.

Long term

Patients with asymptomatic mild/moderate AR with normal ventricular function require regular monitoring only. Antibiotic prophylaxis is required.

Complications

Complications commonly encountered include the following:
- Progressive heart failure
- Mitral regurgitation
- AF
- Sudden death.

Prognosis

The risk of developing symptoms and/or LV dysfunction in severe AR with normal LV function is 4%/year. If there is LV dysfunction, the risk is >25%/year.

Prognosis is excellent in mild or moderate disease. In symptomatic severe AR the yearly mortality rate is >10%.

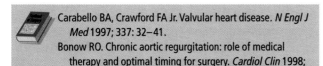

Carabello BA, Crawford FA Jr. Valvular heart disease. *N Engl J Med* 1997; 337: 32–41.
Bonow RO. Chronic aortic regurgitation: role of medical therapy and optimal timing for surgery. *Cardiol Clin* 1998; 16: 449–461.

2.5.3 MITRAL STENOSIS

Aetiology

Most mitral stenosis (MS) is acquired through rheumatic heart disease. It is more common in women, presenting in developed countries in the fourth or fifth decades of life.

Clinical presentation

Mitral stenosis commonly presents with the following:
- Exertional dyspnoea
- Orthopnoea
- Paroxysmal nocturnal dyspnoea
- Haemoptysis
- Palpitations
- Fatigue
- Weight loss
- Embolic phenomena in up to 15%.

Physical signs

Common

When MS becomes haemodynamically significant, common features include the following:
- Malar flush
- AF
- Undisplaced 'tapping' apex
- Left parasternal heave ± palpable opening snap and pulmonary second heart sound
- First heart sound may be loud
- Opening snap and mid-diastolic murmur, with presystolic murmur if in sinus rhythm
- Prominent 'v' waves and murmur suggestive of tricuspid regurgitation.

Uncommon

- Graham Steell murmur (pulmonary regurgitation)
- Presystolic murmur in AF
- Ascites, hepatomegaly, peripheral oedema.

Investigations

ECG

- Normal
- Left atrial enlargement or AF
- RVH.

Chest radiograph

- Normal
- Straightening of left cardiac border as a result of dilated left atrial appendage
- Pulmonary oedema
- Atrial double shadow along right cardiac border (Fig. 49).

Echocardiography

This provides a view of the valve and allows visualization of leaflet mobility, quantification of the valve area (Table 22), left atrial size and RV function. Doppler echocardiography allows assessment of the severity of the lesion, and estimation of the PAP. A transoesophageal study (TOE) is usually required to assess the suitability for valvuloplasty if this is being considered (Fig. 50).

Fig. 49 Chest radiograph showing left atrial enlargement in a patient with mitral valve disease: note the double atrial shadow (left atrial border indicated by broken line) and dilatation of the left atrial appendage (arrow). Reproduced from Axford (ed.) *Medicine*. Oxford: Blackwell Science, 1996.

Fig. 50 Mitral stenosis: the tips of the valve leaflets and subvalvular apparatus have become thickened from rheumatic heart disease. (Courtesy of Dr J Chambers.)

Table 22 Severity of mitral stenosis assessed by mitral valve area.

Severity	Aortic valve area (cm²)
Mild	>1.5
Moderate	1.0–1.5
Severe	<1.0

Cardiac catheterization

This is used only if coexistent coronary artery disease is suspected.

Differential diagnosis

Consider the following:

- Austin Flint murmur
- Left atrial myxoma
- Tricuspid stenosis.

Treatment

Emergency

Treat acute pulmonary oedema with diuretics.

Short term

β Blockers or rate-limiting calcium antagonists may help symptoms. AF may require treatment (see Section 2.2.2, p. 59).

Long term

Formal anticoagulation with warfarin is required. Antibiotic prophylaxis is needed irrespective of severity. Surgical intervention is indicated if there is severe stenosis and > NYHA Class II symptoms: mitral valvuloplasty may be possible, alternatively open valvuloplasty or mitral valve replacement is required.

Complications

The following are possible:
- AF
- Pulmonary hypertension or infarction
- Chest infections
- Tricuspid regurgitation
- RV failure
- Thromboembolic disease.

Prognosis

In severe MS, 5-year survival rates range from 62% with NYHA Class III symptoms to 15% with Class IV. After valvotomy, 5-year survival rates are between 90 and 96%.

 Lawrie GM. Mitral valve repair vs. replacement. Current recommendations and long-term results. *Cardiol Clin* 1998; 16: 437–448.
Bruce CJ, Nishimura RA. Newer advances in the diagnosis and treatment of mitral stenosis. *Curr Prob Cardiol* 1998; 23: 125–192.

2.5.4 MITRAL REGURGITATION

Aetiology/pathophysiology/pathology

Abnormalities of the mitral valve annulus, valve leaflets, chordae tendinae or papillary muscles may cause mitral regurgitation.

Common causes of mitral regurgitation in the adult
- Idiopathic mitral valve prolapse (MVP)—most common cause
- Papillary muscle dysfunction
- Ruptured chordae tendinae
- Annular dilatation
- Rheumatic heart disease
- Infective endocarditis
- ASD
- Failure of valve prosthesis/paraprosthetic leak.

Epidemiology

The prevalence of mitral valve prolapse varies from 1 to 6%, and is twice as common in women.

Clinical presentation

Common symptoms include exertional dyspnoea, orthopnoea, fatigue and lethargy. Occasionally, there are palpitations and, in severe acute mitral regurgitation, the patient may be very unwell with severe dyspnoea.

Physical signs

In mild disease, there are few signs apart from an apical pansystolic murmur radiating to the axilla. In more haemodynamically significant regurgitation, there can be the following:
- AF
- Laterally displaced, hyperdynamic apex beat with systolic thrill
- Left parasternal late systolic heave (atrial filling) in severe mitral regurgitation
- Soft first heart sound, wide splitting of second heart sound, third heart sound
- Late systolic murmur in association with a systolic click suggests MVP.

In acute severe mitral regurgitation, there is poor perfusion with pulmonary oedema.

Investigations

ECG

This may be normal, but look for AF, left atrial enlargement or LV hypertrophy.

Chest radiograph

This can be normal, or may show cardiomegaly with left atrial enlargement or mitral annular calcification (Fig. 51). There is pulmonary oedema in acute mitral regurgitation.

Fig. 51 Mitral annular calcification: a ring of calcification can be seen within the heart shadow.

Echocardiography

Assessment of severity is complex and the subject of some controversy. A transoesophageal study may be necessary to assess the feasibility of repair preoperatively, and in patients with acute mitral regurgitation (Fig. 52).

Coronary angiography

Coronary angiography may be required if there is a suspicion of coronary artery disease.

Treatment

Emergency

Treat acute pulmonary oedema and shock. Vasodilator therapy reduces the afterload and is of benefit. Intravenous nitroprusside may be life saving.

Short term

Symptomatic patients with severe mitral regurgitation who are awaiting surgery should receive diuretic and vasodilator therapy. Digitalis is of particular benefit in the treatment of AF, and anticoagulation will be required.

Long term

All patients must receive antibiotic prophylaxis. Mild-to-moderate disease requires monitoring only. Asymptomatic

(a)   (b)

Fig. 52 (a) Mild and (b) severe mitral regurgitation. Note the difference in size of the regurgitant jets seen mainly as blue. (Courtesy of Dr J Chambers.)

patients with severe mitral regurgitation need closer follow-up to monitor LV function and symptom status.

Indications for surgery in severe mitral regurgitation:
• If surgical repair is possible, it should be considered in all patients aged <75 years who have a flail leaflet or persistent AF
• Deteriorating ventricular function (ejection fraction <60% or end-systolic diameter >45 mm)
• The presence of symptoms, although careful consideration of the aetiology and severity of LV dysfunction is needed in older patients.

Complications

The following are possible:
• LV failure
• AF
• Infective endocarditis
• Pulmonary hypertension
• RV failure
• Thromboembolism (more common in MVP)
• Sudden death (more common in flail leaflet).

Prognosis

Progression of mitral regurgitation depends on the aetiology, but develops in 15% of patients over a 10- to 15-year period with MVP. Without surgery, patients with severe mitral regurgitation have a 5-year survival rate as low as 45%. After surgery, the 5-year survival rates vary from 40% in mitral regurgitation caused by IHD to over 75% in rheumatic mitral valve disease.

Cooper HA, Gersh BJ. Treatment of chronic mitral regurgitation. *Am Heart J* 1998; 135(Pt 1): 925–936.
Quinones MA. Management of mitral regurgitation: optimal timing for surgery. *Cardiol Clin* 1998; 16: 421–435.

2.5.5 TRICUSPID VALVE DISEASE

Aetiology/pathophysiology/pathology

Tricuspid regurgitation (TR) is usually secondary to a combination of right ventricular dilatation and high pressure resulting from severe pulmonary hypertension. Tricuspid stenosis (TS) is almost invariably rheumatic in origin, and accompanies mitral stenosis. In both, right atrial enlargement and hypertrophy occur with the risk of AF.

Less common causes of tricuspid regurgitation:
• Infective endocarditis (especially drug addicts)
• Papillary muscle dysfunction
• Endocardial cushion defects
• Ebstein's anomaly
• Myxomatous degeneration causing prolapse
• Carcinoid syndrome.

Clinical presentation

This is usually asymptomatic, and in the case of TR usually discovered secondary to other more significant cardiac pathology. TR and TS may cause a sensation of neck pulsation, right upper quadrant discomfort and peripheral oedema. Occasionally, a low cardiac output syndrome comprising fatigue, weight loss and syncope may be present.

Physical signs

Tricuspid regurgitation causes prominent 'v' waves in the JVP, whereas TS causes prominent 'a' waves in sinus rhythm. In more severe cases, both cause pulsatile hepatomegaly, ascites and peripheral oedema. In TR, a pansystolic murmur which increases on inspiration and is heard best at the lower left sternal edge is usual. The corresponding murmur in TS is a presystolic murmur in sinus rhythm with mid-diastolic murmur.

Fig. 54 ECG showing changes of acute pericarditis.

with oral NSAIDs given for symptomatic relief. Consider corticosteroids if there is severe pain not responding to NSAIDs after 48 h.

 Stop any oral anticoagulants because of the risk of intrapericardial haemorrhage and tamponade.

Long term

If idiopathic relapsing pericarditis develops, corticosteroids are traditionally used. More recently, colchicine has been gaining favour.

Complications

Beware of the following:
• Pericardial effusion
• Idiopathic relapsing pericarditis
• Cardiac tamponade
• Constrictive pericarditis.

Prognosis

There is complete resolution within 3 months in 80% of patients; 20% develop idiopathic relapsing pericarditis with chronic symptoms of pericardial inflammation. Cardiac tamponade may cause death if untreated, as may some of the precipitating conditions.

 Adler Y, Finkelstein Y, Guindo J *et al.* Colchicine treatment for recurrent pericarditis: a decade of experience. *Circulation* 1998; 97: 2183–2185.
Fowler NO. Recurrent pericarditis. *Cardiol Clin* 1990; 8: 621–626.
Maisch B. Pericardial diseases, with a focus on aetiology, pathogenesis, pathophysiology, new diagnostic imaging methods, and treatment. *Curr Opin Cardiol* 1994; 9: 379–388.

2.6.2 PERICARDIAL EFFUSION

Aetiology/pathophysiology/pathology

Pericardial effusion may develop in acute pericarditis from any cause. The normal pericardial space contains 15–50 mL fluid and can only accommodate a rapid increase in pericardial volume to 150–200 mL before the intrapericardial pressure (IPP) starts to rise. When accumulation of fluid occurs more gradually, volumes of up to 2 L may be present.

Acute cardiac tamponade typically follows cardiac trauma (which may be iatrogenic), aortic dissection, spontaneous bleeding or cardiac rupture after an MI. Chronic tamponade usually results from malignancy, idiopathic pericarditis or uraemia, although almost any cause of acute pericarditis may be responsible.

Clinical presentation

Common

In most cases, the IPP does not rise significantly and the

patient is asymptomatic, although a mild oppressive chest ache is occasionally present.

Uncommon

In a large pericardial effusion without tamponade, compression of adjacent structures may lead to the following:

- Dysphagia (oesophagus)
- Cough (bronchus/trachea)
- Hiccups (phrenic nerve)
- Hoarseness (laryngeal nerve)
- Abdominal bloating and nausea (abdominal viscera).

Physical signs

In most patients, the examination will be normal. In large effusions without tamponade, there may be muffled heart sounds, crackles (compression of lung parenchyma) or Ewart's sign (patch of dullness below the angle of the left scapula caused by compression of the base of the left lung). There may also be pericardial friction rub or signs of cardiac tamponade.

Cardiac tamponade may present in three ways:
1 Cardiac arrest
2 A severely ill patient who is stuporous or agitated and restless (survivor of acute tamponade)
3 With dyspnoea, chest pain, weight loss, anorexia and weakness (more slowly developing tamponade).

Rapid recognition of the clinical signs of tamponade is essential:
- Tachypnoea and tachycardia
- Pulsus paradoxus (pulse becomes impalpable on inspiration in severe cases)
- Elevated jugular venous pressure with prominent systolic x descent and absence of diastolic y descent
- Rarely, normal JVP in severe dehydration.

If you suspect the diagnosis—organize an urgent echocardiogram.

Fig. 55 Pericardial effusion: note the globular shape of the heart shadow.

Investigations

ECG

This is usually normal, although changes of acute pericarditis may be present. There may be a non-specific reduction in QRS voltage and T-wave flattening. Electrical alternans is suggestive of a large effusion.

Chest radiograph

This is often normal; a large effusion may cause an enlarged globular cardiac silhouette with clear lung fields. Look for separation of the pericardial fat lines and a left-sided pleural effusion (Fig. 55).

Echocardiography

Echocardiography is the most sensitive test for detection of pericardial fluid (as little as 20 mL). Diastolic left and right heart collapse suggest tamponade (Fig. 56).

(a) (b) (c)

Fig. 56 Large pericardial effusion. (a) Parasternal long axis, (b) short axis and (c) M-mode views of a large pericardial effusion which appears as an echo-free space immediately adjacent to the heart. (Courtesy of J Harris.)

Pericardiocentesis

Pericardiocentesis is essential and urgent in cardiac tamponade. It is also needed for diagnosis if there is a suspicion of purulent or tuberculous pericarditis or prolonged and otherwise unexplained illness. Details are beyond the scope of this text.

Differential diagnosis

In chronic cases consider the following:
• Constrictive pericarditis
• Restrictive cardiomyopathy.

In those with tamponade, consider causes of circulatory collapse (see *Emergency medicine*, Sections 1.1 and 1.2), in particular massive PE and severe asthma.

Treatment

Consider the following:
• Urgent pericardiocentesis in tamponade
• Symptom relief as for acute pericarditis (see Section 2.6.1, p. 78)
• Recurrent or persistent symptomatic effusions may require balloon pericardiostomy or surgical pericardiectomy.

Complications

Common

Complications arise more commonly from the underlying conditions than from the effusion, although chronic pericardial effusion lasting more than 6 months may be seen. This is more likely after idiopathic, uraemic, myxoedematous or malignant pericarditis.

Uncommon

Uncommon complications are cardiac tamponade and constrictive pericarditis.

Chong HH, Plotnick GD. Pericardial effusion and tamponade: evaluation, imaging modalities, and management. *Compr Ther* 1995; 21: 378–385.

Devlin GP, Smyth D, Charleson HA, Heaven DJ, McAlister HF. Balloon pericardiostomy: a new therapeutic option for malignant pericardial effusion. *Aust NZ Med* 1996; 26: 556–558.

Tsang TS, Oh JK, Seward JB. Diagnosis and management of cardiac tamponade in the era of echocardiography. *Clin Cardiol* 1999; 22: 446–452.

2.6.3 CONSTRICTIVE PERICARDITIS

Aetiology/pathophysiology/pathology

Constrictive pericarditis is characterized by an abnormally thickened and non-compliant pericardium, which limits ventricular filling in mid- to late diastole. This results in elevated cardiac filling pressures and the equalization of end-diastolic pressures of all four chambers. The clinical features are secondary to systemic venous congestion.

Before the 1960s, tuberculous constrictive pericarditis was the most common cause of pericardial constriction worldwide. In the developed world, its importance has declined, and the aetiology is usually idiopathic, postradiotherapy or postsurgical.

Clinical presentation

Common

Oedema, abdominal swelling and discomfort caused by ascites or hepatic congestion are most frequent. Vague abdominal symptoms such as postprandial fullness, dyspepsia, flatulence and anorexia may also be present. Cachexia and fatigue suggest a reduced cardiac output.

Uncommon

Exertional dyspnoea and orthopnoea may occur when ventricular pressures become severely elevated, as may platypnoea (dyspnoea in upright position).

Physical signs

Common

Elevation of the JVP with prominent x and y descents is the most important clinical sign, plus the following:
• AF
• Kussmaul's sign (inspiratory rise in JVP)
• Pericardial knock (third heart sound)
• Hepatosplenomegaly, ascites and peripheral oedema
• Cachexia.

Uncommon

Uncommon complications are pulsus paradoxus and signs of severe liver failure.

Investigations

ECG

This may be normal or show non-specific generalized T-wave changes, low-voltage complexes or AF.

Chest radiograph

This is usually normal, but the cardiac silhouette may be either reduced or enlarged. Left atrial enlargement, pleural effusions and pericardial calcification are non-specific findings.

Echocardiography

Echocardiography shows pericardial thickening and abnormal diastolic filling.

Cardiac catheterization

This is usually needed to confirm the diagnosis, with characteristic equalization of end-diastolic pressures in the two ventricles, persisting with respiration and fluid challenge (Fig. 57).

CT/MRI

These imaging techniques may be used to demonstrate the extent and distribution of pericardial thickening (Fig. 58).

Others

As dictated by clinical suspicion of underlying cause. (See Section 2.6.1, p. 78.)

Differential diagnosis

Consider the following:
- Chronic pericardial effusion
- Restrictive cardiomyopathy: see Section 2.4.3, p. 70
- Superior vena caval obstruction: excluded if there is a pulsatile waveform in JVP
- Congestive cardiac failure
- Nephrotic syndrome
- Malignant hepatic or intra-abdominal disease.

Treatment

A minority of patients may be managed medically with diet and diuretic therapy. Most will require pericardiectomy: early operation is recommended.

Complications

Severe venous congestion with chronic hepatic impairment is common. Death results from the consequences of an inadequate cardiac output.

Prognosis

Morbidity

Without treatment, most patients deteriorate progressively

Fig. 57 Pericardial constriction: the top section of the image contains pressure tracings from catheters placed simultaneously in the left and right ventricles. The pressures from the two chambers are seen to equalize at the end of diastole. (Courtesy of E Tomsett.)

(a)

(b)

(c)

(d)

Fig. 58 Pericardial thickening: these sections (a, b, c and d) through the heart show a markedly thickened pericardium.

with severely limiting symptoms. With pericardiectomy, 90% improve and 50% may gain complete relief of symptoms.

Mortality

The outlook in untreated cases is poor. Hospital mortality rate after pericardiectomy is between 5 and 16%, and 5-year survival rate after surgery is between 74 and 87%.

Mehta A, Mehta M, Jain AC. Constrictive pericarditis. *Clin Cardiol* 1999; 22: 334–344.

Tuna IC, Danielson GK. Surgical management of pericardial diseases. *Cardiol Clin* 1990; 8: 683–696.

Vaitkus PT, Kussmaul WG. Constrictive pericarditis vs. restrictive cardiomyopathy: a reappraisal and update of diagnostic criteria. *Am Heart J* 1991; 122: 1431–1441.

2.7 Congenital heart disease

With advances in paediatric treatment a large number of individuals with congenital heart disease have now survived into adulthood (1 million in the USA). Conditions can be divided into cyanotic and acyanotic (see Table 24).

Particular care should be taken to prevent infective endocarditis associated with dental or surgical procedures using appropriate prophylactic antibiotics. The highest risk is associated with high-pressure jets of blood:

- Tetralogy of Fallot
- Ebstein's anomaly
- VSD
- Patent ductus arteriosus
- Coarctation of the aorta.

Table 24 Congenital heart lesions.

Cyanotic	Acyanotic
Tetralogy of Fallot	Atrial septal defect (ASD)
Eisenmenger's	Ventricular septal defect (VSD)
Transposition of the great arteries	Patent ductus arteriosus
Ebstein's anomaly	Coarctation of the aorta

All lesions require echocardiography to determine anatomy and direction of shunts. MRI also gives detailed anatomical information. Most lesions require cardiac catheterization for calculation of the magnitude of the shunt and pulmonary vascular resistance. These investigations are not listed again under each individual section, unless there is a particular point to note.

The following are the complications of chronic cyanosis (right-to-left shunting causing hypoxaemia):
• Polycythaemia, causing hyperviscosity (symptoms—visual disturbance, headache, dizziness and paraesthesiae) and increased thrombotic risk
• Abnormal haemostasis and thus haemorrhagic risk
• Paradoxical embolism causing cerebral abscess or stroke.

Venesection and isovolumic replacement should be carried out only in patients with symptoms of hyperviscosity, not based on the haematocrit.

Some particular genetic conditions are associated with specific cardiac abnormalities (Table 25).

2.7.1 TETRALOGY OF FALLOT

Aetiology/pathophysiology/pathology

This consists of a large VSD, overriding of the aorta, right ventricular outflow tract obstruction (RVOTO) and RVH (Fig. 59). Left and right ventricular pressures are equal (large VSD) and so RVOTO causes right-to-left

Table 25 Examples of genetic diseases affecting the cardiovascular system.

Syndrome	Inheritance	Gene/chromosome	Cardiac manifestations	Management
Marfan's	AD	Fibrillin/15q	Aortic root dilatation/rupture	Echo surveillance, β blockade, elective aortic root repair when >5.5 cm diameter
Turner's		45 X0	Coarctation of the aorta, bicuspid aortic valve	Echo surveillance of valve, surgery for coarctation
Noonan's	AD	12q24	Pulmonary stenosis most common	
Down's		Trisomy 21	AV canal defects	Surgical
Di George	AD or sporadic	22q deletion	Conotruncal	Surgical
Williams		7 deletion	Supravalvar aortic stenosis	Echo surveillance
Holt–Oram	AD	TBX5/12q	Septal defects (hand–heart)	See Sections 2.7.5, p. 89, and 2.7.6, p. 90
Muscular dystrophies	Various	Various	Conduction defects, cardiomyopathy—may also be seen in female carriers of X-linked	Pacing for heart block, standard treatment for LV dysfunction, echo and ECG screening of carriers

See also cardiomyopathy (see Section 2.4, p. 66 and muscular dystrophies (see *Neurology*, Section 2.2.3). AD, autosomal dominant; LV, left ventricular.

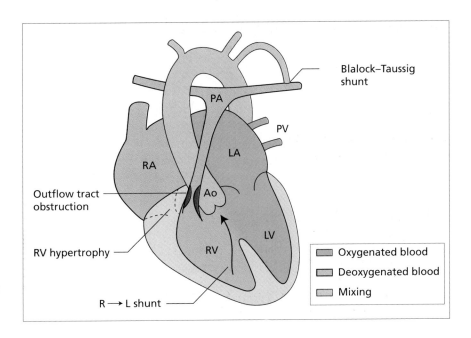

Fig. 59 Tetralogy of Fallot with left Blalock–Taussig shunt. Ao, aorta; LA, left atrium; LV, left ventricle; PA, pulmonary artery; PV, pulmonary veins; RA, right atrium; RV, right ventricle.

shunting (cyanosis), which increases with any decrease in systemic vascular resistance.

Epidemiology

This is the most common cyanotic congenital heart defect after infancy.

Clinical presentation

Presentation is with cyanosis from birth or early infancy; adults have limiting exertional dyspnoea and complications of chronic cyanosis.

Physical signs

Look for the following:
- Cyanosis
- Clubbing (Fig. 60)
- RV heave
- Normal S1, inaudible P2, RV outflow ejection systolic murmur ± thrill.

Investigations

- ECG: R-axis deviation and RVH
- Chest radiograph: boot-shaped heart.

(a)

(b)

Fig. 60 Example of digital clubbing in a patient with cyanotic heart disease.

Treatment

Previously, treatment was with systemic-to-pulmonary artery shunts (e.g. Blalock–Taussig shunt—see Fig. 59) to increase pulmonary blood flow; older adult patients will therefore have these shunts. Currently, complete surgical correction is standard.

Complications

- Ventricular arrhythmias
- AF or atrial flutter
- Pulmonary regurgitation with RV dilatation and failure
- Recurrent RVOTO.

Prognosis

Without surgical repair, the survival rate is 66% at age 1 and 10% at age 20 years.

With complete surgical correction, the mortality rate is <3% in children, slightly higher in adults, with a small excess late mortality as a result of ventricular arrhythmias.

2.7.2 EISENMENGER'S SYNDROME

Aetiology/pathophysiology/pathology

A large left-to-right shunt causes increased pulmonary blood flow, resulting in vascular obstructive disease, pulmonary hypertension and RVH. As the pulmonary vascular resistance exceeds the systemic resistance the shunt is reversed, causing cyanosis (Fig. 61). This usually occurs during or after adolescence.

Clinical presentation

- Cyanosis
- Limiting exertional dyspnoea
- Palpitations (AF or atrial flutter)
- Haemoptysis
- Syncope and sudden death
- RV failure in advanced disease.

Physical signs

Look for the following:
- Cyanosis
- Clubbing
- RV heave and loud P2 (contrast with Fallot's tetralogy), right-sided S4
- Signs of tricuspid or pulmonary regurgitation.

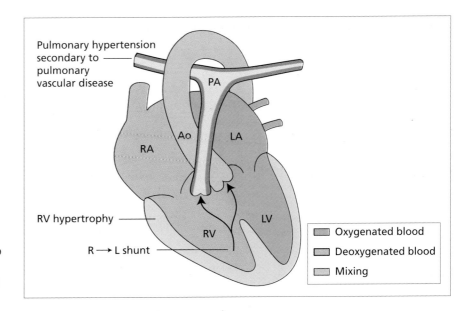

Fig. 61 Eisenmenger's syndrome secondary to ventricular septal defect. Ao, aorta; LA, left atrium; LV, left ventricle; PA, pulmonary artery; RA, right atrium; RV, right ventricle.

In Eisenmenger's syndrome the murmur of the original shunt will have disappeared.

Investigations

- Look for RVH ± atrial arrhythmias on the ECG.
- The chest radiograph may demonstrate prominent central pulmonary arteries and peripheral pruning.
- The response to pulmonary vasodilators on cardiac catheterization should be tested.

Treatment

See Section 2.12.1, p. 101. Avoid anticoagulants (existing coagulation abnormality) unless there is a very compelling indication for them.

Complications

Atrial arrhythmias and the complications of chronic cyanosis.

Prognosis

After diagnosis, the 10-year survival is 80% and the 25-year survival 40%. A poor prognosis is associated with the following:
- Syncope
- Signs of RV failure
- Low cardiac output
- Severe hypoxaemia.

Prevention

By closure of haemodynamically significant left-to-right shunts or protective pulmonary artery banding to reduce pulmonary flow before the development of pulmonary vascular disease.

Important information for patients

Avoid volume depletion, systemic vasodilators, altitude, heavy exertion and pregnancy.

2.7.3 TRANSPOSITION OF THE GREAT ARTERIES

Aetiology/pathophysiology/pathology

The aorta arises anteriorly from the right ventricle (the systemic ventricle) and the pulmonary artery from the left, so the two circulations are completely separate. A communication (foramen ovale, patent ductus arteriosus or septal defect) between them is necessary for survival (Fig. 62).

Clinical presentation

Clinical presentation is with cyanosis from birth, and LVF in infancy if the left-to-right shunt is large.

Physical signs

Signs are of cyanosis and a single loud S2 (anterior aorta).

Investigations

- The ECG may show right axis deviation and RVH.
- Look for cardiomegaly with increased pulmonary vascularity on the chest radiograph.

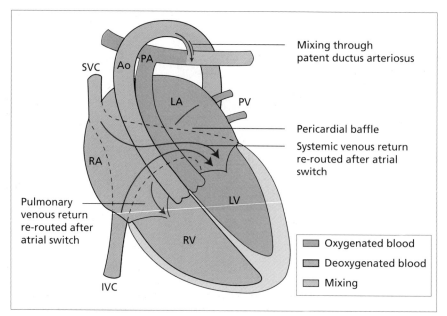

Fig. 62 Transposition of the great arteries with the circulations mixing through a patent ductus arteriosus. The effect of an atrial switch operation is shown in dashed lines, re-routing the venous return to the correct great vessel. In the arterial switch, the great vessels are transected above the valves and switched, with reimplantation of the coronaries. Ao, aorta; IVC, inferior vena cava; LA, left atrium; LV, left ventricle; PA, pulmonary artery; PV, pulmonary veins; RA, right atrium; RV, right ventricle; SVC, superior vena cava.

Treatment

Emergency

The need is to create or increase intracardiac mixing—prostaglandin E to maintain a patent ductus arteriosus and/or atrial septostomy.

Surgery

The treatment was previously by atrial switch (Mustard or Senning) in which the venous returns were re-routed through the atria (Fig. 62), so the physiological circulation was restored, but the right ventricle remained systemic and eventually failed. Currently, treatment is by arterial switch in neonates.

Prognosis

There is a mortality rate of 90% by 6 months without intervention.

2.7.4 EBSTEIN'S ANOMALY

Aetiology/pathophysiology/pathology

The tricuspid valve (regurgitant or stenotic) is displaced down into the right ventricle, leaving a small functional ventricle. Eighty per cent of these patients have an ASD or patent foramen ovale (PFO) and right-to-left shunting occurs if the right atrial pressure rises (Fig. 63).

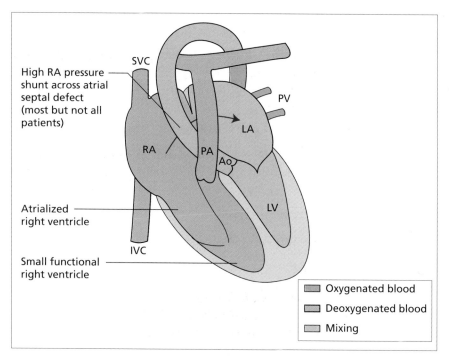

Fig. 63 Ebstein's anomaly with shunting across an associated atrial septal defect. Ao, aorta; IVC, inferior vena cava; LA, left atrium; LV, left ventricle; PA, pulmonary artery; PV, pulmonary veins; RA, right atrium; SVC, superior vena cava.

Clinical presentation

There is a wide spectrum of presentation, from an incidental finding to severe venous congestion and cyanosis.

Physical signs

Signs may include the following:
- Cyanosis
- Tricuspid regurgitation
- Hepatomegaly.

Investigations

Look for the following on the ECG:
- Tall/broad P waves
- RBBB
- First-degree heart block
- δ wave.

Treatment

- Diuretics and digoxin for LV failure
- Antiarrhythmics or ablation for arrhythmias
- Tricuspid repair/replacement and surgical closure of ASD.

Complications

Complications are atrial arrhythmias and/or accessory pathways (the Wolff–Parkinson–White syndrome).

2.7.5 ATRIAL SEPTAL DEFECT

Aetiology/pathophysiology/pathology

Atrial septal defects may be ostium primum, secundum or sinus venosus in type (Fig. 64). The haemodynamic consequences depend on the size of the defect; generally, blood shunts from the left atrium to the right because the right ventricle is more compliant than the left. The right ventricle may dilate and fail, or pulmonary hypertension and possibly Eisenmenger's syndrome develop.

A patent foramen ovale is common in young people. It does not permit left-to-right shunting but allows right-to-left shunting when right atrial pressure exceeds left (e.g. Valsalva manoeuvre); opinion is divided about whether this represents an increased risk of stroke as a result of paradoxical embolism.

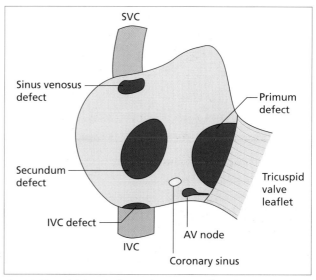

Fig. 64 Sites of defects in the atrial septum seen from the right atrium. AV, atrioventricular; IVC, inferior vena cava; SVC, superior vena cava.

Epidemiology

Atrial septal defects make up 30% of congenital heart disease detected in adults. Female : male = 2 : 1; 75% are ostium secundum.

Clinical presentation

The following are the most common presentations:
- Incidental finding
- Atrial arrhythmias
- Exertional fatigue or dyspnoea
- Right heart failure
- Paradoxical embolism.

Physical signs

Wide fixed splitting of S2 (equalization of RV and LV stroke volumes throughout the respiratory cycle). Pulmonary flow murmur (soft) and RV heave if there is a large shunt.

There is no murmur across the ASD itself.

Investigations

ECG

Look for the following:
- Right axis deviation and RBBB
- Left axis deviation in ostium primum defects
- Atrial arrhythmias.

Fig. 65 Transoesophageal echo image of left-to-right flow across a large atrial septal defect. A denotes the atrial septum, B the left atrium and C the flow into the right atrium. (Courtesy of Dr LM Shapiro.)

Chest radiograph

Prominent pulmonary vasculature.

Echocardiography

Transoesophageal echocardiography is ideal with micro-bubble contrast to visualize shunting (Fig. 65).

Treatment

This consists of closure (surgical or percutaneous device) if the pulmonary : systemic flow ratio (shunt) is >1.5 : 1 and management of the complications, e.g. arrhythmias.

Prognosis

Shunt <1.5 : 1: excellent
Shunt >1.5 : 1: untreated—life expectancy 5th decade (RV failure, rarely Eisenmenger's syndrome).

2.7.6 VENTRICULAR SEPTAL DEFECT

Aetiology/pathophysiology/pathology

A small defect causes a high-pressure left-to-right jet but no haemodynamic abnormality, whereas a large shunt can eventually result in Eisenmenger's syndrome.

Epidemiology

This is the most common congenital heart lesion in children; one-third close by the age of 2 years.

Clinical presentation

Presentation is usually as an asymptomatic pansystolic murmur. If later, it presents with dyspnoea or cyanosis.

Physical signs

- Pansystolic murmur ± thrill at the lower left sternal edge
- Signs of pulmonary hypertension
- Clubbing and cyanosis of Eisenmenger's syndrome.

Treatment

The surgical closure of haemodynamically significant shunts, if the pulmonary hypertension is not already too severe.

2.7.7 PATENT DUCTUS ARTERIOSUS

Aetiology/pathophysiology/pathology

The ductus arteriosus is part of the lung bypass circuit in the fetal circulation, connecting the descending aorta to the left pulmonary artery (see Fig. 62). If it does not close as normal after birth, left-to-right shunting results.

Epidemiology

Patent ductus arteriosus (PDA) accounts for 10% of PDA in cases of congenital heart disease, with a higher incidence in maternal rubella or pre-term infants.

Clinical presentation

Patients present with the following:
- Small PDA: asymptomatic murmur
- Moderate or large shunt: fatigue, dyspnoea, palpitations or eventually Eisenmenger's syndrome.

Physical signs

Signs include the following:
- Continuous machinery murmur in the second left intercostal space
- Significant shunt: wide pulse pressure and hyperdynamic apex or (large shunt) signs of LV failure
- Pulmonary hypertension: machinery murmur shortens (as proportion of cardiac cycle during which pulmonary pressure < systemic reduces) and eventually disappears.

Investigations

ECG

This is abnormal only if there is a large shunt—left atrial (LA) and LV hypertrophy.

Chest radiograph

This is abnormal only if there is a large shunt—prominent proximal pulmonary arteries and ascending aorta, pulmonary plethora.

Treatment

Because of the ongoing risk of endocarditis, closure (surgical or percutaneous) is recommended in all cases except where pulmonary hypertension has already developed.

Complications

Infective pulmonary artery endarteritis and consequent septic pulmonary emboli. Ductal aneurysm and calcification can also occur with risk of rupture.

Prognosis

Without closure, one-third of patients will be dead by the age of 40 and two-thirds by 60.

Surgery generally does not require cardiopulmonary bypass and the mortality rate is very low (<0.5%).

2.7.8 COARCTATION OF THE AORTA

Aetiology/pathophysiology/pathology

A flow-limiting ridge extends into the lumen of the aorta at the site of the fetal ductus arteriosus (see Section 2.7.7, p. 90), usually just distal to the left subclavian artery (Fig. 66). An arterial supply to the lower body is achieved by extensive collateralization.

Epidemiology

This condition is more common in males than in females.

Clinical presentation

Common

• Asymptomatic: incidental finding of murmur or systolic hypertension in the arms.

Fig. 66 Magnetic resonance imaging scan of coarctation of the aorta (arrowed).

Uncommon

• Symptoms of hypertension (epistaxis, headache)
• Palpitations
• Claudication in the legs.

Physical signs

The systolic pressure is usually greater in the arms than in the legs with weak and delayed femoral pulses. A harsh ejection systolic murmur (± thrill in suprasternal notch) may be heard along the left sternal edge and in the back.

Investigations

• Chest radiograph: notching of posterior third to eighth ribs (enlarged intercostal arteries because of collateral flow—Fig. 67), the site of the coarctation with pre- and poststenotic dilatation.
• CT, MRI or angiography to define lesion.

Treatment

• Surgical repair if the transcoarct gradient >30 mmHg
• Balloon dilatation carries a higher risk of aneurysm formation and is not established as a first-line treatment.

Complications

These may include the following:
• LV failure
• Aortic dissection
• Premature coronary disease.

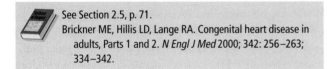

Fig. 67 Chest radiograph of a patient with coarctation of the aorta, showing rib notching (a), the site of the coarct (b) and pre and post stenotic dilatation (c). (Reproduced from Ray, Ryder, Wellings *An Aid to Radiology for the MRCP.* Oxford: Blackwell Science, 1999.)

Prognosis

- Uncorrected: 75% mortality rate by the age of 50 years
- Corrected: survival depends on the age at surgery—the younger the better.

Disease associations

- Turner's syndrome
- Bicuspid aortic valve.

> See Section 2.5, p. 71.
> Brickner ME, Hillis LD, Lange RA. Congenital heart disease in adults, Parts 1 and 2. *N Engl J Med* 2000; 342: 256–263; 334–342.

2.8 Infective diseases of the heart

2.8.1 INFECTIVE ENDOCARDITIS

Aetiology/pathophysiology/pathology

Microbial infection of the endocardium usually affects the heart valves, less often at the site of a septal defect, chordae tendinae or mural endocardium. Prosthetic valves may also be infected. Infective endocarditis (IE) develops as a result of a two-stage process:

1 Non-bacterial thrombotic endocarditis (NBTE): a sterile mass arises from the deposition of platelets and fibrin on areas of endocardium injured from exposure to high-velocity jets, flow from a high- to low-pressure chamber or across a narrow orifice.

2 Trauma to the skin or mucosa, especially the oral mucosa,

precipitates a bacteraemia with organisms that have the capacity to adhere to the NBTE, leading to an infected vegetation. Bacteraemia rates are higher in the presence of diseased mucosa, especially if infected.

The consequences of IE vary from trivial to catastrophic valvular and paravalvular tissue destruction.

Epidemiology

The incidence of IE has declined in recent decades to 2 : 100 000 per year with an increase in average age to 47–64 years. Risk increases with age and IE is more common in men.

Clinical presentation

- Acute IE: rapid onset of high fever, rigors and prostration over days
- Subacute IE: insidious onset over weeks with fever, weight loss, myalgias/arthralgias and malaise.

Infective endocarditis may mimic a broad range of medical conditions that can obscure the diagnosis:

- New or worsening heart failure
- Neurological presentation secondary to cerebral abscess or embolus
- Pneumonia and pulmonary infarction in right-sided IE, or left-sided if a septal defect.

Physical signs

The main sign is fever, which is high grade in acute IE and low grade in subacute infections. Conjunctival, buccal or palatal petechial haemorrhages are quite common, unlike skin petechiae affecting the extremities. A new or changing heart murmur is characteristic. A fluctuating confusional state is frequent, especially in elderly people, and signs of embolization are only too common. The classic skin and nail signs of splinter haemorrhages, finger clubbing, Osler's nodes and Janeway's lesions are quite rare, as are Roth's spots. There may be heart block from the involvement of conducting tissue.

>
> Infective endocarditis must always be considered in a patient presenting with chronic fever, weight loss and malaise, irrespective of the presence of a murmur. Elderly patients may present with little apart from confusion. The absence of the much over-emphasized 'classic' signs of Janeway's lesions etc. does not exclude the diagnosis.

Investigations

Definite pathological diagnosis can be achieved only via isolation or culture of the bacteria from material obtained from a vegetation or abscess. This is not possible in most patients, and diagnosis depends on clinical criteria.

Table 26 Frequency of various organisms in infective endocarditis.

Organism	NVE (%)	IV drug abuse (%)	Early PVE (%)	Late PVE (%)
Viridans streptococci	35	5	<5	25
Enterococci	25	10	<5	<5
Staphylococcus aureus	23	50	20	10
Coagulase-negative staphylococci	<5	<5	30	20
Gram-negative bacteria	<5	5	20	10
Fungi, e.g. *Candida*	<5	5	10	5
Polymicrobial	<1	5	5	5
Other bacteria	<5	5	5	5
Culture negative	5–10	<5	<5	<5

IV, intravenous; NVE, native valve endocarditis; PVE, prosthetic valve endocarditis.

Blood tests

- Mild-to-moderate normochromic/normocytic anaemia
- Leucocytosis is usual in acute IE, but may be absent in the subacute infection
- CRP and ESR are usually elevated
- Positive rheumatoid factor and elevated γ-globulins are common.

Blood cultures

Three sets at least 1 h apart from three sites must be taken as a minimum in all patients (Table 26).

Urinalysis

Microscopic haematuria ± proteinuria are common, with heavy proteinuria and red cell casts an occasional finding, indicating glomerulonephritis.

Echocardiography

For suspected NVE, a transthoracic study is the investigation of choice. If inadequate, negative or non-diagnostic in a patient with a high suspicion of IE, TOE should be performed. TOE is the investigation of choice in suspected PVE (Fig. 68).

Negative blood cultures may indicate suppression as a result of previous antibiotic therapy, fastidious organisms or an alternative diagnosis.

Treatment

Emergency

Treat embolic sequelae, heart failure (see Section 2.3) and septic shock (see *Emergency medicine*, Section 1.28). In an ill patient, antibiotics will need to be started before the culture results are available.

Fig. 68 (Right) Vegetation on mitral valve leaflet and (left) associated mitral regurgitation. (Courtesy of Dr J Chambers.)

Short term

Antibiotic treatment should be determined by the antibacterial sensitivities of the isolated organism with close liaison with your microbiologist (Table 27). Monitor for signs of continued infection—repeating cultures if necessary—changing murmurs, cardiac failure and embolic phenomena, and change venous access sites every 3–4 days. Carry out regular urinalysis and testing of renal and liver function, CRP and ESR, FBC and ECG. Weekly echocardiography should be performed. Check antibiotic levels regularly. Duration of therapy varies according to the severity of infection and organism. A total antibiotic course lasting 4–6 weeks is usually given, the first 2 weeks intravenously. Early valve replacement may be required if there has been severe damage, a compromise having to be made between adequate sterilization of the valve and the haemodynamic compromise secondary to valve destruction.

Long term

Follow-up of valve lesions will be required and patients must be made aware of the need for antibiotic prophylaxis.

Presentation	Antibiotic regimen
Gradual onset	Benzylpenillin 2.4 g 4-hourly i.v. + gentamicin 3 mg/kg/d in one to three divided doses guided by levels
Acute onset	Flucloxacillin 2 g 6-hourly i.v. + gentamicin 3 mg/kg/d in one to three divided doses guided by levels
Recent prosthetic valve	Vancomycin 15 mg/kg 12-hourly i.v. over 60 min guided by levels + gentamicin 3 mg/kg/d in one to three divided doses guided by levels + rifampicin 300 mg 12-hourly p.o.
Intravenous drug abuser	Vancomycin 15 mg/kg 12 hourly i.v. over 60 min guided by levels

Table 27 Antibiotic treatment for infective endocarditis. Modify when microbiological sensitivities are known.

Prognosis

In uncomplicated streptococcal NVE, the mortality rate is <10%, whereas aspergillus PVE is associated with virtually a 100% rate.

Bayer AS. Revised diagnostic criteria for infective endocarditis. *Cardiol Clin* 1996; 14: 345–350.

Barnes PD, Crook DW. Culture negative endocarditis. *J Infect* 1997; 35: 209–213.

Dajani AS, Taubert KA, Wilson W *et al.* Prevention of bacterial endocarditis. Recommendations by the American Heart Association. *Circulation* 1997; 96: 358–366.

Fig. 69 Rheumatic mitral valve disease. The thickened and contracted mitral valve leaflets with the fish-mouth valve orifice can be seen in this postmortem specimen.

2.8.2 RHEUMATIC FEVER

Aetiology/pathophysiology/pathology

Rheumatic fever results from an abnormal immune response to pharyngeal infection with group A β-haemolytic streptococci (GAS). There is evidence of a genetic predisposition with specific B-cell antibody D8/17 in >90%, and linkage with HLA-DR1, -2, -3 and -4.

Characteristic perivascular Aschoff's nodules have a widespread distribution in the connective tissues of joints, tendons and blood vessels. A pancarditis may develop, with endocardial inflammation affecting valve leaflets, chordae tendinae and papillary muscles. Fusion of leaflets and chordae leads most commonly to mitral stenosis, which is worsened further by the progressive fibrosis and eventual calcification that occur after the acute episode. Mitral regurgitation may occur and tricuspid involvement is seen in 10%. Aortic valve involvement more commonly leads to aortic regurgitation (Fig. 69).

Epidemiology

Rheumatic fever is rare in developed countries, with an incidence of <5 per 100 000 per year, usually between the ages of 4 and 18.

Table 28 Duckett–Jones criteria for diagnosis of rheumatic fever.

Major	Minor
Carditis	Fever
Migrating polyarthritis	Previous rheumatic fever
Chorea	Raised CRP or ESR
Erythema marginatum	Arthralgia
Subcutaneous nodules	Long PR interval

Diagnosis is based on evidence of antecedent streptococcal infection, e.g. positive throat swab for group A β-haemolytic streptococci (GAS), elevated streptococcal antibodies or a history of recent scarlet fever, together with either two or more major criteria or one major plus two minor criteria. CRP, C-reactive protein; ESR, erythrocyte sedimentation rate.

Clinical presentation/physical signs/investigations

See Table 28.

Blood cultures

These help to exclude infective endocarditis.

Blood tests

Look for the following:
• Anaemia and leucocytosis

- Elevated ESR and CRP
- Streptococcal serology.

ECG

- Normal
- May show prolonged PR interval.

Chest radiograph

This is either normal or shows cardiomegaly, pericardial effusion, pulmonary oedema or increased pulmonary vascularity.

Echocardiography

Echocardiography helps to exclude infective endocarditis, valvular abnormalities, myocardial dysfunction, pericarditis and pericardial effusion.

Consider the following in your differential diagnosis:
- Infective endocarditis
- Viral infection ± congenital cardiac abnormality
- Non-rheumatic acute streptococcal infections
- Juvenile chronic arthritis
- SLE
- Traumatic or septic arthritis
- Gout.

Treatment

Emergency

Treat heart failure (see Section 2.3, p. 63). Severe valve lesions with deteriorating cardiac function may rarely require valve replacement.

Short term

Bedrest eases joint pains. A 10-day course of oral/intramuscular penicillin (erythromycin in allergic patients) will eradicate the organism. Treatment with salicylates or steroids is symptomatic and does not affect the outcome.

Long term

Duration of anti-inflammatory therapy varies from 1 month in mild cases to 2–3 months in more severe ones. Taper steroid therapy at the end of the course with the substitution of aspirin to reduce rebound inflammation.

Prognosis

Joint pain and fever usually settle within 2 weeks. The risk of residual heart disease increases with the severity of the initial carditis, as does the risk of further damage during any rheumatic recurrence.

da Silva NA, Pereira BA. Acute rheumatic fever. Still a challenge. *Rheum Dis Clin North Am* 1997; 23: 545–568.

2.9 Cardiac tumours

Aetiology/pathophysiology/pathology

The only clinically important cardiac tumours in adults are malignant secondary deposits and myxoma. Cardiac metastases occur most commonly with lung and breast carcinomas and melanosarcomas. Of myxomas, 75% occur in the left atrium, with the remainder being mainly in the right atrium and rarely in the ventricles. They commonly arise from the endocardium at the border of the fossa ovalis as a pedunculated mass that may prolapse through the mitral orifice, mimicking mitral stenosis.

Epidemiology

Remember that myxomas are very rare tumours; they cause left atrial obstruction 200–400 times less commonly than mitral stenosis. It should therefore appear low down on any list of differential diagnoses, particularly as the typical presentation is relatively non-specific.

Prevalence of myxoma is estimated at 2 per 100 000 in the general population, most commonly at age 30–60 years, and with a female : male sex ratio of 2 : 1.

Clinical presentation

Non-specific symptoms such as exertional dyspnoea with fever and weight loss are the most common features of myxoma. Paroxysmal nocturnal dyspnoea, haemoptysis, dizziness and syncope may also occur. Embolic phenomena may lead to an erroneous diagnosis of endocarditis.

Malignant tumours usually present more acutely with the sudden development of heart failure or haemorrhagic pericardial effusion, various arrhythmias or heart block.

Physical signs

Fever, finger clubbing or anaemia reflects the chronic nature of myxoma. Auscultatory findings that mimic

(a)

(b)

Fig. 70 Intracardiac calcification: (a) posteroanterior and (b) lateral views illustrating visible deposition of calcium within the heart.

Fig. 71 Echocardiography: left atrial myxoma. (Courtesy of Dr J Chambers.)

elevated inflammatory markers (ESR/CRP) and increased γ-globulins.

Chest radiograph

A bizarre cardiac contour suggests a tumour. Sudden cardiac or pericardial enlargement, mediastinal lympadenopathy or irregular/indistinct cardiac border indicates malignancy. Intracardiac calcification may be seen in myxoma (Fig. 70).

Echocardiography

Echocardiography is usually diagnostic; occasionally a transoesophageal study may be required (Fig. 71).

Others

Cardiac catheterization and endomyocardial biopsy are occasionally helpful, as are other imaging techniques such as CT or MRI.

Differential diagnosis

Consider endocarditis and mitral valve disease.

Treatment

Palliative therapy is indicated for malignant cardiac deposits, with specific management of cardiac complications. The surgical removal of myxoma is curative.

mitral stenosis, with or without mitral regurgitation, may be present. These characteristically vary with posture, unlike primary valve disease. A friction rub or 'tumour plop' may also help to distinguish myxomas clinically. Clinical findings in malignant tumour deposits are dominated by the manner of acute deterioration.

Investigations

Blood tests

In myxoma these typically show anaemia of chronic disease, elevated white cell count, decreased platelet count,

Complications

Complications are thromboembolic disease and cardiac failure in myxoma. There can also be pericardial disease, heart failure, arrhythmias, or sudden death and heart block in malignant disease.

Prognosis

With complete removal of a myxoma, a normal lifespan should be expected. Recurrences are more likely with 'syndrome myxoma'.

Disease associations

Myxomas are familial, with autosomal dominant transmission in 10%—termed 'syndrome myxoma'.

 McAllister HA Jr, Hall RJ, Cooley DA. Tumors of the heart and pericardium. *Curr Prob Cardiol* 1999; 24: 57–116.

2.10 Traumatic heart disease

Traumatic heart disease is often fatal. Rapid diagnosis and intervention are vital in reducing both mortality and morbidity.

Aetiology

- Road traffic accident
- Assault
- Sports injuries
- Falls
- Kicks from animals.

Pathophysiology/pathology

Virtually all cardiac components may be affected by thoracic trauma. Trauma may cause the following:

Myocardium

Contusion (approximately 20% of patients after blunt trauma), laceration/pericardial tamponade or rupture (ventricles > atria).

Pericardium

Pericarditis, laceration or post-pericardiotomy syndrome.

Endocardium

Ruptured chordae/papillary muscles or valves.

Coronary arteries

Injury/rupture/thrombosis (the LAD artery most commonly).

Conduction system

Bundle-branch block, AV block or atrial/ventricular arrhythmias.

Clinical presentation

The initial insult is usually obvious and leads directly to presentation. Occasionally apparent minor trauma causes significant mediastinal injury, leading to a more insidious presentation:
- Chest pain (including angina)
- Presyncope/syncope.

Physical signs

Look for the following:
- Pulsus paradoxus
- Quiet heart sounds
- Pulmonary oedema
- Murmur/thrill of mitral regurgitation
- Diastolic murmur of aortic regurgitation if ascending aorta involved.

Investigations

ECG

Look specifically for the following:
- ST/T changes (usually non-specific)
- ST elevation secondary to pericarditis
- Acute MI
- Arrhythmias (AF, sinus tachycardia).

Cardiac enzymes

- Elevated CK-MB fraction (may be elevated if huge musculoskeletal trauma)
- Elevated troponin (T/I) (see Section 3.7, p. 136).

Chest radiograph

- Widened mediastinum (Fig. 72)
- Ribs/sternal fracture
- Haemothorax.

Echocardiography (transthoracic and transoesophageal)

- Pericardial effusion
- Abnormal wall motion (contusion)
- TOE best for identifying myocardial injury and valvular involvement.

Fig. 72 Chest radiograph of patient with traumatic aortic rupture. Note the widened mediastinum and abnormal descending aortic outline.

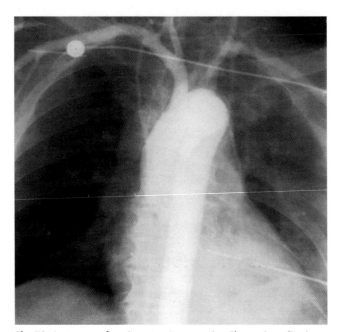

Fig. 73 Aortogram of aortic rupture/trans-section. The aortic outline is clearly irregular, representing aortic rupture.

TOE is contraindicated in the following:
- Severe facial trauma
- Cervical spinal injury
- Possible oesophageal injury.

Aortography

Aortography is usually considered the 'gold standard' for diagnosing aortic trauma (Fig. 73). Damage is most commonly seen in the upper descending aorta—the site of the ligamentum arteriosum.

Computed tomography

Computed tomography may identify surrounding haematoma, but will not always establish the integrity of the aorta.

Radionuclide imaging

Reduced myocardial perfusion with contusion or ischaemia secondary to coronary thrombosis may be demonstrated.

Treatment

Emergency

If there is haemodynamic compromise, consider urgent pericardiocentesis/operative intervention for pericardial tamponade. If there is any doubt, seek immediate contact with a cardiothoracic surgical centre.

Short term

High risk

Monitor initially and mobilize gently.

Low risk

Early gentle mobilization.

Long term

Long-term treatment may require further cardiac evaluation with radionuclide imaging/cardiac catheterization.

Risk stratification after chest trauma
- Minor trauma and normal/abnormal ECG: relatively low risk
- Major trauma with associated thoracic or extrathoracic injuries and normal/abnormal ECG: relatively high risk.

Always consider aortic rupture when serious thoracic injuries have occurred

- 80% mortality rate
- often have back pain as well as chest pain
- high risk group: head-on collision at speed, ejection from vehicle, death of other person involved, fall from great height
- >50% have the following triad: increased arterial pressure/pulse amplitude in upper limbs; reduced arterial pressure/pulse amplitude in lower limbs; widened mediastinum on chest radiograph
- definitive investigation is aortography
- immediate surgical repair required
- intravenous β blockers reduce aortic wall stresses as interim measure before surgery.

Banning AP, Pillai R. Non-penetrating cardiac and aortic trauma. *Heart* 1997; 78: 226–229.

Olsovsky MR, Wechsler AS, Topaz O. Cardiac trauma diagnosis, management, and current therapy. *Angiology* 1997; 48: 423–432.

Pretre R, Chilcott M. Blunt trauma to the heart and great vessels. *N Engl J Med* 1997; 336: 626–632.

2.11 Diseases of systemic arteries

2.11.1 AORTIC DISSECTION

Aetiology/pathophysiology/pathology

The aortic intima tears, exposing a diseased media that is split in two longitudinally by the force of blood flow. This dissection usually progresses distally for a variable distance. Medial degeneration is often idiopathic but may be the result of cystic medial necrosis, especially in Marfan's syndrome. There is also an association with the following:

- Hypertension (history of hypertension in 80% of cases)
- Pregnancy
- Trauma.

Aortic dissection is classified according to whether or not there is involvement of the ascending aorta (Stanford classification—Fig. 74). This has practical and prognostic implications.

Epidemiology

- Peak age >60 years
- Male : female = 2 : 1.

Clinical presentation

Common

There is central chest pain in 90%—classically a tearing pain that migrates to the back (interscapular) as dissection proceeds. A dissected aorta found incidentally in a patient without pain is usually chronic and therefore low risk. Thoracic back pain of sudden onset is also common.

Uncommon

- Syncope
- Stroke
- Acute pulmonary oedema
- Electromechanical dissociation (EMD) arrest.

Physical signs

Common

- Hypotension
- Unequal radial pulses or brachial blood pressures (found in 50% of proximal dissections)
- Aortic regurgitation
- Pericardial rub
- Pleural effusion

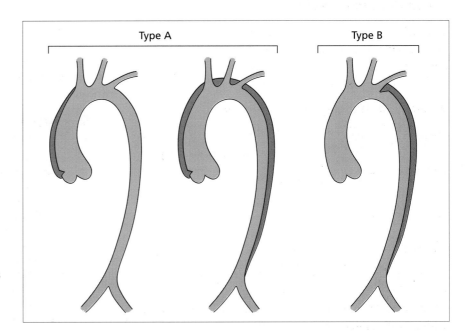

Fig. 74 Stanford classification of aortic dissection. Type A refers to dissection of the ascending aorta, with or without involvement of the descending aorta. In type B, dissection is confined to the descending aorta. This classification has implications for prognosis and treatment.

Fig. 75 Chest radiograph showing widened mediastinum. Blood in the pleural space from a leaking aorta may show as an effusion.

Fig. 76 Transoesophageal echocardiogram of aortic dissection demonstrating the true (T) and false (F) lumina in the descending aorta. (From Armstrong P, Wastie ML. *Diagnostic Imaging* (4th edn). Oxford: Blackwell Science, 1998.)

• Tamponade (see Section 2.6.2, p. 80)
• Hemiplegia.

Investigations

ECG

The ECG may reveal inferior MI (if dissection extends to the right coronary artery). Anterior infarction is rarely seen, perhaps because occlusion of the left main coronary artery results in such a big infarct that the patient does not reach hospital alive.

Chest radiograph

This may show widened mediastinum (Fig. 75), but an absence of this does not rule out aortic dissection. Blood in the pleural space from a leaking aorta may show as an effusion.

Echocardiography

The diagnosis is suggested by the following:
• Dilated aortic root
• Aortic regurgitation
• Pericardial effusion
• Dissection flap in the ascending aorta (unusual).

Other investigations

Consider the following:
• CT scan of the chest with contrast
• Aortography
• MRI
• TOE (Fig. 76).

 The differential diagnosis of aortic dissection should include the following:
• MI/unstable angina
• Thoracic vertebral pathology, e.g. fracture, discitis
• Pulmonary embolism.

Treatment

Emergency

• Do not await confirmation of diagnosis before starting medical treatment
• Transfer to the CCU
• Lower systolic blood pressure to <120 mmHg with intravenous labetolol or sodium nitroprusside
• If confirmatory imaging cannot be obtained quickly, arrange urgent transfer to cardiothoracic centre
• Type A dissection requires emergency repair unless chronic (>2 weeks)
• Type B dissection is generally managed medically because risks of surgery outweigh benefits. Consider surgery if there is a rupture or vital organ/limb ischaemia.

Short term

After 24 h, begin transfer of blood pressure control to oral agents, e.g. β blocker, ACE inhibitor or calcium antagonist.

Complications

Death caused by aortic rupture or tamponade is common. Occlusion of any of the major aortic branches may occur, producing the following:
- Hemiplegia
- Acute renal failure
- Mesenteric ischaemia
- Lower limb ischaemia.

Prognosis

There is an early mortality rate of 1% per hour if left untreated. The mortality rate in the first 2 weeks is about 80%, after which a dissection would be classed as chronic.

 Treasure T, Raphael MJ. Investigation of suspected dissection of the thoracic aorta. *Lancet* 1991; 338: 490–495.

2.12 Diseases of pulmonary arteries

2.12.1 PRIMARY PULMONARY HYPERTENSION

Primary pulmonary hypertension is defined as a sustained elevation of pulmonary artery pressure (PAP) to a mean of more than 25 mmHg at rest or 30 mmHg with exercise, in the absence of a demonstrable cause.

Aetiology/pathophysiology/pathology

The aetiology is unknown. The following have been suggested:
- Genetic: 10% of cases are familial (localized to chromosome 2) with autosomal dominant inheritance and genetic anticipation (a feature of trinucleotide repeat sequence disorders).
- Autoimmune.
- Pulmonary vascular endothelial dysfunction: this may be cause or effect.

Similar pulmonary vascular disease is seen in patients with portal hypertension, HIV infection or a history of cocaine or appetite-suppressant use.

Increased pulmonary vascular resistance is produced by:
- Vasoconstriction (increased thromboxane and endothelin, decreased prostacyclin and nitric oxide)
- Vascular wall remodelling (medial hypertrophy and smooth muscle proliferation)
- Thrombosis *in situ*.

This results in right ventricular hypertrophy (RVH), then failure, as a result of increased afterload.

Epidemiology

Incidence is about 1 per million per year, with use of appetite suppressants associated with a greater than 20-fold increased risk. Female : male is 2 : 1, with most diagnoses made in the fourth decade.

Clinical presentation

 Early symptoms of primary pulmonary hypertension (PPH) are non-specific.

Common

- Exertional dyspnoea
- Fatigue
- Angina (right ventricular ischaemia)
- Syncope/near syncope, especially exertional.

Uncommon

- Peripheral oedema
- Raynaud's phenomenon—mostly in women
- Haemoptysis.

Physical signs

- Loud P2 (pulmonary component of second heart sound)
- S4 originating from the right ventricle (pressure overload)
- Left parasternal heave
- Pansystolic murmur, prominent jugular 'v' waves and pulsatile liver of tricuspid regurgitation
- Peripheral oedema and elevated JVP of RV failure (RVF).

 Clubbing is not a feature of PPH and, if present, may indicate lung disease or cyanotic congenital heart disease as the underlying cause of the pulmonary hypertension.

Investigations

To confirm pulmonary hypertension, determine prognosis and guide therapy.

Echocardiogram

- Dilated and/or hypertrophied right heart
- Measurement of PAP

Fig. 77 ECG of patient with pulmonary hypertension, showing right ventricular hypertrophy and right axis deviation. The patient is also in atrial fibrillation. (Courtesy of the Pulmonary Vascular Disease Unit at Papworth Hospital.)

• Exclusion of shunts, valvular and left ventricular abnormalities

• A transoesophageal study may be necessary to see an ASD.

ECG

Look for (Fig. 77):
• Tall P waves
• Right axis deviation
• RV hypertrophy.

Chest radiograph

Look for prominent pulmonary arteries with peripheral pruning, and for features of underlying lung disease (Fig. 78).

Left and right heart catheterization

Measure pressures and saturations (prognosis and shunt calculation) and assess response to acute vasodilators such as prostacyclin, adenosine or inhaled nitric oxide.

To exclude secondary causes

• Blood: FBC (for secondary polycythaemia), liver function tests, ESR, rheumatoid factor and autoantibody screen, and consider HIV test

Fig. 78 Posteroanterior chest radiograph of a patient with pulmonary hypertension, showing prominent pulmonary arteries (arrowed) and cardiomegaly. (Courtesy of the Pulmonary Vascular Disease Unit at Papworth Hospital.)

• Pulmonary function tests to exclude obstructive or restrictive lung disease

• Sleep study if there is a suspicion of obstructive sleep apnoea

• Exclusion of pulmonary thromboembolism by: ventilation–perfusion ($\dot{V}/\dot{Q}$) scan, spiral CT scan of the chest with contrast, or pulmonary angiography (Fig. 79).

Fig. 79 Left pulmonary angiogram of a patient with thromboembolic pulmonary hypertension, showing (B) the characteristic bands and cut-offs of vessel occlusion and (A) lack of perfusion in the left lower lobe. (Courtesy of the Pulmonary Vascular Disease Unit at Papworth Hospital.)

Primary pulmonary hypertension—consider the following in your differential diagnosis:
- Secondary pulmonary hypertension
- LV outflow tract obstruction
- IHD.

Treatment

- Anticoagulation
- Diuretics with daily weight avoiding excessive fluid depletion
- Oxygen for hypoxaemia
- High-dose calcium channel blockers in those who have a significant fall in pulmonary vascular resistance on acute vasodilator testing
- Consideration of intravenous/nebulized prostacyclin therapy in those of poor functional class who fail to respond to acute vasodilator testing
- Consideration of atrial septostomy to decompress the right ventricle and improve left-sided filling pressures
- Lung or heart–lung transplantation in those who fail to respond to any other treatment.

Prognosis

Survival depends on right ventricular function and can be predicted by:
- Mixed venous oxygen saturation (adverse if <60%)
- Right atrial pressure (adverse if >15 mmHg)
- Cardiac index (adverse if <2 L/min/m^2)
- Exercise tolerance (6-min walk test)
- Response to vasodilators.

Overall 5-year survival is 20%, but the subgroup with adverse haemodynamics have a 20% 3-year survival. Responders to chronic calcium channel blocker therapy have a 95% 5-year survival.

Anticoagulation, prostacyclin and heart–lung transplantation (5-year survival of 50–60%) all confer a survival benefit.

Important information for patients

Strongly advise against pregnancy. Avoid the oral contraceptive pill if possible—it may exacerbate pulmonary hypertension.

Gaine SP, Rubin LJ. Primary pulmonary hypertension. *Lancet* 1998; 352: 719–725.

2.12.2 SECONDARY PULMONARY HYPERTENSION

Secondary pulmonary hypertension is defined as sustained elevation of the mean PAP to >25 mmHg at rest or 30 mmHg on exercise, with an identified cause.

Aetiology/pathophysiology

Causes of secondary pulmonary hypertension are shown in Table 29.

Vascular wall remodelling and vasoconstriction increase pulmonary vascular resistance and therefore PAP, with resulting RVH and right ventricular failure (RVF). When the primary cause is respiratory, this is known as cor pulmonale.

Table 29 Causes of secondary pulmonary hypertension.

Mechanism	Cause
Increased left atrial pressure	Aortic/mitral valve disease
	Left ventricular dysfunction
Left-to-right shunts	ASD, VSD, PDA
Chronic pulmonary disease	COAD
	Bronchiectasis
	Pulmonary fibrosis
Chronic venous thromboembolism	–
Chronic hypoventilation/hypoxia	Kyphoscoliosis
	Respiratory muscle weakness
	Obstructive sleep apnoea

ASD, atrial septal defect; COPD, chronic obstructive pulmonary disease; PDA, patent ductus arteriosus; VSD, ventricular septal defect.

Clinical presentation

- Ankle oedema
- Dyspnoea (may be associated with the underlying primary condition)
- The primary condition.

Physical signs

The signs of the primary condition, including cyanosis if present, and then of pulmonary hypertension, RVH, dilatation and failure:
- Left parasternal heave
- Loud P2
- Elevated JVP with prominent 'v' wave
- Pansystolic murmur of tricuspid regurgitation
- Pulsatile liver
- Ankle oedema.

Investigations

See Section 2.12.1, p. 101.

Differential diagnosis

Consider left ventricular dysfunction and primary pulmonary hypertension.

Treatment

General

- Optimize treatment of the underlying condition
- Diuretics
- Calcium channel blockers
- Consideration of prostacyclin therapy
- Lung or heart–lung transplantation.

Specific

Shunts

Consideration of defect closure or pulmonary artery banding (some protection of pulmonary vasculature against high right-sided flow), if pulmonary hypertension not already too severe.

Chronic obstructive pulmonary disease

Long-term oxygen therapy benefits selected patients with chronic obstructive pulmonary disease. (See *Respiratory medicine*, Section 2.12.1.)

Thromboembolism

Anticoagulation and consideration of IVC filter or pulmonary thromboendarterectomy.

Ventilatory disorders

Consideration of nocturnal continuous positive airway pressure (CPAP) or nasal positive pressure ventilation. (See *Respiratory medicine*, Section 2.12.2.)

Prognosis

The prognosis is related to the underlying condition and the severity of the pulmonary hypertension. The 5-year survival rate of COPD with oedema is 30%.

 Ricciardi MJ, Rubenfire M. How to manage secondary pulmonary hypertension. *Postgrad Med* 1999; 105: 183–190.

2.13 Cardiac complications of systemic disease

2.13.1 THYROID DISEASE

Clinical presentation

Hyperthyroidism

A patient with hyperthyroidism may have:
- Sinus tachycardia
- Sustained or paroxysmal AF
- Hyperdynamic left ventricle.

Hypothyroidism

A patient with hypothyroidism may have:
- Bradycardia with prolonged QT interval
- Cardiac enlargement
- Pericardial effusion.

Treatment

Hyperthyroidism

Short term

- β Blockers for symptomatic relief until rendered euthyroid

- AF generally reverts to sinus rhythm with treatment of thyroid disease.

Long term

- Cardioversion after anticoagulation if AF persists.

Hypothyroidism

Treat with thyroxine, starting in very small doses to avoid precipitation of myocardial ischaemia. The effusion resolves and drainage is hardly ever required.

 See *Endocrinology*, Section 2.3.

2.13.2 DIABETES

Aetiology/pathophysiology/pathology

Accelerated atherogenesis

This is the result of the following:
- Dyslipidaemia: enhanced atherogenicity of low-density lipoprotein (LDL), increased triglyceride and decreased high-density lipoprotein (HDL)
- Hypercoagulable state and increased platelet aggregation
- Hyperinsulinaemia (in type 2 diabetes) promoting vascular smooth muscle proliferation
- Glycosylated proteins promoting the production of oxidants.

Autonomic neuropathy

This causes impairment of the protective sensation of angina (silent ischaemia) and thus causes prolonged ischaemia, arrhythmias and sudden death.

Diabetic cardiomyopathy

There is impairment of systolic and diastolic function independent of macroscopic coronary artery disease, possibly secondary to microvascular disease.

Epidemiology

In people with diabetes the risk of acute MI is increased by 50% for a man and 150% for a woman. Mortality and the rate of all major complications are also increased.

Clinical presentation

Silent ischaemia may lead to atypical presentations, e.g. acute MI as ketoacidosis.

Treatment

Acute MI

Standard treatment plus an insulin infusion ('sliding scale'). The absolute benefit of all standard interventions is greater in people with diabetes.

Coronary revascularization

Diabetic coronary disease is more diffuse and distal, so that both CABG and angioplasty have poorer outcomes than in people without diabetes, although recent work suggests that coronary stenting plus the use of a glycoprotein IIb/IIIa receptor blocker (antiplatelet) may improve results.

Prevention

Primary

Good glycaemic and blood pressure control, and avoidance of smoking.

Secondary

Treatment with a statin and an ACE inhibitor, though most of this high-risk group should now be on these drugs as primary prevention.

2.13.3 AUTOIMMUNE RHEUMATIC DISEASES

Clinical presentation

The autoimmune rheumatic diseases have the following cardiac associations.

Systemic lupus erythematosus (SLE)

- Premature atherosclerosis: important to differentiate, if possible, from coronary vasculitis (also in SLE) because the latter needs steroids
- Pericarditis ± effusion: clinically in 30%; at post-mortem examination in 60%
- Sterile valvular vegetations (Libman–Sachs) in 60%, rarely clinically significant
- Myocarditis
- Conduction defects.

Primary antiphospholipid syndrome

- Pulmonary thromboembolism (also in SLE if anticardiolipin antibody positive)
- Degenerative mitral valve disease.

Rheumatoid arthritis

- Pericarditis: often clinically silent but may lead to symptomatic effusion or constriction
- Rheumatoid nodules causing valvular regurgitation and AV block
- Coronary vasculitis (rare).

Systemic sclerosis

- Pulmonary hypertension: the major cause of death in systemic sclerosis
- Pericarditis and chronic effusions
- Myocardial fibrosis causing ventricular dysfunction and conduction abnormalities.

Investigations

Coronary angiography

Coronary angiography may help to distinguish between vasculitis and atheromatous disease.

Echocardiography

Transoesophageal echocardiography should be used if necessary for close inspection of valve abnormalities.

Treatment

Pericarditis

Non-steroidal anti-inflammatory drugs (NSAIDs) and steroids are used if necessary for symptomatic relief. Tamponade requires immediate pericardiocentesis followed by steroids.

Myocarditis

The standard management of LV dysfunction and consideration of anticoagulation (see Section 2.3, p. 63).

Pulmonary hypertension

The standard management (see Section 2.12, p. 101).

2.13.4 RENAL DISEASE

Aetiology/pathophysiology/pathology

Features of end-stage renal failure/renal replacement include:
- Uraemia
- Elevated serum phosphate and calcium phosphate product
- Anaemia
- Electrolyte imbalance
- Hypertension
- Dyslipidaemia
- Amyloidosis (β_2 microglobulin).

These result in the following cardiovascular complications via the mechanisms shown in Fig. 80:
- Myocardial ischaemia
- Ventricular arrhythmias and sudden death
- Impaired ventricular function
- LV hypertrophy
- Valvular calcification, aortic > mitral, with rapidly progressive stenosis in a small proportion and the risk of endocarditis.

The heart in renal failure

Do not confuse fluid overload with LV dysfunction, although the two often coexist. LV function is impaired by uraemia and improves with dialysis, not just with the removal of fluid.

Epidemiology

Cardiovascular disease is much commoner in patients receiving renal replacement than the general population and is the most common cause of death (40–50%). Those in whom renal failure is associated with diabetes are at particularly high risk.

Investigations

- Myocardial ischaemia: coronary angiography if intervention or renal transplantation is being considered; nuclear perfusion imaging has a poor predictive value in these patients.
- Consider echocardiography for assessment of valves, LV function and pericardial effusion.

Treatment

Aim to normalize the haemoglobin and blood pressure and, if possible, to dialyse as well. If coronary artery disease is present, bypass grafting is the treatment of choice

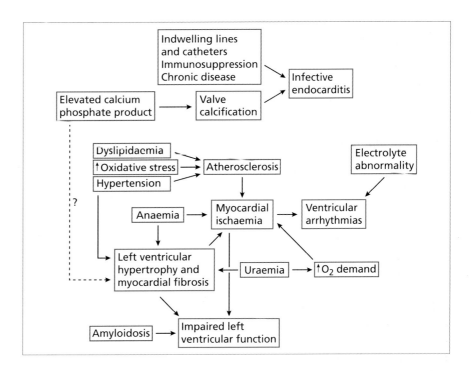

Fig. 80 The pathogenesis of cardiac complications of renal failure.

because the post-angioplasty re-stenosis and coronary event rate are very high. The indications for surgery in calcific valve disease and endocarditis are the same as in a patient without renal disease. Uraemic pericarditis is an absolute indication for dialysis; cardiac tamponade (of any cause) requires immediate pericardiocentesis. Recurrent effusions may warrant pericardiectomy (a 'window' to allow drainage into the pleural space).

 Prescribing in renal failure: see *Clinical pharmacology*, Section 5.6.
Be aware that a patient on dialysis may have large fluctuations in serum potassium, with effects on antiarrhythmic therapy.

Prognosis

The presence of LV dysfunction in a dialysis patient reduces the 2-year survival rate from 80 to 33%. Acute MI and cardiac surgery have a higher mortality than in the general population, but CABG and valve surgery are still an acceptable risk when indicated.

Prevention

Careful control of phosphate and calcium phosphate product reduces valve calcification. Good aseptic technique is essential when inserting and using dialysis catheters to minimize the risk of infective endocarditis. Aim for good control of blood pressure and serum cholesterol and maintenance of haematocrit at about 35%. Stop smoking!

 Hussain S, Isenberg DA. Autoimmune rheumatic diseases and the heart. *Hosp Med* 1999; 60: 95–99.
Hyde T, Timmis AD. Diabetes and the heart. *Hosp Med* 1999; 60: 90–94.
Staffeld CG, Pastan SO. Cardiac disease in patients with end-stage renal disease. *Cardiol Clin* 1995; 13: 209–223.
Woolfson RG. Renal disease and the heart. *Hosp Med* 1999; 60: 85–89.

2.14 Systemic complications of cardiac disease

2.14.1 STROKE

Aetiology

There are many cardiac causes of stroke:
- AF
- MI (acute/chronic)
- Dilated cardiomyopathy
- Infective endocarditis
- Valvular disease
- Prosthetic mechanical valve
- Intracardiac mass
- Hypertension
- Aortic dissection.

Physical signs

Common

- AF (up to 25%)
- Murmurs (particularly mitral predisposing to AF).

Uncommon

- Pulmonary oedema
- Added hearts sounds.

Investigations

ECG

There is a significant chance that, if there is underlying cardiac pathology resulting in thromboembolism, the ECG will be abnormal.

Examination of the ECG for cardiac cause of stroke:
- AF
- Previous MI (in 90% of cases the MI is anterior)
- Persistent ST elevation suggestive of LV aneurysm
- LVH suggestive of hypertension or aortic stenosis.

Chest radiograph

Look for abnormal cardiac shape/size, pulmonary oedema and wide mediastinum suggestive of enlarged aorta.

Echocardiography

If any possible cardiac cause has been identified from the history, examination or ECG/chest radiograph, it is reasonable to examine the structure and function of the heart for the following:
- Structural abnormalities
- Intracardiac thrombus
- TOE: particularly suited for examination of the left atrial appendage
- Consider paradoxical embolus: look for intracardiac shunts, if necessary using contrast.

Treatment

In general, correct the underlying abnormality and aim for restoration of sinus rhythm where possible. (See Section 2.2.2, p. 59.)

Complications

The risk of haemorrhage into an ischaemic stroke if anticoagulated usually outweighs the benefit of secondary prevention.

Prevention

Anticoagulation in atrial fibrillation/flutter should be considered in all patients as follows.

Primary prevention of stroke/TIA

In patients who do not have a history of stroke/TIA:
- Structurally abnormal heart—warfarin
- Structurally normal heart, age <65 years, no hypertension, no previous stroke/TIA, no diabetes—aspirin
- Structurally normal heart, age >65 years—warfarin.

Secondary prevention after stroke/TIA

In patients who have had a previous stroke/TIA:
- Exclude haemorrhagic stroke—warfarin
- If warfarin contraindicated—aspirin
- Warfarin therapy—aim for an international normalized ratio (INR) of 2.0–3.0. This will give satisfactory protection while minimizing the risks of haemorrhage. A number of near patient monitoring devices are now available, so specifically selected patients may be able to monitor the level of anticoagulation themselves.

Barnett HJM, Eliasziw M, Meldrum HE. Evidence based cardiology: prevention of ischaemic stroke. *BMJ* 1999; 318: 1539–1543.

2.15 Pregnancy and the heart

Aetiology

Normal physiological changes in pregnancy include the following:
- Decrease in systemic and pulmonary vascular resistance
- Increase in heart rate, blood volume (large shifts after delivery) and cardiac output
- No significant change in blood pressure
- Anaemia (caused by increased blood volume and/or haematinic deficiency).

These can all cause problems in women with cardiovascular disease.

Clinical presentation

Fatigue, mild dyspnoea, ankle oedema, palpitations (usually ectopics) and postural dizziness are all common in normal pregnancy, but likely to be more severe in those with cardiac disease.

Physical signs

An S3, a soft systolic murmur at the lower left sternal edge and mild ankle oedema are all common in normal pregnancy. Look for signs of worsening cardiac failure and/or exacerbation of the physical signs of particular cardiac lesions.

Investigations

Exclude cardiac disease:
• Echocardiography for ventricular function and murmurs
• ECG/24-h tape for palpitation
• Chest radiograph rarely clinically indicated, but should be performed if it is, because the dose to a screened fetus is negligible.

Prognosis/treatment

In a patient with pre-existing cardiac disease the ability to tolerate pregnancy is related to the following:
• Cyanosis
• Pulmonary hypertension
• Haemodynamic significance of the lesion
• Pre-pregnancy functional status.

High risk

Primary pulmonary hypertension/Eisenmenger's syndrome

There is a 50% maternal mortality rate and patients should be strongly advised to undergo sterilization.

Mitral stenosis

Mitral stenosis may present for the first time in pregnancy with pulmonary oedema secondary to increased cardiac output or an episode of AF. Treatment consists of diuretics to clear the pulmonary oedema and digoxin or β blockers to control heart rate and thereby improve atrial emptying. Mitral valvuloplasty may be necessary.

Aortic/pulmonary stenosis

Gradients are exacerbated by decreased vascular resistance and there is no effective medical therapy.

Marfan's syndrome

There is an increased risk of aortic dissection; those who already have echocardiographic evidence of aortic root dilatation >4.5 cm should be advised against pregnancy.

Intermediate risk

• Coarctation of the aorta (risk of aortic dissection)
• Hypertrophic cardiomyopathy
• Cyanotic congenital heart disease without pulmonary hypertension—note increased risk (40%) of fetal death if mother is cyanotic.

Low risk

• Well-tolerated valvular regurgitation
• Septal defects without pulmonary hypertension
• Totally corrected congenital heart disease
• Prosthetic valves: bioprostheses do not require anti-coagulation but pregnancy reduces their lifespan. There is no consensus of opinion on the optimum management of anticoagulation in pregnant women with mechanical valves. In addition to the issues discussed in *Clinical pharmacology*, Section 5.3, there is the concern that heparin is not as effective as warfarin in preventing valve thrombosis.

 Antibiotic prophylaxis is recommended for vaginal delivery in cases at high risk of endocarditis (prosthetic valves, prior subacute bacterial endocarditis [SBE], complex cyanotic congenital heart disease and surgical shunts) and for instrumented delivery in any cardiac lesion, but not for caesarean section.

New cardiac disease in pregnancy

Thromboembolic disease

Thrombolysis should be used for a massive life-threatening PE, as in the non-pregnant patient.

Peripartum cardiomyopathy

This presents as dilatated cardiomyopathy in the third trimester or in the first 6 months postpartum.

Hypertension

Hypertension may be chronic (i.e. predates the pregnancy or develops before 20 weeks) or pregnancy induced (part of a spectrum that includes pre-eclampsia).

Fig. 81 Pulmonary oedema.

Indications to look for a secondary cause of hypertension

- Any evidence of underlying cause in history or examination (Table 30).
- Accelerated (malignant) hypertension.
- Hypokalaemia (not diuretic induced).
- Young age (<35 yr).
- Resistant hypertension (uncontrolled by 3 drugs).

To pursue the possibility of secondary causes, do the following:
- 24-h urine collection: may require creatinine clearance, urinary protein excretion, catecholamines.
- Renal ultrasonography: the presence of two small kidneys indicates chronic renal disease; marked asymmetry of renal size (more than 2 cm difference in length) increases the probability of renal artery stenosis.
- Doppler ultrasonography of renal arteries, captopril renography or renal angiography (conventional, digital subtraction, MRI) to look for renal artery stenosis.
- Test of plasma renin and aldosterone.
- Other investigations as led by clinical suspicion.

Differential diagnosis

Consider the following:
- Essential hypertension
- Secondary hypertension
- Erroneous reading of elevated blood pressure as a result of an inadequate cuff size
- Isolated clinic hypertension ('white coat hypertension').

Treatment

Secondary causes of hypertension may require specific treatment. In essential hypertension, advise lifestyle modi-fication (see key point below) and monitor blood pressure. In mild hypertension (diastolic BP <105 mmHg), check blood pressure on another occasion before initiating treatment; in moderate (diastolic BP >105 mmHg) or severe (diastolic BP >115 mmHg) hypertension, commence drug therapy. Tailor the choice of initial drug according to associated medical conditions. Review every 4–6 weeks. Aim for blood pressure of <140/85 mmHg.

Advice regarding lifestyle modifications for patients with hypertension

- Stop smoking
- Appropriate weight loss
- Moderation of alcohol intake (<14 units/week for women, <21 units for men)
- Dietary changes: lower saturated fat, increase oily fish, fruit and vegetable intake
- Limit salt intake
- Sensible exercise.

Drug treatment of hypertension

Points to remember:
- Tailor initial therapy, based on coexistent medical conditions, e.g. ACE inhibitor in heart failure, β blocker in IHD
- Remember evidence of variation in response with age and some races, e.g. thiazide and calcium antagonists tend to be more effective than β blockers and ACE inhibitors in elderly and Afro-Caribbean individuals
- Be prepared to use combination therapy to allow low dosages, reducing the side effects.

Complications

- Retinopathy, LVH, proteinuria
- Vascular events: stroke, MI, peripheral arterial disease
- Cardiac failure, worsening of pre-existing renal failure
- Worsening hypertension (especially if poorly treated).

Prognosis

Morbidity

Essential hypertension increases the risk of stroke sixfold, of coronary artery disease and heart failure threefold, and doubles the risk of peripheral vascular disease. Renal failure usually occurs only in malignant hypertension, but elevated blood pressure increases the progression of renal failure from other causes. Treatment of hypertension is well established to reduce the incidence of cardiovascular disease.

Mortality

- At an age <50 years, both diastolic and systolic hypertension are risk factors for cardiovascular death. A reduction of 5–6 mmHg in diastolic pressure is associated with a 12% reduction in mortality rate over 5 years.

(a)　　　　　　　　　　　　　　(b)

Fig. 82 Hypertensive retinopathy: (a) grade IV showing mild papilloedema, hard exudates (12 o'clock), cottonwool spots and flame haemorrhages (4 o'clock); (b) grade III showing extensive flame-shaped haemorrhages. (Courtesy of Professor J Ritter.)

• At an age >50 years, evidence suggests that the systolic blood pressure is the important determinant of risk, with an inverse relationship with diastolic blood pressure, i.e. the greater the pulse pressure for a given value of systolic pressure, the higher the risk.

Anonymous. Tight blood pressure control and risk of macrovascular and microvascular complications in type 2 diabetes: UKPDS 38. UK Prospective Diabetes Study Group. *BMJ* 1998; 317: 703–713.

Franklin SS, Khan SA, Wong ND, Larson MG, Levy D. Is pulse pressure useful in predicting risk for coronary heart disease? The Framingham heart study. *Circulation* 1999; 100: 354–360.

Hansson L, Zanchetti A, Carruthers SG *et al*. Effects of intensive blood-pressure lowering and low-dose aspirin in patients with hypertension: principal results of the Hypertension Optimal Treatment (HOT) randomised trial. HOT Study Group. *Lancet* 1998; 351: 1755–1762.

Ramsay LE, Williams B, Johnston GD *et al*. British Hypertension Society guidelines for hypertension management 1999: summary. *BMJ* 1999; 319: 630–635.

2.17.1 ACCELERATED PHASE HYPERTENSION

Aetiology/pathology

The aetiology is unknown, but patients with accelerated phase hypertension are more likely than those with 'benign' (not accelerated phase) hypertension to have a secondary cause. Pathological hallmark is the presence of fibrinoid necrosis in the arterioles.

Epidemiology

The incidence is around 1–2 : 100 000 per year.

Clinical presentation

• Hypertensive encephalopathy: visual disturbance, headaches, drowsiness, epileptic fits

• Other hypertensive emergencies: pulmonary oedema, acute renal failure, aortic dissection, pre-eclampsia.

Physical signs

Common

The diagnosis cannot be made without high blood pressure and evidence of fibrinoid necrosis of the vessels, which can be viewed directly only in the fundi:

• Grade III retinopathy: flame-shaped superficial haemorrhages or 'dot-and-blot' haemorrhages deeper within the retina, cottonwool spots (retinal microinfarcts); hard exudates (Fig. 82).

• Grade IV retinopathy: haemorrhages and exudates with papilloedema (Figs 82 and 83).

Attempts used to be made to distinguish between accelerated (grade III) and malignant (grade IV) hypertension because prognosis used to be worse in grade IV. This is no longer the case, and the term 'malignant hypertension' (originally coined because of the dire prognosis before effective antihypertensive treatment was

Fig. 83 Hypertensive retinopathy: grade IV showing florid papilloedema, haemorrhages and cottonwool spots. (Courtesy of Mr H Towler.)

113

Fig. 84 CT scan of aortic dissection. The descending aorta is enlarged and contrast shows a double lumen.

available) should be avoided—it makes patients think that they have cancer.

Uncommon

Drowsiness, coma, epileptic fitting, stroke, pulmonary oedema, aortic dissection.

Investigations

Immediate

Check urine for blood, protein and red cell casts. Perform ECG, chest radiograph, FBC, electrolytes, renal and liver function tests. If there is a clinical suspicion of aortic dissection (Fig. 84), urgent CT scan of the chest or TOE is needed. If there is a clinical suspicion of renal inflammatory condition, e.g. SLE, vasculitis or scleroderma, specific serological tests will be needed.

Elective

When blood pressure has been controlled, all patients with accelerated phase hypertension require a thorough work-up for secondary causes of hypertension. Renal biopsy may be required.

Differential diagnosis

The differential diagnosis is of acute glomerulonephritis or renal vasculitis, or scleroderma renal crisis.

Treatment

All patients with accelerated phase hypertension should be admitted to hospital for blood pressure control. General management consists of the following:
• Bedrest.

• No smoking: cigarettes cause an acute rise in blood pressure in accelerated hypertension!
• Monitor blood pressure regularly: every hour to start with, then less frequently.
• Monitor fluid input/output, daily weight and renal function (serum creatinine).
• Intravenous furosemide (frusemide) if there is pulmonary oedema.
• Aim to lower diastolic pressure by 15–20 mmHg over 24 h with oral atenolol 50–100 mg daily or nifedipine 10–20 mg 8-hourly (tablets, not sublingual formulation). Alternatively, intravenous therapy may be required: labetolol or nitroprusside. Most would avoid ACE inhibitors in the acute setting in case the patient had renal artery stenosis.
• Avoid rapid reduction in blood pressure—cerebral autoregulation is impaired and there is a substantial risk of causing ischaemic 'watershed' stroke. In most cases, aim to reduce the diastolic blood pressure to 100–105 mmHg over 2–3 days.
• Consult renal team if there is renal impairment or other suspicion of primary renal condition: patients with presenting creatinine <300 μmol/L are likely to recover renal function; those with creatinine >300 μmol/L are likely to progress to end-stage renal failure and require long-term renal replacement therapy.

Complications will require specific management:
• Hypertensive encephalopathy: coma—check airway, breathing, circulation; protect airway; give high-flow oxygen. Epileptic fits—anticonvulsants.
• Aortic dissection: use intravenous β blockade to slow heart rate; urgent imaging; urgent cardiothoracic surgical consultation.
• Renal failure: may require urgent dialysis/ultrafiltration to remove fluid if pulmonary oedema present.
• Pre-eclampsia: delivery of child.

Complications

Stroke, aortic dissection, chronic renal failure.

Prognosis

If untreated, 80% will die within 2 years. One recent series reported a 69% survival rate at 12 years.

Ahmed MEK, Walker JM, Beevers DG, Beevers M. Lack of difference between malignant and accelerated hypertension. *BMJ* 1986; 292: 235–237.
McGregor E, Isles CG, Jay JL, Lever AF, Murray GD. Retinal changes in malignant hypertension. *BMJ* 1986; 292: 233–234.
Webster J, Petrie JC, Jeffers TA, Lovell HG. Accelerated hypertension—patterns of mortality and clinical factors affecting outcome in treated patients. *Q J Med* 1993; 86: 485–493.

2.18 Venous thromboembolism

2.18.1 PULMONARY EMBOLISM

Embolism can be from any source (e.g. tumour, air, amniotic fluid), but this section will consider only thrombotic venous thromboembolism.

Aetiology/pathophysiology/pathology

Virchow's triad (local trauma to the vessel wall, hypercoagulability and venous stasis) causes thrombosis in the deep veins of the legs, pelvis or (more rarely) arms, which may propagate and extend proximally. Thrombus may dislodge and embolize to the pulmonary arterial tree, causing physical obstruction and the release of vasoactive substances, elevating pulmonary vascular resistance and resulting in the following:
• Redistribution of blood flow, causing ventilation–perfusion mismatch and impairment of gas exchange
• Increased RV afterload, causing dilatation and dysfunction of the right ventricle.

Epidemiology

The incidence of venous thromboembolism in the general population (in the USA) is 0.1% per year. Pulmonary embolism is the cause of 10% of all deaths in hospital.

The following are risk factors (found in 80–90% of patients with PE):
• Thrombophilia: factor V Leiden; deficiencies of antithrombin III, protein C and protein S; hyperhomocysteinaemia; antiphospholipid antibodies or lupus anticoagulant. (See *Haematology*, Section 1.20.) Ask about personal and family history of thromboembolism.
• Surgery/trauma/fractures (especially lower limb).
• Immobilization of any cause.
• Obesity.
• Smoking.
• Hypertension.
• Old age.
• Pregnancy/postpartum.
• Current (not prior) use of combined oral contraceptive or HRT—minor risk only.
• Malignancy.
• Chronic cardiorespiratory disease.

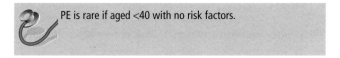
PE is rare if aged <40 with no risk factors.

Clinical presentation

Common

• Isolated dyspnoea
• Pulmonary infarction: pleuritic pain, cough or haemoptysis
• Massive PE: severe dyspnoea, syncope and haemodynamic collapse
• Deep venous thrombosis (DVT): swollen, firm, tender calf.

A young woman with isolated pleuritic chest pain and no risk factors except the oral contraceptive pill is extremely unlikely to have a PE if she has a respiratory rate of <20/min and a normal chest radiograph. But the risk of missing a life-threatening condition means that you should pursue investigation unless you can make a confident alternative diagnosis.

Uncommon

• Progressive ankle oedema and dyspnoea (secondary pulmonary hypertension)
• Pyrexia of unknown origin
• AF.

Physical signs

Common

• Tachypnoea
• Tachycardia
• Crackles on auscultation
• Pleural rub.

Uncommon

• Cyanosis
• Raised JVP, left parasternal heave, loud P2, pansystolic murmur of tricuspid regurgitation
• Swollen, firm calf of DVT.

Investigations

Investigations must be used in conjunction with an assessment of the clinical probability of PE.

ECG

Most commonly the ECG shows sinus tachycardia, sometimes anterior T-wave inversion. Atrial fibrillation, new RBBB, right axis deviation, RVH and S1Q3T3 are rare.

Chest radiograph

This may be normal, but common findings in PE include focal infiltrate, segmental collapse, raised diaphragm and pleural effusion. Wedge-shaped infarct and focal oligaemia are less common. A useful investigation in exclusion of differential diagnoses.

Arterial blood gases

Hypoxaemia and hypocapnia increase the suspicion, but normal gases do not exclude a diagnosis of PE.

Venous ultrasonography

This is used if there is clinical suspicion of a current DVT, although normal results do not exclude a PE.

Ventilation–perfusion lung scanning

This is useful if it is normal, or indicates a high probability of PE, correlated with clinical suspicion. Other results are difficult to interpret, especially in the presence of pre-existing cardiorespiratory disease. Perfusion scanning alone gives comparable diagnostic yield (Fig. 85).

Spiral chest CT with contrast

Increasingly used in the diagnosis of pulmonary emboli (Fig. 86). Clearly the imaging technique of choice when there is pre-existing cardiorespiratory disease.

Pulmonary angiography

Pulmonary angiography remains the 'gold standard', but with spiral chest CT, indications are diminishing.

Echocardiography

Echocardiography identifies RV pressure overload and dysfunction, as well as excluding other causes of haemodynamic collapse. It is useful as a quick source of information in a critically ill patient.

Plasma D-dimer enzyme-linked immunosorbent assay (ELISA)

This test is sensitive but not specific, i.e. it helps to exclude the diagnosis.

Consider the following in the differential diagnosis of PE:
- Pleurisy/breathlessness
- Pneumothorax
- Pneumonia
- Musculoskeletal pain
- Rib fracture
- Asthma/chronic airflow obstruction

Circulatory collapse
- MI
- Cardiac tamponade.

Treatment

Emergency

For massive PE with hypotension, treatment should be one of the following:
- Thrombolysis: different protocol from MI, via a peripheral vein or pulmonary artery catheter—as successful as embolectomy
- Embolectomy: transvenous catheter or open surgical—only if thrombolysis contraindicated or patient fails to respond
- Colloid to maintain right-sided filling in hypotension.

Short term

- Analgesia.
- Heparin: unfractionated or low molecular weight. Prevents further thrombus formation and permits endogenous fibrinolysis. Continue until INR >2.0.
- Oxygen.
- Warfarin, once heparinized.

Paradoxically, warfarin without heparin may initially increase hypercoagulability.

Long term

Continue warfarin for 6 weeks to 3 months if the risk factor is temporary; consider long term for recurrent embolism and persisting risk factors such as thrombophilia. Consider thrombophilia screening—especially if there is a family history. (See *Haematology*, Section 1.20.) Inferior vena caval (IVC) filters are indicated for recurrent PE in the presence of adequate anticoagulation or if anticoagulation is contraindicated.

Complications

The most significant complication is secondary pulmonary hypertension.

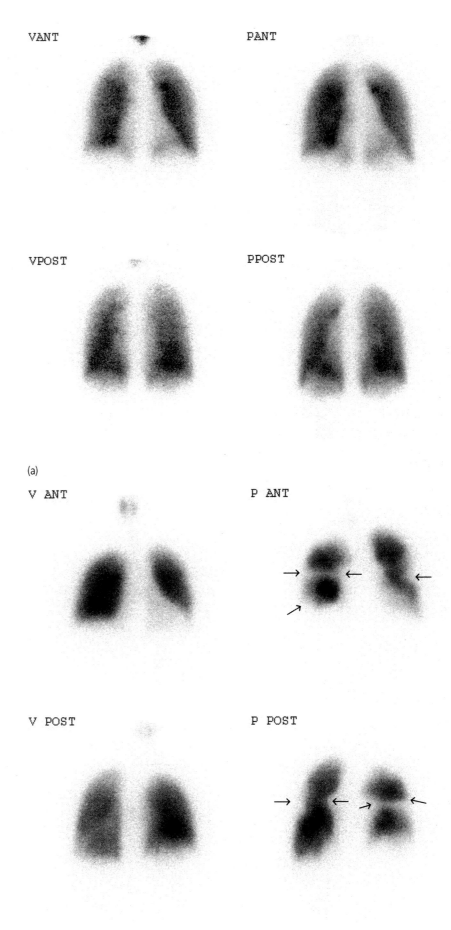

Fig. 85 (a) Normal ventilation–perfusion ($\dot{V}/\dot{Q}$) scan. Anterior and posterior views are shown. (b) Multiple perfusion defects (arrowed) which are not matched by ventilation defects and therefore indicate a high probability of pulmonary embolism.

117

Fig. 86 Contrast CT scan of a patient with a large pulmonary embolus visible as a grey filling defect (arrowed) against the white contrast in the pulmonary artery.

Prognosis

Overall mortality rate at 3 months is 15.0–17.5%, reflecting in large part the underlying conditions. Right ventricular dysfunction on echocardiography predicts an adverse outcome. Note that the mortality associated with anticoagulation (following established guidelines) is very low at 0.1% of cases.

Prevention

Primary

• Consideration of compression stockings and prophylactic heparin in hospitalized patients, especially those with trauma, the critically ill and general and orthopaedic surgery
• Discourage smoking

Secondary

• Thrombophilia screening and consideration of the duration of anticoagulation
• Discourage smoking and advise alternatives to the oral contraceptive pill
• Weight loss and blood pressure control if necessary
• Consideration of IVC filter in selected cases.

Disease associations

• Thrombophilia
• Malignancy

• Antiphospholipid syndromes
• Hypertension.

 Goldhaber SZ. Pulmonary embolism. *N Engl J Med* 1998; 339: 93–104.

2.19 Driving restrictions in cardiology

Group 1 entitlement (normal driving)

Angina

Patients may drive providing that there are no symptoms at rest or at the wheel.

Angioplasty

Patients must not drive for 1 week.

MI/CABG

Patients must not drive for 1 month.

Arrhythmia

Patients must not drive if the arrhythmia has caused, or is likely to cause, incapacity. If AV block documented, patients must not drive until 4 weeks after the cause has been identified and controlled.

Pacemaker

Patients must not drive for 1 week.

Syncope

Patients must not drive until the cause has been identified and controlled.

Heart failure, valvular heart disease and cardiomyopathy

Patients may continue to drive provided that there is no other disqualifying condition.

Group 2 entitlement (vocational driving)

Angina/MI/angioplasty/CABG

Patients must stop driving and inform the DVLA.

Relicensing is permitted once the patient is free of angina for 6 weeks with a satisfactory exercise test (see below).

Arrhythmia

Patients must not drive if the arrhythmia has caused, or is likely to cause, incapacity. Driving is permitted when the arrhythmia has been controlled for at least 3 months, provided that the LV ejection fraction is >0.4 and a satisfactory exercise test has been done.

Pacemaker

Patients must not drive for 6 weeks.

Syncope

Patients must not drive after single or recurrent episodes. Relicensing may be permitted after 3 months if specialist review and investigations are satisfactory.

Heart failure, valvular heart disease and cardiomyopathy

Patients must not drive if symptomatic. Relicensing possible if symptoms controlled and specialist review satisfactory.

Exercise test requirements

The patient must be off antianginal medication for 48 h.

The patient must complete the three stages of the Bruce protocol without any of the following:
- Angina
- Syncope
- Hypotension
- Sustained VT
- Horizontal or down-sloping ST segment shift >2 mm. Repeat every 3 years.

Angiography

This is not required for relicensing. If angiography has been undertaken, relicensing will not normally be permitted if the ejection fraction is ≤0.40 on ventriculography, or if there is significant proximal unrelieved coronary arterial stenosis (left main and proximal LAD ≥30% or proximal >50% elsewhere, unless subtending a completed infarction).

 http://www.dvla.gov.uk/at_a_glance/ch2_cardiovascular.htm.

3 Investigations and practical procedures

3.1 ECG

Principle

The ECG is a graphic representation of the electrical potentials of the heart. Each deflection represents electrical activity in the cardiac cycle:
- P wave: atrial depolarization. A further deflection that represents atrial repolarization is usually hidden within the QRS complex.
- PR interval: atrioventricular conduction time.
- QRS complex: ventricular depolarization. Q is the first negative deflection, R the first positive deflection and S the first negative deflection following a positive deflection.
- ST segment: from the end of the QRS to the start of the T wave.
- T wave: ventricular repolarization.
- U wave: after or in the end portion of the T wave. Cause unknown.

Adopting a systematic method of interpreting an ECG will enable you to approach the most complex of ECGs with confidence. If you approach all ECGs in this manner, certain patterns will become familiar, enabling rapid diagnosis of arrhythmias and possible structural cardiac abnormalities.

ECG interpretation scheme

After establishing the basic parameters, start at the P wave and progress through to the QRS and finally the T wave:
- What is the rhythm? (regular/irregular)
- What is the rate? [300/number of large squares between each QRS] (normal/bradycardia/tachycardia)
- What is the QRS axis?
- What is the P-wave axis?
- Is the P-wave morphology normal?
- Is the PR interval short/long?
- Are there any δ waves?
- Are there any Q waves?
- Is the QRS morphology normal? (RBBB/LBBB)
- Does the ST segment look normal in every lead?
- Are any T waves inverted?
- What is the QT interval?
- Are there any additional features? (U waves)

QRS axis

To establish the QRS axis you need to do the following:

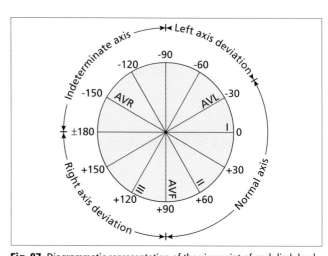

Fig. 87 Diagrammatic representation of the viewpoint of each limb lead.

- Identify the limb lead where the QRS is isoelectric—the axis will be 90° from this.
- Look at the limb lead whose axis is at 90° to the lead where the QRS is isoelectric (Fig. 87)—if deflection is positive, the axis is directed towards the positive pole of that lead (and if negative, away from it).

The normal axis is from −30° to +90°. Figure 88 demonstrates examples of the normal axis and right and left axis deviation.

Normal intervals

1 small square = 0.04 s

- PR interval (onset of P wave to first deflection of QRS) = 0.12 – 0.20 s
- QRS duration (<0.12 s)
- QT interval (onset of QRS complex to end of T wave) = 0.35 – 0.45 s
- QTc = QT adjusted for rate = $(QT/\sqrt{[R-R \text{ interval}]})$ = 0.38 – 0.42 s.

Bradyarrhythmias/conduction disturbances

The key to identification of bradyarrhythmias is in establishing the relative relationship of the P wave and QRS complex. The following are the key features to identify:
- Rate
- Identify whether irregular/regular P waves/QRS complexes
- Plot all P waves and all QRS complexes
- No P wave before normal QRS suggests junctional rhythm
- No P wave before wide QRS suggests ventricular escape rhythm.

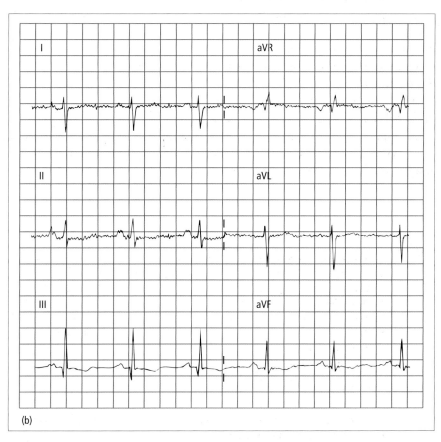

Fig. 88 Examples of (a) normal axis, (b) right and (c) left axis deviation.

(c)

Fig. 88 *Continued*

Fig. 89 Example of first-degree heart block. The PR interval is in excess of 0.20 s.

Fig. 90 Second-degree heart block (Wenckebach's or Mobitz, type I) with progressively increasing PR interval before failure of conduction with no QRS complex.

Fig. 91 Second-degree heart block (2 : 1): only alternate P waves are followed by a QRS complex. When there is failure of conduction without progressive increase in the PR interval, this is known as Mobitz, type II.

Fig. 92 Complete heart block: P waves and QRS complexes are not related. There is a slow ventricular escape rhythm (wider QRS complexes).

Fig. 93 Junctional bradycardia: slow ventricular rate with no discernible P waves.

Fig. 94 Complete heart block in patient with atrial fibrillation as the underlying atrial rhythm.

Figures 89–94 illustrate varying degrees of atrioventricular block.

Conduction abnormalities occur because of abnormalities of the normal depolarization from the AV node to the His bundle and bundle branches.
• Abnormalities in AV node/His bundle conduction lead to degrees of heart block, e.g. coronary artery disease, myocarditis, digoxin toxicity, electrolyte abnormalities.
• Abnormalities in conduction in the bundle branches leads to widened QRS complexes. Block of both bundles has the same effect as block of the His bundle, causing complete heart block (Table 31).

Table 31 Some key causes of bundle-branch block.

RBBB	LBBB
May be normal	Coronary artery disease
Coronary artery disease	Cardiomyopathy
Cardiomyopathy	Left ventricular hypertrophy
Atrial septal defect	(hypertension, aortic stenosis)
Ebstein's anomaly	Conduction system fibrosis
Massive pulmonary embolism	

LBBB, left bundle-branch block (wide [>0.12 s] notched, M- or plateau-shaped QRS complex in leads orientated to the left ventricle—V5, V6, AVL and I); RBBB, right bundle-branch block (M-shaped QRS complex in leads orientated to the right ventricle—V1 and V2).

Tachyarrhythmias

Find out whether there are any of the following:
• Narrow/broad complex?
• Identify whether irregular/regular.
• 'Saw-tooth' appearance of baseline suggests atrial flutter (ventricular rate may be irregular if variable block).
• Regular narrow complex tachycardia with no P waves seen suggests AVNRT (see Section 2.2.2).
• Consider differential diagnosis of SVT with aberration (Fig. 95) (Table 32).

Specific morphological changes in the ECG

Left ventricular hypertrophy

There are several criteria:
• Usually left axis deviation (>−30°)
• Amplitude of V1 or V2 + V5 or V6 >40 mm
• Note in young men with thin chest wall, criteria may be met without LVH.

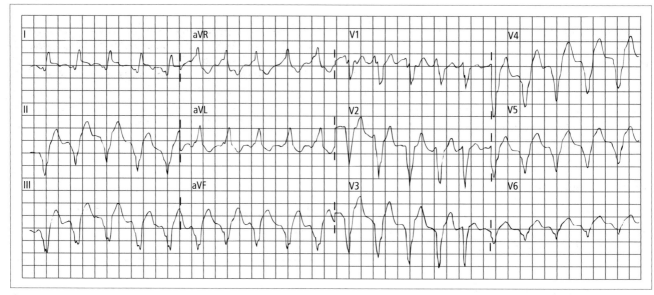

Fig. 95 Twelve-lead ECG of ventricular tachycardia with significant axis deviation, broad complexes and concordance across the chest leads.

Table 32 Differentiating ventricular tachycardia (VT) and supraventricular tachycardia (SVT).

Features supporting VT	Features supporting SVT
Very broad QRS complexes (>140 ms)	Termination with Valsalva manoeuvre/adenosine
Fusion beats	
Capture beats	Association of 'p' waves and QRS complexes
AV dissociation	
Significant axis deviation (right or left)	Onset following premature atrial beat
Concordance of the QRS deflexions in V1–6	
Onset following R on T	

Right ventricular hypertrophy

Criteria are the following:
- Right axis deviation (>90°)
- R V1 + S V6 >11 mm
- R V1 or S V6 >7 mm.

Metabolic abnormalities

- Hypercalcaemia: short QT, prominent U wave
- Hypocalcaemia: long QT
- Hyperkalaemia: flat/lost P waves, increased PR interval, wide QRS, tented T wave, arrhythmias
- Hypokalaemia: first-degree heart block, ST depression, U waves.

3.1.1 EXERCISE ECGs

Excercise ECGs are an extremely useful non-invasive investigation in appropriate clinical circumstances, but it is always important to remember that it can produce both false negatives and false positives. If significant diagnostic doubt remains in a patient who gives a good history of angina, further investigation should be considered (coronary angiography/myocardial perfusion imaging). Exercise testing in asymptomatic patients is of limited value.

Principle

The aim of the study is to document the electrophysiological and haemodynamic response to physical stress.

Indications

Exercise ECGs are indicated for the following:
- Establishing a diagnosis of angina in a patient with chest pain
- Obtaining a measure of exercise tolerance
- Evaluating a haemodynamic response to exercise
- Evaluation of exercise-induced arrhythmias.

Contraindications

There is a very low mortality if the test is used in appropriate patients: <1 : 20 000. The following are contraindications:
- Significant aortic stenosis
- Hypertrophic obstructive cardiomyopathy (for relative contraindications see Section 2.4.1)
- Acute pericarditis/myocarditis
- Acute MI/unstable angina
- Acute aortic dissection
- Systemic infection
- Physical impairment restricting patient from exercising.

Practical details

Before investigation

Omit antianginal medication if the test is for diagnostic reasons. Continue if a functional assessment on treatment is required. Note that β blockers and antihypertensives will mask the haemodynamic response.

The investigation

Close observation of the patient is required with full resuscitation facilities to hand. At least two qualified people should supervise the test.

After investigation

Continue to observe the patient closely. Dramatic haemodynamic changes can occur during the recovery period. Terminate the investigation only when all the parameters have returned to their normal level.

Results

Response to exercise

Normal ECG response to exercise:
• Ventricular rate increases
• P wave: increase in amplitude
• PR: shortens
• QRS: R-wave amplitude decreases
• ST: sharply up-sloping
• QT: shortens
• T wave: decrease in amplitude.
  Abnormal ECG response to exercise (Fig. 96):
• No increase in ventricular rate
• ST depression >1 mm (horizontal/down-sloping): myocardial ischaemia (the greater the degree and the longer it persists into recovery the greater the probability of coronary heart disease)
• ST elevation (horizontal/up-sloping): where previous MI suggests dyskinetic ventricle/aneurysm
• QRS: bundle-branch block may suggest ischaemia
• QT: prolongation of QTc may be a risk marker for *torsade de pointes*
• T wave: inversion suggests ischaemia
• Arrhythmias: ventricular arrhythmia suggests ischaemia.

 Cleland JGF, Findlay IN, Gilligan D, Pennell DJ. *The Essentials of Exercise Electrocardiography.* London: Current Medical Literature Ltd, 1993.
Hampton JR. *The ECG Made Easy.* Edinburgh: Churchill Livingstone, 1997.
Xiao HB, Spicer M. How to do electrocardiography. *Br J Cardiol* 1996; 3: 148–150. (Seven part series).

3.2 Basic electrophysiology studies

Principle

Pace/sense electrodes are placed transvenously via the femoral vein and/or subclavian vein to various intracardiac locations. Electrograms are recorded during sinus rhythm. Arrhythmias are induced using pacing protocols with programmed extra stimuli.

Indications

Electrophysiology studies (EPS) may be helpful in the following circumstances:
• Narrow complex tachyarrhythmias: assessing for radio-frequency ablation
• Broad complex arrhythmias: assessing for radio-frequency ablation or implantation of an ICD
• Establishing a diagnosis in patients with palpitations/syncope
• Assessing bradyarrhythmias (limited value)
• Assessing effectiveness of antiarrhythmic to suppress arrhythmia.

Contraindications

EPS are not indicated for patients with the following:
• Reversible aetiology for arrhythmia
• Severe electrolyte abnormality.

Practical details

Before investigation

Antiarrhythmic medication is usually stopped 48 h before study.

The investigation

Intravenous sedative (often benzodiazepine) may be used before the procedure because some pacing protocols

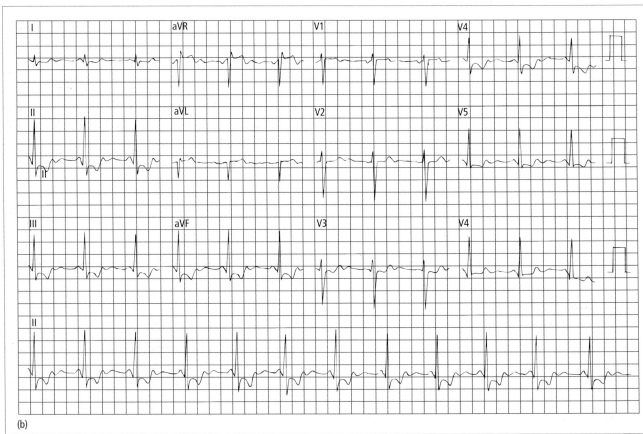

Fig. 96 Positive exercise ECG: note (a) the significant ST changes in the inferolateral leads which (b) become more marked in recovery.

Fig. 97 Radiograph demonstrating electrodes placed in the high right atrium, right ventricular outflow tract and His bundle during an electrophysiological test. Sternal wires present from previous coronary bypass grafting.

produce extremely rapid heart rates. Bipolar electrodes are placed to obtain intracardiac electrograms (high right atrium, RV apex/outflow tract and His–Purkinje system) (Fig. 97). A multipolar electrode placed in the coronary sinus records electrograms from the left atrium. Arrhythmias are induced by delivering extra pacing beats after a train of paced beats in the atrium and ventricle. These extra stimuli are timed to occur during the refractory period in an attempt to establish a possible re-entry mechanism (Fig. 98). The timing of the individual electrograms will indicate whether there is a possible electrophysiological substrate for arrhythmias. Assessment of the function of the SA and AV nodes indicates whether permanent pacing might be required.

After investigation

Patients are observed for 24 h. Drug therapy may be changed as a result of the EPS.

Complications

- Femoral vein/subclavian vein (haematoma)
- Incessant arrhythmias requiring cardioversion, e.g. AF.

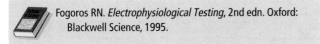
Fogoros RN. *Electrophysiological Testing*, 2nd edn. Oxford: Blackwell Science, 1995.

3.3 Ambulatory monitoring

Principle

Documenting a single-channel electrocardiogram over 24 h can provide useful information in the investigation of patients with palpitations, arrhythmias and syncope. It is non-invasive and, with current analysis hardware/software, tapes can be analysed rapidly and accurately. It is always important when using Holter monitoring to appreciate that this provides only a brief snapshot of the patient's heart rhythm, and that a negative result does not mean that the patient's symptoms are not secondary to an arrhythmia.

Indications

Ambulatory monitoring is indicated for the following:
- Evaluation of patients with palpitations and syncope
- Monitoring the efficacy of antiarrhythmic therapy
- Evaluation of heart rate variability.

Practical details

There are a number of different methods by which heart rate and rhythm can be observed.

Twenty-four-hour Holter monitoring

This is used for patients with frequent symptoms. Even some patients who have infrequent symptoms may have asymptomatic arrhythmic episodes on a 24-h recording that may provide valuable information (Fig. 99).

Patient-activated devices

These are used for less frequent symptoms, e.g. Cardiomemo recorder. However, the efficacy of these devices relies on the patient activating the device, which is not always possible during or shortly after a symptomatic episode.

Implantable loop recorders

These are used for infrequent symptoms. They enable the patient to activate the device up to 40 min after the event and still record the heart rhythm (Figs 100 and 101).

(a)

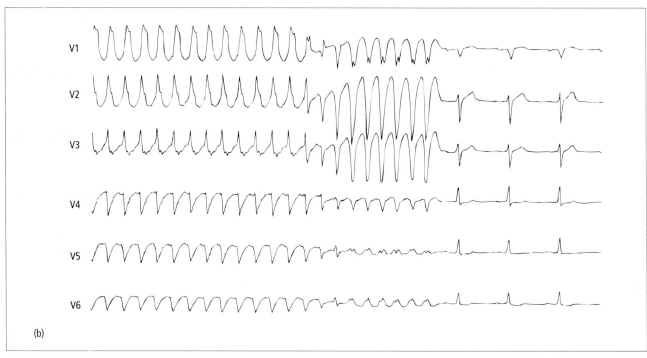

(b)

Fig. 98 Induction of ventricular tachycardia. (a) Note the train of paced beats followed by earlier extra stimuli and then onset of monomorphic ventricular tachycardia. (b) Ventricular tachycardia is then terminated with nine beats of overdrive pacing.

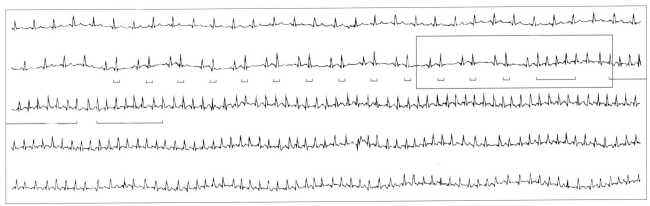

Fig. 99 Holter monitor recording demonstrating atrioventricular nodal re-entry tachycardia (AVNRT)/atrioventricular re-entry tachycardia (AVRT). Note the sudden onset after a short period of ventricular bigeminy.

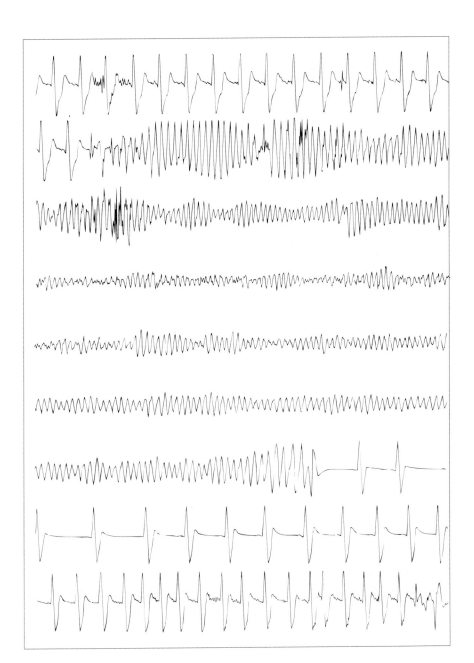

Fig. 100 Loop recording showing sinus tachycardia followed by *torsades de pointes* with spontaneous resolution.

3.5 Pacemakers

Pacing of patients with non-reversible significant brady-arrhythmias can restore life expectancy to close to that of the normal population. Pacemakers have improved considerably over the last two decades. Devices have increased in longevity and been reduced in size. In addition, many technical innovations have resulted in pacemakers that are more physiological in their mode of action. The simplest of pacemakers consists of a single lead, with its tip in the right ventricular apex connected to the pulse generator in the subcutaneous tissue of the chest wall. Dual-chamber devices have a further lead with its tip positioned in the right atrial appendage (Fig. 103). Pacemakers have a designated terminology which describes the pacing and sensing functions of the device (Table 33).

Indications

Temporary pacemaker

Temporary pacing is useful in the following circumstances:
• As an interim measure before permanent pacemaker
• Inferior MI: second-/third-degree block and hypotension/heart failure
• Anterior MI: second-/third-degree block (usually large infarct to involve the AV node)
• Symptomatic/asymptomatic patients with trifascicular block undergoing general anaesthesia (should be assessed for permanent pacemaker)
• Drug overdose, e.g. digoxin, β blockers, verapamil.

Temporary pacing is not indicated for asymptomatic patients with bifascicular block who are undergoing general anaesthesia.

Fig. 103 ECG demonstrating dual-chamber pacing. Note the pacing 'spike' before most P waves and QRS complexes.

Table 33 Algorithm used to describe pacemaker function*.

Paced chamber	Sensed chamber	Effect of sensing	Programming/rate responsiveness
0 = none	0 = none	0 = none	0 = none
A = atrium	A = atrium	T = triggered	P = simple
V = ventricle	V = ventricle	I = inhibited	M = multiprogrammable
D = dual (A + V)	D = dual (A + V)	D = dual (T + I)	C = communicating
			R = rate responsive

*For example, a DDDR pacemaker both senses and paces in the atrium and ventricle, and triggers and inhibits, depending on what is or is not sensed. It also has a rate response which means that the heart rate will be paced faster if appropriate, e.g. during exercise.

Permanent pacemaker

The permanent pacemaker is useful for the following:
- Third-degree heart block
- Symptomatic, second-degree block
- Asymptomatic, type II, second-degree block
- AF with pauses >3.0 s
- Symptomatic documented sinus node dysfunction
- Recurrent syncope associated with >3.0 s pause with carotid sinus stimulation.

Practical details

Before procedure

Patients should give informed consent and be fasted.

The procedure

The procedure is usually performed under local anaesthesia. The pacemaker leads are placed transvenously via the cephalic/subclavian routes into the right ventricular apex and right atrial appendage under fluoroscopic guidance. The leads are checked to ensure correct pace/sense functions and the pulse generator is implanted subcutaneously.

After procedure

After a satisfactory pacemaker check the following day, most patients may be discharged from hospital, usually with 5 days of antibiotic therapy and after a lateral and posteroanterior chest radiograph (Fig. 104). For driving regulations, see Section 2.19, p. 118. Pacemakers can be programmed and interrogated by placing a 'wand' over the device; using electromagnetic induction, information can be received or transmitted to the pacemaker. Patients are usually seen every 6–12 months to monitor the pacemaker and re-program if necessary. The expected life of the battery is 8–12 years.

Complications of pacemakers

Although complications are rare, the following may occur.

Common

- Pneumothorax
- Pacemaker lead displacement (Fig. 105)
- Haematoma.

(a)

(b)

Fig. 104 Chest radiograph of dual-chamber pacemaker: (a) anteroposterior and (b) lateral.

Uncommon

- Local infection
- Pericardial effusion
- Thrombosis and thromboembolism
- Infective endocarditis
- Pacemaker syndrome: single-chamber pacing, leading to symptoms as a result of loss of AV synchrony.

Fig. 105 Chest radiograph showing displacement of ventricular lead through ventricle to pericardial space.

Fig. 106 Schematic diagram of cardiac silhouette on chest radiograph. AA, arch aorta; Asc A, ascending aorta; LA, left atrial appendage; LV, left ventricle; PA, pulmonary artery; RA, right atrium; SVC, superior vena cava.

Rare

• Twiddler's syndrome: patient consciously/subconsciously turns the pacemaker generator, leading to retraction and eventual displacement of the pacing lead
• Component failure: lead/pulse generator.

Schilling R, Peters N. Insertion of permanent pacemakers. *Br J Cardiol* 1999; 6: 550–556.
Lamb D, Schilling R. Who's for a pacemaker? *Br J Cardiol* 1999; 6: 580–582.

3.6 The chest radiograph in cardiac disease

Commonly encountered abnormalities

The normal cardiac silhouette is shown in Fig. 106. Below are the most commonly encountered abnormalities.

Cardiomegaly

Cardiothoracic ratio >0.5 on posteroanterior projection is a fairly specific indicator of cardiac disease, but may be falsely increased in pes excavatum and very thin patients. Echocardiography is much more sensitive.

Aortic enlargement

This is seen in hypertension, atherosclerosis or aortic regurgitation:
• Prominent aortic arch
• Ascending aorta protrudes further to the right side
• Tortuous descending aorta.

Mediastinal widening

This may indicate an aortic dissection.

Enlarged pulmonary artery

This is seen in the following:
• Pulmonary hypertension: COAD, primary pulmonary hypertension, Eisenmenger's syndrome
• Pulmonary stenosis: poststenotic dilatation as a result of turbulent blood flow
• Collagen disorders, e.g. Marfan's syndrome.

Left atrial enlargement

This is seen in mitral disease or replacement and LV impairment. It may be mimicked by mediastinal or pleural neoplasm. Occasionally, the left atrium may be so grossly enlarged that it forms the right heart border (i.e. lateral to the right atrium). In this situation, left atrial enlargement may be recognized by following the superior border of the left atrium, which will cross the midline. If the prominent right heart border is caused by right atrial

Fig. 107 Globular cardiomegaly caused by a large pericardial effusion. Note sternal wires from recent cardiac surgery.

enlargement, the contour is continuous with the superior vena cava.

Left ventricular enlargement

- Pressure overload: apex elevated and more rounded
- Volume overload: widening of cardiac shadow.

Right ventricle enlargement

The right ventricle does not normally form a cardiac border, but enlargement pushes the LV posteriorly and to the left, causing widening of the heart shadow.

Pericardial effusion

This may produce massive cardiomegaly, giving the cardiac contour a globular appearance, with clear lung fields (Fig. 107).

Common abnormalities of pulmonary vasculature

Increased pulmonary blood flow

- Enlarged pulmonary arteries
- Recruitment of upper lobe vessels.

Pulmonary hypertension

- Peripheral vasoconstriction (pruning)
- Further enlargement of pulmonary arteries
- Pulmonary artery calcification.

Pulmonary venous hypertension and oedema

In increasing order of severity:
- Upper lobe blood diversion
- Interlobular septal thickening (Kerley B lines): thin horizontal lines at lung bases
- Alveolar oedema, typically involving the inner two-thirds of the lung ('bat wing' hilar shadowing).

Pulmonary oedema is occasionally unilateral. After treatment, the radiographic appearances often lag behind clinical improvement. Prominent interstitial lines also occur in the following:
- Fibrosis
- Tumour infiltration
- Interstitial pneumonia.

3.7 Cardiac biochemical markers

Principle

Heart muscle damage, usually caused by acute ischaemia, causes release of proteins that can be detected in the blood stream.

CK-MB

This cardiospecific isoenzyme of creatine kinase (CK):
- is the most widely used marker of heart muscle damage
- has a reasonable specificity but only a moderate sensitivity
- an arbitrary cut-off point is used for retrospective diagnosis of MI
- is used in conjunction with the ECG to make the diagnosis of non-Q-wave (or subendocardial) infarction
- gives results that are often equivocal and may be uninterpretable in some circumstances, e.g. very high CK caused by coexisting skeletal muscle damage.

Troponin tests

These tests are now superseding CK-MB assays. Troponins are regulatory elements of the contractile apparatus in muscle; they exist in cardiac-specific isoforms and are highly sensitive. Rapid bedside assays for cardiac troponins T and I are available. They are normally very low/ undetectable in the blood and appear 4–6 h after myocardial damage, peak at 24 h and persist for up to 14 days. In addition, they are raised in 30% of patients with unstable angina. A positive test is associated with a higher risk of death or MI—the higher level indicating a worse prognosis. They may be used to select high-risk unstable angina

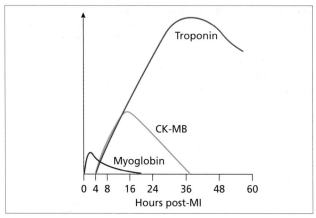

Fig. 108 Time course of cardiac markers after heart muscle damage. MI, myocardical infarction.

patients who would benefit from more aggressive treatment, e.g. low-molecular-weight heparin, glycoprotein IIb/IIIa receptor antagonists or early revascularization. A negative test may be used in conjunction with clinical and ECG criteria to identify low-risk patients who are suitable for early discharge without the need for overnight stay.

Myoglobin

Myoglobin is present in both skeletal and cardiac muscle, and released about 30 min after heart muscle damage. Elevated values may detect infarction much sooner after the onset of chest pain than CK-MB or troponins (Fig. 108). However, as a result of the poor specificity of myoglobin measurement, a positive test must be confirmed by troponin or CK-MB.

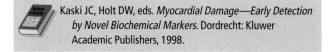

Kaski JC, Holt DW, eds. *Myocardial Damage—Early Detection by Novel Biochemical Markers.* Dordrecht: Kluwer Academic Publishers, 1998.

3.8 Cardiac catheterization, percutaneous transluminal coronary angioplasty and stenting

3.8.1 CARDIAC CATHETERIZATION

Principle

Catheters are introduced into the arterial or venous system and advanced to the left or right heart, respectively, allowing the following:
• Pressure measurements in the cardiac chambers and major vessels.

• Injection of radiographic contrast into cardiac chambers, major vessels or coronary arteries. Digital cineangiography provides a permanent versatile record of cardiac anatomy.
• Oxygen saturation measurements in blood sampled from the cardiac chambers and major vessels.

Indications

Left heart catheterization

• Angina (stable or unstable) not controlled by medical therapy, or with positive stress test at low/moderate workload. (See Section 2.1, p. 51.)
• Proposed heart valve surgery
• Suspected aortic dissection not clearly seen by other imaging methods. (See Section 2.11.1, p. 99.)

Right heart catheterization

This is indicated in suspected primary pulmonary hypertension and selected cases of pulmonary embolism.

Combined left and right heart catheterization

• Mitral stenosis and selected cases of mitral regurgitation before surgery
• Congenital heart disease: to confirm diagnosis and assess severity
• Pre-transplantation assessment.

Contraindications

Severely impaired coagulation. Pulmonary oedema and cardiogenic shock are relative contraindications because radiographic contrast may lead to haemodynamic deterioration, even death.

Practical details

Before investigation

• FBC, urea and electrolytes, INR if on warfarin
• ECG
• Informed consent
• Premedication with oral benzodiazepine.

The investigation

Lead aprons are worn to protect staff from radiation. Aseptic procedures are followed. Usually the right femoral artery and/or vein is punctured under local anaesthetic (but patients on warfarin with an INR of 1.5–3.0 may be safely catheterized from the arm). A 5–7 French gauge sheath (incorporating a haemostatic valve) is introduced

(a)

(b)

Fig. 109 Normal coronary angiogram: the right coronary artery is small (non-dominant) and shown in (a) with the left coronary demonstrated in (b). LAD, left anterior descending; LCx, left circumflex; RCA, right coronary artery.

Table 34 Normal intracardiac pressure values.

Pressure	Range (mmHg)
Right atrium mean	1–5
Right ventricle systolic	15–30
Right ventricle end-diastolic	1–8
Pulmonary artery systolic	15–30
Pulmonary artery diastolic	5–12
Pulmonary artery mean	9–16
Pulmonary capillary wedge mean	5–13
Left atrium mean	2–12
Left ventricle systolic	90–140
Left ventricle end-diastolic	5–12

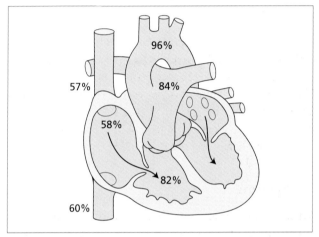

Fig. 110 Oxygen saturation measurements showing a 'step up' in the right ventricle, indicating a ventricular septal defect with left-to-right shunt.

The size of the shunt can be estimated from the ratio of pulmonary to systemic blood flow, using the following formula (derived from the Fick equation):

$$\frac{Qp}{Qs} = \frac{Ao - MV}{PV - PA}$$

where Qp = pulmonary flow; Qs = systemic flow; Ao = aortic saturation; MV = mixed venous saturation; PV = pulmonary venous saturation; PA = pulmonary arterial saturation. Pulmonary venous saturation is not usually measured directly, but is assumed to be 97%. From Fig. 110, the ratio of pulmonary to venous flow is calculated to be 2.9 : 1. A shunt >1.5 : 1 is regarded as significant.

After investigation

- Remove the sheath and press on the vessel to achieve haemostasis (arterial at least 10 min, venous 5 min). During this time, preliminary results may be given to the patient.
- Instruct patients on how to press on the vessel themselves.
- Arrange for return to the ward.
- Bedrest for 2–4 h after femoral artery puncture.
- Review and report catheter data.
- Review patient on the ward.
- Explain full results and plan.

using the Seldinger technique. Pre-shaped catheters are passed through the sheath (on a long J-tipped guidewire in the arterial system) and guided using continuous pressure monitoring and fluoroscopic imaging. A three-lead ECG is also monitored continuously.

Examples of images obtained from a left heart catheter are shown in Fig. 109. Normal values for pressure data are given in Table 34. Oxygen saturation measurement from a case of left-to-right shunting is illustrated in Fig. 110.

Complications

Minor

- Bruising in 50%
- Haematoma in 5%.

Major

- Femoral arterial damage requiring repair
- Stroke, MI or death.

Each of these complications has an incidence of about 1 per 1000.

Important information for patients

While obtaining consent, ensure that the patient understands why the procedure is being carried out, what is involved and what the risks are.

Patients should not drive for 24 h afterwards, and must have someone staying with them if they are going home after a day-case procedure.

Miller GAH. *Handbook of Cardiac Catheterization.* Oxford: Blackwell Scientific Publications, 1990.

3.8.2 PERCUTANEOUS TRANSLUMINAL CORONARY ANGIOPLASTY AND STENTING

Principle

Angina is relieved by inflating a catheter-delivered balloon within a coronary artery at the site of stenosis.

Indications

- Patients with suitable stenoses in one or two coronary arteries who have angina (stable or unstable) that is not adequately controlled by medical therapy
- Recurrent angina after CABG (selected patients)
- Acute MI as primary treatment (primary angioplasty)
- Acute MI after unsuccessful thrombolysis (rescue angioplasty).

Contraindications

PTCA should not be undertaken in the following:
- Patients who would benefit prognostically from coronary bypass grafting. (See Section 2.1, p. 51.)
- Patients without angina (no evidence that life expectancy improved).

Practical details

Before procedure

This is as for cardiac catheterization (see Section 3.8.1, p. 136), but in addition insert an intravenous cannula.

The procedure

Usually a right femoral arterial approach is used. The coronary ostium is intubated with an angioplasty guide catheter. Heparin 10 000 units as an intravenous bolus is given at this stage. A guidewire is introduced through the guide catheter into the coronary artery lumen; it is advanced beyond the lesion using fluoroscopy and injections of radiographic contrast, given as necessary. A balloon catheter is passed over this guidewire, positioned at the site of narrowing and inflated for approximately 1 min. If a satisfactory result cannot be obtained using the balloon alone, a coronary stent may be deployed (Fig. 111). This is a latticework stainless steel tube mounted on a deflated balloon. After positioning at the site of narrowing, the balloon is inflated so that the stent is expanded and embedded in the coronary artery wall. When the balloon is deflated, the stent remains as a 'scaffold' to hold the artery open. If a stent is used, the activated clotting time (ACT) is checked and further heparin given if necessary to achieve an ACT of >350 s.

After procedure

The sheath is removed 4–6 h after the procedure, once the heparin has worn off. If a stent has been used, prescribe clopidogrel 300 mg stat dose, and 75 mg daily thereafter for 4 weeks, to reduce the risk of stent thrombosis. Patients may go home the day after an uncomplicated procedure.

Outcome

- The success rate is 95%
- The chance of re-stenosis in 6 months is 30% (slightly less if stented)
- If occlusion is chronic, there is a 50% chance of success and 50% chance of re-occlusion.

Complications

- Coronary dissection, acute vessel closure: usually controlled by stenting.
- Coronary thrombosis: most commonly seen in unstable angina. The glycoprotein IIb/IIIa receptor antagonists (e.g. abciximab) are intravenous antiplatelet agents which may be given to protect against this complication.

(a)

(b)

(c)

(d)

Fig. 111 Coronary artery stenting: (a) left coronary angiogram showing a tight stenosis in the left anterior descending coronary artery. (b) Positioning of a stent mounted on an angioplasty balloon. (c) Inflation of balloon to deploy stent. (d) Final result.

- Death, MI, emergency CABG, stroke about 1 per 200. (See also Section 3.8.1, p. 138.)

 Landau C, Lange RA, Hillis LD. Percutaneous transluminal coronary angioplasty. *N Engl J Med* 1994; 330: 981–983.

 Important information for patients

- Expect transient angina during balloon inflations
- Get consent from all patients for angioplasty ± stent ± emergency CABG.

3.9 Computed tomography and magnetic resonance imaging

3.9.1 COMPUTED TOMOGRAPHY

Principle

Multiple radiography views are processed and a digital cross-sectional image produced, with different tissue densities displayed as different grey-scale values. In spiral CT the radiography tube rotates continuously around the slowly moving patient, scanning a large volume in a single breathhold and reducing artefacts. These images can be reconstructed in other (non-axial) planes.

Indications

- Pericardial disease: thickening, infiltration or effusion
- Spiral CT: contrast angiography of pulmonary vasculature down to the level of segmental branches ($\dot{V}/\dot{Q}$ or invasive pulmonary angiogram still better for smaller branches), aorta for aneurysms or dissection, renal or carotid stenoses.

Contraindications

- Contrast: known sensitivity or renal impairment (relative contraindication)
- Pregnancy: relative contraindication—large radiation dose but depends on risk/benefit balance and uterus can be shielded.

3.9.2 MAGNETIC RESONANCE IMAGING

Principle

The human body is about 60% hydrogen atoms. Inside a strong magnetic field, hydrogen nuclei (protons) align like small magnets. A further oscillating perpendicular magnetic field excites the protons and they move out of alignment. As they return to the equilibrium state they emit signals that are processed into images, reflecting different tissue characteristics.

Indications

Anatomy

- Aortic aneurysms, dissection or coarctation, and large arteries, e.g. carotid
- Congenital heart disease: very detailed three-dimensional anatomy

- Cardiomyopathies, ventricular mass and tumours
- Pericardial disease.

Function

- LV regional wall motion
- Myocardial perfusion.

Future clinical use—not currently

- Native coronaries and grafts.

Contraindications

- Embedded ferromagnetic objects: intracranial clips, foreign bodies, early Starr–Edwards valves
- Permanent pacemakers or implantable defibrillators (affects function)
- Later prosthetic valves and sternal wires safe, but cause an artefact.

Practical details

All ferromagnetic or magnetized objects (e.g. credit cards) must be removed. The ECG is used to 'gate' the image, i.e. it is only acquired during diastole when the heart is relatively still. ST-segment changes seen are artefactual. Irregular rhythms result in a poorer image quality. The magnet makes a knocking sound and a claustrophobic patient may find the experience unpleasant. A scan takes 30–60 min.

3.10 Ventilation–perfusion isotope scanning ($\dot{V}/\dot{Q}$)

Principle

The principle of this investigation is comparison of ventilation and perfusion in the lungs to detect areas of mismatch (i.e. ventilated but not perfused), which occur in acute pulmonary embolism. Many other conditions (e.g. tumour or consolidation) cause perfusion defects, but these are generally matched by ventilation defects and associated with chest radiograph abnormality.

Indication

A suspected pulmonary embolism, preferably with a normal chest radiograph. Ventilation–perfusion scan reports are useful if perfusion is normal and PE therefore excluded, or if definite unmatched defects are seen and the diagnosis confirmed; however, many scans do not produce clear-cut results and are reported as being of intermediate probability. The diagnostic yield is improved by correlation with clinical suspicion, but there are still many cases where other imaging modalities are required.

Contraindications

There are none. It is safe in pregnancy, although some centres modify the dose.

Practical details

• Inhalation of radioisotope (krypton-81m, xenon-133 or technetium-99m [^{99m}Tc]): patient needs to be able to inhale sufficiently
• Injection of ^{99m}Tc-labelled albumin macroaggregates or microspheres
• Scanning after each; some centres only perform a ventilation scan if the perfusion is abnormal
• Duration of about 40 min.

 PIOPED Investigators. Value of the ventilation/perfusion scan in acute pulmonary embolism. *JAMA* 1990; 263: 2753–2759.

3.11 Echocardiography

Principle

Ultrasonic waves are generated in pulses. As the ultrasonic wave travels through tissues, some of it is reflected back towards the transducer as an echo every time the sound crosses an interface—typically the junctions between blood and the heart valves or myocardium. Several modes of imaging are recognized.

M-mode

Ultrasonic pulses are directed along a single line and the interfaces displayed as a graph of depth against time. It allows detailed evaluation and measurement of particular structures (Fig. 112).

Two-dimensional echocardiography

The information is displayed as a fan-shaped image. Detailed information about cardiac structures and their movement can be observed. Standard transthoracic views

Fig. 112 Parasternal long axis M-mode at the level of the mitral valve leaflets. 1, at the end of systole the mitral valve begins to open; E, maximum excursion of anterior mitral leaflet; 2, initial diastolic closing wave; D, diastole; A, reopening of mitral valve caused by atrial systole; 3, mitral valve closes at onset of ventricular systole. (Courtesy of Dr J Chambers.)

include the parasternal short and long axes, and the apical long axis (Fig. 113).

Doppler echocardiography

Quantitative measurements of velocity can be made (continuous and pulsed-wave Doppler), allowing the estimation of pressure gradients, intracardiac pressures and valve areas, on which the determination of the severity of valve lesions depends. Qualitative information can be obtained by colour coding velocity information and displaying this superimposed on a two-dimensional image. Detection of abnormal flow patterns within the heart is made possible with this technique (see Fig. 53).

In some patients and indications, transthoracic images may not be of sufficient quality to allow diagnosis. TOE, where the ultrasonic transducer is positioned in the oesophagus, behind and close to the heart, allows much better image quality. This can be combined with exercise or dobutamine to assess reversible areas of hypokinesia, which suggest ischaemia if they occur on stress. The development of intravenous contrast agents, allowing echocardiographic imaging of perfusion, has enormous potential in this respect.

Dobutamine stress echocardiography can also be used to assess myocardial viability, and is finding an increasing role in the assessment of the functional significance of valve lesions.

(a)

(b)

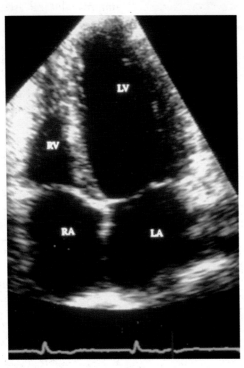

(c)

Fig. 113 Parasternal long (a) and short (b) axes (at the level of the aortic valve) and four-chamber views (c) of a normal heart. LA, left atrium; LV, left ventricle; RA, right atrium; RV, right ventricle; Ao, aorta. (Courtesy of Dr J Chambers.)

Indications

Echocardiography forms an essential part of the non-invasive assessment of valvular and structural heart disease, ventricular function and myocardial ischaemia viability.

Contraindications

• Unstable angina at the time of stress echocardiography.
• TOE: known pharyngeal pouch or severe oesophageal disease. If there is unexplained dysphagia, arrange barium swallow before considering TOE.

Practical details

Transoesophageal echocardiography

• Nil by mouth for at least 4 h; consider antibiotic prophylaxis if prosthetic valve
• Obtain written consent
• Insert intravenous cannula
• Check for loose teeth; remove false teeth
• Position patient
• Give sedation—e.g. midazolam 4 mg i.v. or diazepam 5–10 mg i.v.
• Monitor peripheral oxygen saturation continuously
• Insert mouth guard and perform test, ensuring that mouth secretions cleared using suction
• Monitor recovery; allow home with escort once free of sedation.

Stress echocardiography

Intravenous access is required for administration of dobutamine. Resting echocardiogram followed by stress with exercise or dobutamine, noting symptoms ± ECG changes. Monitor echocardiogram to assess development of wall motion abnormality (ischaemia) or recovery of function (viable myocardium). Monitor to ensure disappearance of symptoms and resolution of any ECG changes.

Complications

Transoesophageal echocardiography

- Oesophageal trauma ranging from inflammation to rupture
- Aspiration.

Important information for patients

Explain the following:
- The benefits and risks of the procedure
- The need for sedation, such that they may not remember the test
- That they will be drowsy afterwards, should not drive for the rest of the day and will need to be escorted home
- That they may have a sore throat for 1–2 days.

Stress echocardiography

- Supraventricular tachyarrhythmia
- VT/VF: 1 : 5000 treadmill tests
- Death as a result of resistant VF—1 : 10 000 treadmill tests
- Precipitation of acute coronary syndrome.

Important information for patients

Stress echocardiography
Stop β blockers for 48 h before test. Inform patients about the procedure and chosen stress modality. Make sure that they are aware that they may experience their angina pain during the test. Explain risk of arrhythmias.

Bach DS, Armstrong WF. Dobutamine stress echocardiography. *Am J Cardiol* 1992; 69: 90.

Chambers J. *Clinical Echocardiography.* London: BMJ Publishing Group, 1995.

Sanderson JE, Chan WW. Transoesophageal echocardiography. *Postgrad Med J* 1997; 73: 137–140.

3.12 Nuclear cardiology

3.12.1 MYOCARDIAL PERFUSION IMAGING

Thallium-201 is actively taken up by myocardial cells in a manner similar to potassium. Its concentration in the myocardium depends on both perfusion and integrity of the myocardial cell membrane. A graded colour representation of perfusion is obtained, allowing comparison between regions. Absolute values of blood flow are not obtained.

A scan after exercise or pharmacological stress with dipyridamole or adenosine is followed by a resting scan at 2–4 h. Defects seen during stress, which are not present at rest, represent ischaemia. Defects present in both scans ('fixed perfusion defect') usually indicate infarction (Fig. 114). The sensitivity for detection of significant coronary artery disease is 80–85% and specificity >90%.

(a)

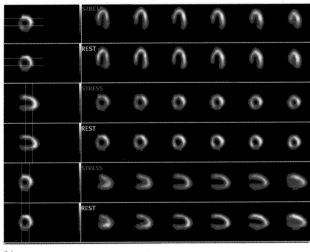

(b)

Fig. 114 (a) Normal and (b) abnormal stress thallium-201 perfusion scan, showing inferior ischaemia (b). (Courtesy of Dr Jan.)

Indications

Nuclear techniques are expensive. In most cases, myocardial perfusion imaging should be used when ECG morphology or patient morbidity precludes the interpretation or use of exercise ECG testing. Indications in common with exercise testing include the following:

• Prognostic stratification after MI
• Identification of ischaemia in symptomatic patients, especially atypical pain
• Risk stratification in patients with known or high risk of coronary artery disease before non-cardiac surgery.

3.12.2 POSITRON EMISSION TOMOGRAPHY

This technique uses positron-emitting radionuclides to produce tomographic images of coronary flow and metabolism. The technique also allows quantification of blood flow within specified regions of the heart. Rest and pharmacological stress scans are performed in a similar manner to thallium imaging. Myocardial viability is suggested by maintained glucose metabolism in an area with a fixed perfusion defect.

Dilsizian V, Bonow RO. Current diagnostic techniques of assessing myocardial viability in patients with hibernating and stunned myocardium. *Circulation* 1993; 87: 1–20.
Kotler TS, Diamond GA. Exercise thallium-201 scintigraphy in the diagnosis and prognosis of coronary artery disease. *Ann Intern Med* 1990; 113: 684–702.

Acknowledgements

The authors and editor would like to thank: Dr L.M. Shapiro, Dr R. Coulden, and the Pulmonary Vascular Diseases Unit, Papworth Hospital, Cambridge for their help in the preparation of this module.

4 Self-assessment

Answers are on pp. 261–265.

Question 1
Raised cardiac troponin levels in the blood (T/F):
A Are often found in unstable angina
B Can be used to distinguish subendocardial from transmural myocardial infarction
C Are often seen after elective DC cardioversion
D Indicate that the patient's chest pain must be the result of coronary artery disease
E Are of limited value in the presence of skeletal muscle injury.

Question 2
The following drugs have been shown to improve prognosis after a myocardial infarction (T/F):
A Atenolol
B Intravenous glyceryl trinitrate
C Nifedipine
D Sotalol
E Insulin.

Question 3
A Chest radiograph
B Tilt-table test
C 24-h ECG monitor
D Transthoracic echocardiography
E Resting 12-lead ECG
F Exercise ECG
G Transoesophageal echocardiography
H Stress echocardiography.
For each of the conditions listed below, select the investigation in the list above that is most likely to establish the diagnosis. Each option may be used once, more than once or not at all:
1 Acute myocardial infarction
2 Aortic dissection
3 Hypertrophic cardiomyopathy
4 Pulmonary oedema.

Question 4
A Intravenous amiodarone
B DC cardioversion
C Emergency coronary angioplasty
D Emergency cardiac surgery
E Pericardiocentesis
F Oral nifedipine
G Intravenous nitrate infusion

H Oral angiotensin-converting enzyme (ACE) inhibitor
I Intravenous fluids.
For each of the conditions listed below, select the most appropriate emergency treatment from the list above. Each option may be used once, more than once or not at all:
1 Acute myocardial infarction
2 Acute pulmonary oedema
3 Aortic dissection (type A)
4 Unstable angina.

Question 5
A Percutaneous transluminal coronary angioplasty (PTCA)
B Diltiazem
C Furosemide (frusemide)
D Cardiac surgery
E Permanent pacemaker
F Flecainide
G β Blocker.
For each of the conditions listed below, select the most appropriate treatment from the list above. Each option may be used once, more than once or not at all:
1 Coronary vasospasm
2 Left main-stem stenosis
3 Aortic dissection (type B)
4 Restrictive cardiomyopathy.

Question 6

A 67-year-old retired farmer presented with a severe episode of central chest pain, which came on suddenly while lying in bed. After about 15 min, he noticed that the pain had moved to the left shoulder. He felt sweaty and nauseated. He got up to make a cup of tea and collapsed. According to his wife he was unconscious for about 2 min, and he quickly recovered. The pain subsided to a dull ache.
• Past medical history: duodenal ulcer diagnosed 20 years previously; hypertension treated with bendrofluazide for 15 years.
• On examination he had a regular tachycardia of 112 beats/min, BP 120/60 mmHg in both arms, jugular venous pressure (JVP) elevated at 5 cm above sternal angle, soft pericardial rub with a short early diastolic murmur.
• His chest radiograph is shown in Fig. 115.
1 What is the most likely diagnosis?
2 What investigations should be carried out?
3 What should be the initial management?

Question 23

The ECG in acute pulmonary embolism characteristically shows (T/F):

A Sinus tachycardia

B Right axis shift

C Changes that may disappear in a few days

D Right bundle-branch block

E Prolonged QT interval.

Question 24

Randomized trials have shown that the following treatments improve life expectancy in patients with stable angina (T/F):

A Statins

B Hormone replacement therapy

C Vitamin E

D Long-acting nitrates

E Percutaneous transluminal coronary angioplasty (PTCA).

Question 25

In patients presenting with chest pain (T/F):

A A chest radiograph is the most important initial test

B Thrombolysis should be given if cardiac troponin levels are elevated

C A negative troponin test rules out significant coronary disease

D The exercise test is the best predictor of risk

E A chest radiograph is useful to screen for aortic dissection.

Question 26

A Cytoskeletal protein

B Intracellular signalling protein kinase

C Membrane receptor

D Fibrillin

E Contractile protein

F Nuclear receptor

G Cardiac ion channel

H Mitochondrial.

For each condition listed below, select the gene mutation most likely to be found from the list above.

1 Hypertrophic cardiomyopathy

2 Familial dilated cardiomyopathy

3 Aortic dissection

4 Long QT syndrome.

Question 27

In patients with heart failure (T/F):

A The detection of bilateral crackles on auscultation of the lung bases is unreliable as an indicator of pulmonary oedema

B The history and physical examination will be sufficient for diagnosis in most cases

C Digoxin is useful even if the patient is in sinus rhythm

D β Blockers must be avoided

E Oral drug treatment can improve symptoms but cannot improve the ejection fraction.

Question 28

In heart muscle (T/F):

A Myofibres are bundles of cardiac myocytes

B Thick filaments are made up of actin

C Both intracellular and extracellular calcium are important for initiation of cardiac contraction

D The energy required for relative motion of thick and thin filaments is provided by the Na^+/K^+ ATPase

E The sarcoplasmic reticulum has an important role in the initiation of cardiac contraction.

Question 29

With regard to cardiac hypertrophy (T/F):

A Aortic regurgitation typically gives rise to concentric left ventricular hypertrophy (LVH)

B Eccentric LVH is the hallmark of hypertrophic cardiomyopathy

C Hypertensive LVH is not altered by drug treatment

D LVH is an independent risk factor for cardiovascular death

E Assessment of the apex beat helps distinguish pressure overload from volume overload.

Question 30

Coronary stenting (T/F):

A Improves life expectancy for patients with stable angina

B Is the initial treatment of choice for patients presenting with unstable angina

C Is useful for patients with coronary bypass grafts and recurrent angina

D Reduces re-stenosis rates

E Has reduced the proportion of angioplasty patients requiring emergency bypass grafting.

Question 31

The following are clinical features of a normal pregnancy (T/F):

A Anaemia

B Atrial fibrillation

C A third heart sound

D A diastolic murmur at the lower left sternal edge

E Hypotension.

Question 32

1 Pulmonary hypertension is associated with significant mortality

2 Marfan's syndrome is low risk if hypertension is not present

3 Any cyanotic congenital heart disease is associated with unacceptable maternal mortality
4 Pre-pregnancy New York Heart Association (NYHA) functional class is irrelevant because individual physiological changes are unpredictable
5 Pregnancy is a major risk factor for thromboembolism.
For the statements about maternal risk in pregnancy in the list above, select which are true from the list below:
A All
B 1, 2, 3 and 5
C 3, 4 and 5
D 1 and 5
E 3 only.

Question 33
The following are good indications for cardiac magnetic resonance imaging (MRI) (T/F):
A Coarctation of the aorta
B Arrhythmogenic right ventricular dysplasia
C Björk–Shiley prosthetic valve dysfunction
D Severe coronary artery disease
E Complex congenital heart disease.

Question 34
1 End-stage renal failure
2 Rheumatoid arthritis
3 Thyrotoxicosis
4 Systemic lupus erythematosus
5 Mitral valve prolapse.
Is pericarditis associated with the above conditions? Select an answer from the options below:
A All
B 1, 2 and 4
C 2, 3 and 5
D 1 and 4
E 2 only.

Question 35
Therapy for primary pulmonary hypertension includes (T/F):
A Calcium channel blockers
B ACE inhibitors
C Intravenous prostacyclin by continuous infusion
D Loop diuretics
E Nitrates
F Oxygen
G Hydralazine
H Anticoagulation
I Heart–lung transplantation.

Respiratory Medicine

AUTHORS:
P. Bhatia, M.I. Polkey and V.L.C. White

EDITOR:
M.I. Polkey

EDITOR-IN-CHIEF:
J.D. Firth

1 Clinical presentations

1.1 New breathlessness

Case history

A 52-year-old man presents with a 2-month history of increasing breathlessness.

Clinical approach

Breathlessness or dyspnoea is defined as difficult, laboured or uncomfortable awareness of breathing. It is a feature of many cardiac and respiratory conditions. The physician must seek to make a clinical diagnosis before attempting a definitive test. The main diagnostic categories are shown in Table 1. An important concern is to identify malignant disease as early as possible.

History of the presenting problem

> Listen to your patient. He is telling you the answer. (René Laënnec)

When and how?

A careful description of the dyspnoea is required. Let patients tell their story in their own words, but clarify the following points if they do not emerge spontaneously.

Table 1 Causes of slow onset new breathlessness.

Common
Airways disease
Cardiac disease
Pleural effusion/disease
Lobar/lung collapse (from obstructing tumour)

Must consider
Thromboembolic disease
Anaemia

Other conditions
Pulmonary artery hypertension
Interstitial lung disease
Neuromuscular disease
Chest wall disease

• Is the dyspnoea really new or is this a progression of previous mild symptoms? Airways disease in particular often becomes a 'new' problem when the patient is unable to perform a particular task?
• When is it worse? Exertional dyspnoea is a non-specific symptom, but the specific complaint of orthopnoea suggests heart failure (or rarely bilateral diaphragm paralysis).
• If the symptoms are worse lying on one side, this may suggest unilateral lung disease, e.g. a patient with right lung collapse may report a preference for sleeping on the right side.
• Nocturnal dyspnoea usually makes the clinician think of heart failure, but asthma is also worse at night.

Is the patient a smoker?

Is the patient a smoker—currently or previously? Does the patient have cancer? These points needs to be clarified early. In a smoker, lung cancer requires positive exclusion if there are ominous associated symptoms (particularly weight loss or haemoptysis). New breathlessness may also indicate a new perception of previously unrecognized airflow obstruction.

What is the patient's job?

The incidence of mesothelioma is set to peak in 2015. These symptoms could fit, especially if associated with unilateral pain and if the employment history indicates asbestos exposure. Some periods of such employment may have been temporary, hence—when relevant—it is necessary to reconstruct the patient's full work CV. (See Section 1.11, p. 178.)

Pets or unusual hobbies

Although the answer is usually 'no', this question is quick to ask.

Features to suggest infection

Infection would not be a common cause of dyspnoea of 2 months' duration. The exceptions to this are tuberculosis or lung abscess and you should therefore ask about fever, shivering attacks and sputum production. Is the patient at high risk of tuberculosis (for example an immigrant from an endemic area, or living on the streets).

153

Inhaled foreign body. Patients often have to be prompted to enable this diagnosis, which is suggested by lobar collapse or persistent cough.

Relevant past history

Previous pulmonary disease

A previous history of asthma, wheeziness or colds 'going to my chest' clearly raises the likelihood of airflow obstruction being the diagnosis. Remember that the patient may have had undiagnosed asthma at school (and therefore been unable to play sport or have disliked the playground in the winter) and grown out of it, only to have it relapse.

Examination

Always note the general appearance, followed by a full cardiac and respiratory examination.
- General appearance—breathless at rest; weight loss; pale (anaemic); jaundiced; can the patient lie supine?
- Give a cough—normal in character; productive
- Take big breath—stridor (a 'wheezing' found on inspiration)
- Hands—clubbing; muscle wasting
- Pulse rate—regular
- Eyes—anaemia; Horner's syndrome (if complaining of apical pain)
- Tongue—central cyanosis
- Lymph nodes—palpable; axillary examination not mandatory unless lymph nodes are palpable elsewhere or history of breast cancer
- Jugular venous pressure (JVP)—elevated?
- Apex—position
- Heart auscultation—added sounds and murmurs
- Tracheal position—centred
- Chest wall—scoliosis (may be surprisingly hidden by clothes); movement equal and adequate; paradoxical abdominal movement
- Tactile vocal fremitus—normal and equal
- Percussion—not forgetting the apices and lateral chest wall
- Auscultation—not forgetting the apices and lateral chest wall
- Ankles—swelling.

The measurement of peak expiratory flow (PEF), and ideally spirometry, should form part of the outpatient assessment unless a clear-cut diagnosis (e.g. large pleural effusion) is made on examination.

Approach to investigations and management

Investigations

Chest radiograph

The chest radiograph is almost an extension of physical examination. Most new patients attending the chest clinic have a chest radiograph before seeing the doctor. Frequently this will show an abnormality that initiates a standard diagnostic pathway, e.g. pleural effusion, a solitary lung mass or apical alveolar shadowing. It is important to check for cardiac enlargement.

If the chest radiograph appears to be normal, then carefully review the apices, the mediastinum and the bony structures.

A patient with dyspnoea and pain may have a pneumothorax. This is usually of sudden onset, but not always, and may be forgotten by the patient. A chest radiograph taken in expiration may demonstrate the condition, as shown in Fig. 1.

Blood tests

These are of limited value in the assessment of slow onset of new dyspnoea. The haemoglobin will exclude anaemia (and polycythaemia if there has been long-standing hypoxia). Blood tests may be diagnostic where the history and/or examination suggests a specific diagnosis, e.g. in avian extrinsic alveolitis, and clinical clues of malignancy should be pursued (e.g. measurement of liver function tests).

Sarcoid is notoriously variable in its presentation: measurement of serum angiotensin-converting enzyme (ACE) and calcium are indicated where this diagnosis is entertained.

Lung function

Lung function measurements are the next investigation for the breathless patient in whom the chest radiograph is non-contributory. Look for evidence of airflow obstruction or a restrictive lung defect. Lung volumes and gas transfer measurements are required where the diagnosis is genuinely uncertain.

Additional investigations

Further investigations are guided by the clinical features and results of the radiograph and lung function, but might include:
- high-resolution computed tomography (CT) of the thorax
- spiral protocol CT of the thorax
- ECG and echocardiogram (possibly with contrast)

(a)

(b)

Fig. 1 A pair of radiographs taken in a patient with a right-sided pneumothorax. In the inspiratory film (a) the pneumothorax is around 20% which increases to around 60% in the expiratory film (b).

- bronchoscopy
- thoracoscopy
- lung biopsy
- respiratory muscle function tests.

Consider respiratory muscle weakness if there is a restrictive defect with a normal or supernormal gas transfer in the presence of a normal chest radiograph [1]. A good screening test is to compare the erect and supine vital capacity, when a drop of >20% suggests bilateral diaphragm paralysis.

1 Polkey MI, Green M & Moxham J. Measurement of respiratory muscle strength. *Thorax* 1995; 50: 1131–1135.

Fig. 2 Chest radiograph of patient showing right upper lobe nodule.

1.2 Solitary pulmonary nodule

Case history

A 48-year-old executive has a chest radiograph as part of his company's health screening programme. It shows a pulmonary nodule in the right upper lobe (Fig. 2).

Clinical approach

The most important differential is lung cancer. Other possibilities would be an old tuberculous (TB) nodule, a benign adenoma or a lung secondary (rarer possibilities are shown in Table 2).

History of the presenting problem

Any old radiographs are extremely helpful: ask the patient—they may have had a chest radiograph performed previously, perhaps in another hospital, e.g. before elective surgery.

Table 2 Differential diagnosis of a solitary pulmonary nodule.

Common
Lung cancer
Lung secondary
Old tuberculous nodule

Uncommon
Infection, e.g. lung abscess
Benign tumour, e.g. adenoma, hamartoma, carcinoid
Arteriovenous malformation
Active granulomatous disease, e.g. tuberculosis, sarcoid, Wegener's granulomatosis, rheumatoid nodule

Is this lung cancer?

Find out the following.
- Smoking history—never, ex- or current smoker?
- Occupational history—the patient may not always have been an executive. (See Section 1.11, p. 178.)
- Is there any history of cough and/or haemoptysis?
- Any chest wall pain, brachial plexus symptoms or shortness of breath?
- Any recent weight loss or anorexia?
- Enquire about symptoms that might arise from systemic manifestations of cancer (e.g. bone pains from hypercalcaemia or metastases, weakness from Eaton–Lambert syndrome).

Could it be tuberculosis?

The lesion may be active TB or an old nodule. Check the following:
- ethnic origin, foreign travel or residence
- personal or family history of TB
- recent fevers or night sweats
- haemoptysis.

Other considerations

- Benign tumour—history of haemoptysis would make this less likely
- Lung secondary—any history of other tumours, weight loss or anorexia (Fig. 3).

Fig. 3 Chest radiograph of a patient with a malignant salivary gland tumour showing multiple nodular pulmonary secondaries.

Relevant past history

Previous tuberculosis

Is there a history of prolonged hospital stays as a youngster? If treated for TB, were they given antibiotics, and if so, which ones and for how long (it may be impossible to find this information, but important to ask)?

Examination

General

Does the patient look unwell? Do they appear to have lost weight recently? Do they look pale? Is there ptosis or jaundice?

Respiratory

Look carefully for the following:
- cough—is this of normal character? Is it productive?
- stridor
- clubbing
- lymphadenopathy—both cervical, supraclavicular and axillary
- superior vena cava obstruction
- position of trachea
- chest expansion
- percussion
- breath sounds
- vocal and tactile fremitus
- dependant oedema
- hepatomegaly
- neurological signs
- telangectasia—may suggest arteriovenous malformations (AVMs).

A lung secondary

Feel for an abdominal mass and for groin lymphadenopathy. Examine the thyroid gland, and do not forget to examine the breasts in women and testes in men.

Breast examination

- If a woman presents with a mass on her chest radiograph, explain why you need to examine her breasts: 'sometimes problems with the breasts can show up on a chest radiograph'.
- Do not forget to reassure if you find nothing abnormal: 'your breasts feel entirely normal, I don't think that they are the cause of the problem'.
- Ask for a chaperone if you think this appropriate.

Approach to investigations and management

Investigations of solitary pulmonary nodule
- Computed tomography scan of chest, liver and adrenals—preferably before bronchoscopy
- Bronchoscopy—ideally within a week: lateral chest radiograph is essential if computed tomography scan is not available beforehand
- Sputum for cytology, microbiology (including acid-fast bacilli (AFB))
- Blood tests for routine haematology, coagulation screen, electrolytes, calcium and liver function tests.

Investigations

Computed tomography scan of chest

This must include the liver and adrenals when lung cancer is in the differential. Normally both lung and soft tissue views are obtained; the former looking at the lung parenchyma, the latter for mediastinal lymphadenopathy (Fig. 4) (see *Haematology*, Sections 1.16 and 2.2).

Bronchoscopy

Seventy per cent of lung cancers are visible bronchoscopically. Endobronchial lesions should be biopsied if there are no contraindications and routine blood tests do not demonstrate coagulopathy. Most operators also brush the lesion and send washings for cytological analysis.

Fig. 4 Computed tomography scan showing a solitary pulmonary nodule in the posterior aspect of the right lower lobe, which was difficult to view on the plain chest radiograph. This patient was later diagnosed as having lymphoma.

- Bronchial biopsies should be sent for histology in formalin and for microscopy and culture in saline if TB is suspected.
- Bronchial washings and brushings should be sent for cytology and washings for microscopy and culture.
- Remember to request AFBs specifically when appropriate—they are not carried out automatically.

Cytological examination of sputum

This can yield a diagnosis in some patients but, because bronchoscopy is also required as a prelude to surgery, this approach is usually reserved for patients whose general health means that they will not receive active treatment for a tumour if one is found.

It is worth asking the physiotherapist to help obtain induced samples. Do not forget to send for microscopy and culture (specifically including AFB) as well as for cytology.

Blood tests

These should include a full blood count (FBC), erythrocyte sedimentation rate (ESR) (may be raised in active TB), clotting (before bronchoscopy or biopsy), blood biochemistry including electrolytes, calcium and liver function tests.

Do not miss hypercalcaemia associated with malignancy. (See *Endocrinology*, Section 1.2; *Emergency medicine*, Section 1.18.)

Computed tomography-guided biopsy

For peripheral lesions where bronchoscopic results are negative, percutaneous biopsy is the next procedure of choice. Lung function needs to be carefully assessed beforehand as there is a 10% chance of a pneumothorax: patients should be warned of this complication when they are consented.

Positron emission tomography

Fluorodeoxyglucose (FDG) positron emission tomography (PET) can be useful in the management of a solitary nodule. The principle is that metabolically active diseases will take up labelled glucose that can then be identified on images obtained by the PET scanner. The main indications are to provide reassurance if deciding against an open surgical biopsy or resection for undiagnosed nodules, or to look for otherwise covert metastases in patients being considered for a curative resection of a proven tumour.

Management

- Lung cancer: see Section 2.9.1, p. 220
- Chest infection/abscess
- Tuberculosis: see *Infectious diseases*, Section 2.6.1
- Sarcoidosis: see Section 2.8.2, p. 208
- Wegener's granulomatosis: see *Rheumatology and clinical immunology*, Section 2.5.2
- Benign tumour—resection is normally recommended to avoid the complications of bronchial obstruction, haemoptysis and possible mitotic transformation (2% of adenomas). However, the rate of growth of the tumour and general condition of the patient enter the risk–benefit equation and need to be taken into account.
- Pulmonary AVMs—only need to be treated if symptomatic. When part of an hereditary syndrome, bleeding elsewhere may cause greater problems. Pulmonary AVMs may be locally embolized using catheter techniques under radiological guidance. Occasionally lung resection may be necessary [1,2].

1 Temes RT, Paramsothy P, Endara, SA, Wernly JA. Resection of a solitary pulmonary arteriovenous malformation by video-assisted thoracic surgery. *J Thorac Cardiovasc Surg* 1998; 116: 878–879.
2 Puskas, JD, Allen MS, Moncure AC *et al.* Pulmonary arteriovenous malformations: therapeutic options. *Ann Thorac Surg* 1993; 56: 253–258.

1.3 Exertional dyspnoea with daily sputum

Case history

A 24-year-old man attends the chest clinic with a 7-month history of worsening exertional dyspnoea and coughing up a cupful of sputum daily. He remembers that as a child he was a frequent visitor to his general practitioner with cough. There is no history of wheeze. He also complains of intermittent abdominal pain for the last 12 months. He has smoked over 40 cigarettes daily since the age of 15 years.

Clinical approach

This young man has both pulmonary and abdominal symptoms. He is a very heavy smoker and coughing up excessive amounts of phlegm, which suggests an inflammatory process. Bronchiectasis, lung abscess and pneumonia can produce purulent sputum, which may be offensive

and blood tinged. Mucoid or mucopurulent sputum is characteristic of chronic bronchitis. In cystic fibrosis (CF), there may be copious purulent phlegm and frequent haemoptysis.

He is very young to be suffering from chronic bronchitis and emphysema, even if he has α_1-antitrypsin deficiency.

In any patient presenting with chronic exertional dyspnoea and sputum production, consider:
- chronic obstructive pulmonary disease (COPD) (history of smoking, wheeze, check spirometry)
- bronchiectasis (and any condition associated with bronchiectasis): see Section 2.4, p. 197
- bronchial asthma (history of wheeze, episodic)
- lung abscess, pneumonia (usually of acute onset, accompanied by fever)
- congestive cardiac failure.

History of the presenting problem

Extent of history

Was he perfectly well before this 7-month history of breathlessness? He remembers frequent visits to his general practitioner for treatment of cough. He could be suffering from asthma, but he denies wheeze. A 7-month history suggests a chronic disorder, but was respiratory function really normal prior to this? Could he play games at school? Could he keep up with his friends when he played football or went cycling?

Amount and character of sputum

He is coughing up a cupful (approximately 200 mL) of sputum in 24 h. Normally the mucous glands of the respiratory tract produce 100 mL of sputum daily and most of this is swallowed.

Abdominal pain related to pulmonary problem

Intermittent abdominal pain could be caused by a variety of problems (see *Gastroenterology and hepatology*, Sections 1.2 and 1.14), but might indicate underlying gallstone or a partial intestinal obstruction—meconium ileus equivalent in CF. Is he well built for his age? Malabsorption caused by CF may result in failure of linear growth in childhood and short stature in later life.

Nasal or sinus problems

This may suggest hypogammaglobulinaemia (see *Rheumatology and clinical immunology*, Sections 1.1 and 2.1.1).

Relevant past history

Childhood diseases

Did he suffer from measles, pneumonia or pertussis as a child? This may suggest underlying bronchiectasis.

Family history

This man is young to develop a chronic respiratory disorder. Is there a family history of such problems?
• Does he have any brothers or sisters, and do they (or could they) have CF—an autosomal recessive disorder with a carrier frequency of 1 in 22 in caucasians?
• Is there a family history of COPD? This might indicate α_1-antitrypsin deficiency—autosomal dominant and usually presenting at 20–40 years of age: smokers develop emphysema; 10–15% develop cirrhosis.

In a young patient with chronic exertional dyspnoea and sputum production, consider:
• bronchiectasis—may be caused by CF
• α_1-antitrypsin deficiency
• hypogammaglobulinemia—may be suggested by recurrent pneumonia or sinusitis.

Examination

Full general, respiratory and cardiac examinations are required (see Sections 1.1, p. 153 and 1.2, p. 155), but in this case pay particular attention to the following aspects.

General

• Look in the sputum pot: note quantity and character of sputum.
• Is the patient cachexic, of short stature, clubbed, cyanosed or oedematous (hypoproteinaemic/cor pulmonale) (CF)?

Respiratory

The auscultatory findings are only part of the picture, but concentrate on the following:
• Are the breath sounds vesicular or bronchial (underlying consolidation)?
• Is expiration prolonged (COPD)?
• Are crackles persistently heard over the same area (bronchiectasis)?
• Are breath sounds impaired over a specific area (lung abscess)?

Abdominal

As this patient could be suffering from CF, it is essential to examine the abdomen carefully. A mobile right lower quadrant mass may be palpable. Intermittent abdominal pain in CF can be caused by intermittent partial obstruction, low-grade appendicitis, duodenal irritation as a result of failure to buffer gastric acid, or cholelithiasis.

Look for signs of cirrhosis, which can occur in both CF and α_1-antitrypsin deficiency (see *Gastroenterology and hepatology*, Sections 1.4, 1.6 and 2.10).

Approach to investigations and management

Investigations

Blood tests

A raised white cell count with neutrophilia suggests underlying bacterial infection. Secondary polycythaemia suggests chronic hypoxia. Serum α_1-antitrypsin level may be low suggesting its deficiency and underlying emphysema. Liver function tests can exclude hepatic involvement in both CF and α_1-antitrypsin deficiency.

Chest radiograph

A chest radiograph is helpful to exclude an acute infection. It may also reveal features of COPD, bronchiectasis, lung abscess or cardiomegaly in congestive cardiac failure. Dextrocardia may be present.

Sputum examination

Send for microscopy, culture and sensitivity, including AFB.

Lung function tests

These will determine if there is airway obstruction, and in cases of COPD will help evaluate treatment. It is important to request full lung function tests comprising static lung volumes, spirometry and transfer factor.

Other investigations

• Arterial blood gases—indicated if fingertip SaO_2 <94% to check whether there is any respiratory failure (type I or II)
• Electrocardiogram—is there cor pulmonale?
• Sweat sodium concentration—in CF the sweat sodium concentration is usually high (>60 mmol)
• High-resolution CT scan of the lungs—can diagnose bronchiectasis, emphysema or presence of bullae
• Ultrasound examination of the hepatobiliary system—looking for cirrhosis and/or gall stones.

Management

- Cystic fibrosis: see Section 2.5, p. 199
- Bronchiectasis: see Section 2.4, p. 197
- COPD: see Section 2.3, p. 194
- Pulmonary infections (lung abscess/pneumonia): see *Infectious diseases*, Sections 1.5 and 2.5
- Hypogammaglobulinaemia: see *Rheumatology and clinical immunology*, Section 2.1.1.

 MacNee W. Chronic obstructive pulmonary disease: causes and pathology. *Medicine* 1999; 27(9): 68–72.
Calverley, PMA. Management of chronic obstructive pulmonary disease. *Medicine* 1999; 27(9): 73–78.
Peckham DG, Conway S. Cystic fibrosis. *Medicine* 1999; 27(9): 82–87.

1.4 Dyspnoea and fine inspiratory crackles

Case history

A 53-year-old retired car salesman presents with a history of breathing difficulty. He has long-standing atrial fibrillation and is on amiodarone 200 mg once daily and warfarin. On examination he is dyspnoeic on transferring to the couch and has fine bibasal crackles.

Clinical approach

Breathlessness is a cardinal symptom of both cardiac and pulmonary disease. In this case it is obviously critical to determine whether the main cause is cardiac or pulmonary. Note that myocardial ischaemia may be silent and hence this cause of impaired left ventricular function and breathlessness may not be obvious.

History of the presenting problem

History of sputum production

Dyspnoea along with bibasal crackles may be a feature of bronchiectasis, which is typically accompanied by copious sputum. Chronic bronchitis and emphysema are also characterized by dyspnoea and bibasal crackles may represent superadded infection. Diffuse interstitial lung diseases may be accompanied by a dry cough.

Swelling of the ankles

Congestive cardiac failure or cor pulmonale may be accompanied by pedal and sacral oedema.

History of wheeze

Obstructive airways disease is accompanied by wheeze, but wheeze can also be a feature of cardiac failure.

Is breathlessness cardiac?

Can the patient sleep lying flat? Does the patient wake up with breathing difficulty at night? Orthopnoea and paroxysmal nocturnal dyspnoea suggest cardiac failure. When the patient gets breathless, is there any tightness in the chest? Breathlessness of many sorts can be associated with chest discomfort, but this might indicate angina and ischaemic left ventricular failure as the cause of breathing difficulty in this case. (See *Cardiology*, Sections 1.6, 2.3 and 2.4.)

Exercise tolerance limited by dyspnoea?

What activities are limited by breathlessness? This is not helpful in arriving at a differential diagnosis, but provides an estimate of disability and is essential in monitoring the response of disease to treatment.

Relevant past history

- This man has long-standing atrial fibrillation. This may be 'lone' (when by definition there is no other evidence of cardiac disease), but any history of cardiac disease (the most common form of which is ischaemic heart disease) makes breathlessness resulting from cardiac failure more likely than otherwise.
- Childhood pneumonia, measles, mumps or pertussis could cause bronchiectasis.
- A history of painful nodules on the shins (erythema nodosum) may point to sarcoidosis.
- Associated rheumalogical disease suggests pulmonary fibrosis.

Occupational and drug history

A detailed occupational and drug history is important to determine whether the patient has been in contact with any agent associated with diffuse interstitial lung disease (Table 3). Amiodarone is an obvious worry in this case.

Recreational history

Does the patient breed pigeons or keep a budgerigar? (Bird fancier's lung).

Family history

A family history of dyspnoea in young adults might

Table 3 Classification of interstitial lung disease.

Classification	Examples
Connective tissue disorder	Rheumatoid arthritis, scleroderma, systemic lupus erythematosus, ankylosing spondylitis, mixed connective tissue disorder, Sjögren's syndrome, polymyositis–dermatomyositis
Occupational/environmental	Silicosis, asbestosis, berylliosis, coal worker's pneumoconiosis, siderosis, stanosis, aluminium oxide fibrosis, bird fancier's lung, farmer's lung, malt worker's lung, mushroom worker's lung, humidifier lung, bagassosis
Autoimmune	Inflammatory bowel disease, primary biliary cirrhosis, Wegener's granulomatosis
Idiopathic	Cryptogenic fibrosing alveolitis, bronchiolitis obliterans organizing pneumonia, sarcoidosis
Drug induced	Antibiotics (sulfasalazine, furantoin), antiarrythmics (amiodarone, propranolol), anti-inflammatory (gold, penicillamine), anticonvulsants (phenytoin), chemotherapeutic agents (busulfan, bleomycin, cyclophosphamide), paraquat, crack cocaine inhalation
Rarities	Irradiation, amyloidosis, postinfectious, lymphangioleiomyomatosis, neurofibromatosis, Gaucher's disease, lipoid pneumonia, tuberous sclerosis, acquired immune deficiency syndrome, eosinophilic pneumonia, adult respiratory distress syndrome

suggest α_1-antitrypsin deficiency. Cryptogenic fibrosing alveolitis may be familial.

Examination

Full general, respiratory and cardiac examinations are required (see Sections 1.1, p. 153 and 1.2, p. 155), but in this case pay particular attention to the following aspects.

General

• Finger clubbing (cryptogenic fibrosing alveolitis, bronchiectasis, CF)
• Erythema nodosum (sarcoid—rare)
• Side effects of amiodarone (slate grey discoloration of the skin, signs of hypo/hyperthyroidism).

Cardiovascular

Does the patient have cardiac failure? If yes: is it right ventricular (cor pulmonale or disease of heart alone), left ventricular or biventricular (both suggesting heart disease other than cor pulmonale)?

Note the following:
• Pulse rate, rhythm and character (does the patient still need to be on amiodarone?)
• JVP—is this elevated?
• Cardiac apex—is this displaced? (Suggests cardiac disease other than cor pulmonale)
• Left or right ventricular heaves—are these present?

(Left ventricular heave suggests cardiac disease other than cor pulmonale)
• Cardiac murmurs or added sounds—are these present? (Murmurs or added sounds loudest at the apex suggest cardiac disease other than cor pulmonale)
• Palpate for the liver—is this enlarged? Is it pulsatile?
• Peripheral oedema.

Respiratory

Take special care to note the following.

Palpation

The movement of the thoracic cage is symmetrically diminished in diffuse fibrosis. The trachea may be pulled to the affected side if fibrosis is unilateral or asymmetrical.

Percussion

The percussion note at the bases is dull with pleural effusions (perhaps caused by cardiac failure in this case), but is normal in fibrosis.

Auscultation

Bilateral fine end-inspiratory crackles are characteristic of cryptogenic fibrosing alveolitis. Ask the patient to cough. The crackles of alveolitis are not influenced by cough, whereas they often lessen in pulmonary oedema.

Fig. 5 Plain chest radiograph of a woman with fibrosing alveolitis; there is bilateral alveolar shadowing.

Approach to investigations and management

Investigations

Chest radiograph

Look for honeycomb appearance of diffuse lung fibrosis (Fig. 5), bilateral hilar lymphadenopathy in sarcoidosis, pleural plaques in asbestos exposure and asbestosis. Look for an enlarged heart and Kerley B lines, which would suggest cardiac failure.

Spirometry

In fibrosis both forced expiratory volume in 1 s (FEV_1) and forced vital capacity (FVC) are reduced and hence their ratio remains constant. The total lung capacity (TLC) and the transfer factor are both reduced.

High-resolution computed tomography scanning

High-resolution CT (2–3 mm slices) is superior to conventional CT scanning (Fig. 6). It helps to diagnose the presence of lung fibrosis and may also determine the aetiology in some cases, avoiding lung biopsy.

Echocardiography

The finding, by echocardiography or other means, of good left ventricular function can be helpful in excluding heart failure as a cause of dyspnoea and crackles.

Blood tests

Check full blood count for anaemia, or for polycythaemia caused by hypoxia. It is appropriate to test for inflammatory markers (C-reactive protein (CRP), ESR), rheumatoid factor, antinuclear antibodies, serum ACE and calcium level (sarcoidosis), antineutrophil cytoplasmic antibodies (Wegener's granulomatosis) and relevant precipitins (extrinsic allergic alveolitis).

Arterial blood gases

If SaO_2 <94% when breathing air, measure arterial blood gases to assess severity.

Electrocardiogram

Look for features of pulmonary hypertension—right axis deviation, P pulmonale in lead II (in patient who is not in atrial fibrillation), dominant R in V1.

Fig. 6 High-resolution computed tomography scan of a patient with fibrosing alveolitis.

Lung biopsy

This may have to be performed to determine the aetiology if all other tests are unhelpful. Transbronchial biopsy is helpful if sarcoidosis is suspected, but as the sample size is small it may not be of use in other causes of lung fibrosis. Open lung biopsy or video-assisted thoracoscopic biopsy may be required.

Management

Whether or not amiodarone is the culprit, the strength of the indication should be reviewed and the drug stopped if possible.

• If the diagnosis is amiodarone pneumonitis, high-dose oral prednisolone is indicated.

• If the diagnosis is left ventricular failure, the management is of this condition. (See *Cardiology*, Sections 1.6, 2.3 and 2.4.)

Otherwise management depends on the final diagnosis reached.

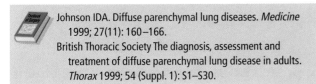

Johnson IDA. Diffuse parenchymal lung diseases. *Medicine* 1999; 27(11): 160–166.
British Thoracic Society The diagnosis, assessment and treatment of diffuse parenchymal lung disease in adults. *Thorax* 1999; 54 (Suppl. 1): S1–S30.

1.5 Pleuritic chest pain

Case history

A 54-year-old previously fit woman is admitted with left-sided pleuritic chest pain that began suddenly 8 h ago. On examination she is tachypnoeic at rest, with a respiratory rate of 28/min. She also gives a history of recent constipation and digital examination reveals a hard mass in the rectum.

Clinical approach

The visceral and parietal pleurae consist of single layers of cells separated by the pleural space. Pleuritic pain is characteristically triggered by deep inhalation, cough or movement of the thorax. It is usually unilateral, sharp, and can be referred to the shoulder, neck or abdominal wall. The following diagnoses should be considered:

• pulmonary embolism with pulmonary infarction (sudden onset, risk factors for thromboembolism)

• pneumothorax (sudden onset)

• pneumonia with infective pleurisy (recent history of purulent phlegm, fever)

• musculoskeletal causes (history of trauma or osteoporosis)

• malignant disease (often a duller and steady pain of some duration)

• non-infective pleurisy (systemic lupus erythematosus (SLE), rheumatoid arthritis).

In most cases, including this, the first priority is to exclude pulmonary embolism.

History of the presenting problem

Pain

Is the pain really pleuritic? Did it develop suddenly? Sudden pleuritic chest pain is most likely to be due to a pulmonary embolus with pulmonary infarction or a pneumothorax. Sudden onset of unilateral chest pain/discomfort and breathlessness should make you think immediately of pneumothorax, particularly in a tall, thin 'Marfanoid' man.

What was the patient doing in the hours before and at the moment when the pain came on? Unaccustomed or vigorous activity, e.g. painting the ceiling, is likely to precipitate musculoskeletal pain.

Breathlessness

Was the breathlessness sudden? Sudden onset of breathlessness with tachycardia and light-headedness caused by hypotension are suggestive of substantial pneumothorax or major pulmonary artery embolism.

Was there any haemoptysis? Haemoptysis occurs because of pulmonary infarction and strongly supports the diagnosis of pulmonary embolism.

Thromboembolic risk factors

Are there any risk factors for thromboembolism? In this case clearly the findings on rectal examination suggest the possibility of a rectal tumour. Cancer is a risk factor for thromboembolic disease. Other risk factors are:

• previous thromboembolism

• recent surgery: particularly major abdominal, pelvic, hip or knee surgery

• immobility, e.g. long haul aeroplane flights

• pregnancy/puerperium

• thrombophilia: protein C, protein S or antithrombin III deficiency; factor V Leiden mutation; family history of thromboembolism

• obstruction to venous flow (may be present if there is local spread of a tumour)

• smoking

• obesity

• age over 40 years.

Fever

Has there been fever? It is probable that this woman has had a pulmonary embolus, but ask about fevers, sweats or rigors. Most patients with pulmonary embolism are feverish, but high fever ($T > 38.5°C$), sweats or rigors make the diagnosis of pneumonia more likely.

Contraindications to anticoagulation

It is unlikely that this woman will have any contraindications to anticoagulation, but ask about these, the most common being a history of gastrointestinal bleeding. It is probable that you would decide to anticoagulate someone proven to have pulmonary embolism, but in the presence of a relative contraindication you would advise particularly close monitoring and counsel the patient to report problems immediately, e.g. change in colour of bowel motions, feeling of dizziness.

Examination

Full general, respiratory and cardiac examinations are required (see Section 1.1, p. 153 and 1.2, p. 155), but in this case pay particular attention to the following aspects.

General

Is the patient seriously ill? Does the patient need resuscitation of airway, breathing and circulation? If yes, resuscitate and seek immediate help from intensive care (see *Emergency medicine*, Sections 1.2 and 1.8).

If the patient is not gravely ill, note respiratory rate (tachypnoea is defined as a respiratory rate >20/min) and look for central cyanosis. Is there any evidence of deep venous thrombosis? Is there any evidence of metastatic spread (nodes)?

Cardiovascular

There should be particular emphasis on signs of acute pulmonary artery obstruction and/or pulmonary hypertension, which would be likely to be caused by subacute or chronic pulmonary embolism in this case:
- tachycardia
- hypotension
- elevated JVP
- right ventricular heave (along the left sternal border)*
- loud P2 and right ventricular S3.*
(*Features more typical of pulmonary hypertension.)

Respiratory

Respiration may be entirely normal, but listen carefully for a pleural rub. This can be very localized: ask the patient to put a finger on the spot that hurts most and listen carefully at and around that point. Consolidation typically gives bronchial breathing and dullness to percussion.

Musculoskeletal

Can the pain be reproduced by any movement or by localized pressure? If it can, then this supports a musculoskeletal cause of pleuritic pain. However, remember that pleurisy is exacerbated by anything that causes pleural movement. If in doubt, assume pulmonary embolism: be safe and not sorry.

Pulmonary embolism

- Sudden unexplained dyspnoea is the most common and often the only symptom.
- The combination of dyspnoea plus tachypnoea is present in 90% of patients.
- Only 3% of patients do not have one of the following: dyspnoea, tachypnoea or pleuritic chest pain.
- Examination may be normal.
- Tachycardia is a consistent but non-specific finding.
- Carefully search for risk factors for thromboembolism.

Approach to investigations and management

Investigations

Chest radiograph

This may be normal, but common findings in pulmonary embolism are linear infiltrates, segmental collapse, raised hemidiaphragm and pleural effusion. Look for other causes of pleuritic chest pain, in particular pneumothorax, but also for pneumonic consolidation. Remember that a normal chest radiograph in an acutely breathless hypoxic patient increases the likelihood of pulmonary embolism.

Electrocardiogram

The most common abnormalities are tachycardia and non-specific ST/T wave changes. Look for acute right heart strain with tall P waves, right axis deviation and ST/T wave changes in right ventricular leads (V1 and V2), and remember that the 'classical' S1Q3T3 pattern is seen in fewer than 10% of cases of proven pulmonary embolism.

Arterial blood gases

Occlusion of a pulmonary artery or its branches results in an area of lung that is ventilated but not perfused. This part of the lung does not then participate in gas exchange and hence results in wasted ventilation. Because of this ventilation–perfusion mismatching and hyperventilation the arterial blood gases in pulmonary embolism frequently show arterial hypoxaemia, hypocapnia and respiratory alkalosis. However, do not forget that a normal PaO_2 does not exclude pulmonary embolism.

Plasma D-dimer

D-dimer is a breakdown product of cross-linked fibrin and is elevated in active venous thromboembolism. A normal value can be used to exclude thromboembolism. The enzyme-linked immunosorbent assay (ELISA) is more accurate than the rapid latex test.

Echocardiography

In pulmonary embolism this is only helpful if a large embolus is suspected, when there may be right ventricular dilatation and hypokinesis, pulmonary artery enlargement, tricuspid regurgitation, abnormal septal movement, and failure of the inferior vena cava to collapse during inspiration.

Specific tests for pulmonary embolism

VENTILATION–PERFUSION ISOTOPE SCANNING

Ventilation scans are obtained using krypton-81m, technegas or xenon-133 and perfusion scans with intravenous ^{99m}Tc-labelled macroaggregates of albumin (Fig. 7). Scanning should ideally be performed within 24 h of clinical suspicion as appearances can revert to normal within a few days, and 50% do so within a week. The scans are interpreted as being normal, or of low, intermediate or high probability: reports need to be interpreted in the clinical context.

PULMONARY ANGIOGRAPHY

This is not routinely available in most hospitals in the UK. It is regarded by some as the 'gold standard' for diagnosing pulmonary embolism, but is invasive—with major or fatal complications in 0.5–1.3% of investigations, and minor complications in 2%—and interpretation is not always straightforward, particularly for those who do not perform the test regularly. The most common finding is a filling defect in the pulmonary artery as the radio-opaque dye flows around the embolus (Fig. 8).

SPIRAL COMPUTED TOMOGRAPHY

This can detect intravascular clot from the pulmonary trunk down to the segmental arteries, but unlike pulmonary angiography it cannot visualize emboli in the subsegmental arteries. In many centres this has become the investigation of choice, particularly for patients with pre-existing lung disease, which renders the interpretation of ventilation–perfusion scans difficult or impossible.

Investigations relevant to the rectal mass

Most cases of pulmonary embolism will not have a rectal mass, but in this case appropriate investigation would include sigmoidoscopy and biopsy. (See *Gastroenterology and hepatology*, Sections 1.5, 1.11 and 2.7.2.)

Management

If the patient is in shock administer high-flow oxygen and intravenous fluids, and immediately seek intensive care help.

Anticoagulation reduces the incidence of fatal recurrent embolism, and heparin should be started immediately pending the results of investigations when there is high or intermediate clinical suspicion.

Low-molecular-weight heparin is as effective as standard unfractionated heparin in non-life-threatening pulmonary embolism and has the advantages of rapid anticoagulation, simple once-daily administration and no need for laboratory monitoring.

Warfarin should be started once the diagnosis is confirmed.

 In patients without a contraindication to warfarin it is reasonable to start this at the same time as heparin, even in patients in whom the diagnosis is unsure. It can be stopped if the diagnosis of pulmonary embolism is subsequently excluded. If pulmonary embolism is confirmed, then the patient may be able to return home earlier.

Thrombolytic treatment is recommended for patients who are haemodynamically unstable. This is given peripherally, the doses used often being different from those used in myocardial infarction [1].

Pulmonary embolectomy is now reserved for patients who do not respond to thrombolysis or who have a contraindication to thrombolysis. Active bleeding from a rectal tumour would be a contraindication in this case.

Inferior vena caval filters should be considered in patients at high risk of emboli in whom anticoagulation is contraindicated and in those with recurrent embolism despite adequate anticoagulation.

(a)

(b)

Fig. 7 Ventilation–perfusion scan showing right mid zone pulmonary embolism (arrowed): (a) perfusion; (b) ventilation images.

Fig. 8 Pulmonary angiogram showing large right pulmonary embolus (arrow). There are also clear abnormalities of perfusion in the left middle and lower zones.

See *Emergency medicine*, Sections 1.2 and 1.8
See *Haematology and oncology*, Section 3.6
See *Cardiology*, Sections 1.9, 2.18 and 3.10
British Thoracic Society. Suspected acute pulmonary embolism: a practical approach. *Thorax* 1997; 52: Supplement 4.
Arcasoy SM, Kreit JW. Thrombolytic therapy of pulmonary embolism: a comprehensive review of current evidence. *Chest* 1999; 115(6): 1695–1707.
1 The PIOPED investigators. Value of the ventilation/ perfusion scan in acute pulmonary embolism. *JAMA* 1990; 263: 2753–9.

1.6 Unexplained hypoxia

Case history

A 44-year-old man has been admitted with a 2-week history of non-specific symptoms of tiredness and being

Table 4 Pathophysiologic processes leading to hypoxia.

Process	Example
Insufficient inspired oxygen	Altitude, anaesthetic mishaps
Right-to-left shunt	Anatomical shunts (cardiac, AVM), physiological shunts (e.g. resulting from atelectasis)
V/Q imbalance	Many causes, e.g. asthma, pneumonia, fibrosis, thromboembolic disease
Alveolar hypoventilation	Severe obstructive sleep apnoea, neurological/neuromuscular disease
Impaired diffusion	Fibrosis

AVM, arteriovenous malformation.

unwell. His chest radiograph is reported as normal but he is found to be hypoxic with a PaO_2 of 8.4 kPa.

Clinical approach

It is reasonable to assume that the patient has new-onset hypoxia, given that he is experiencing new symptoms. There are five physiological processes that can give rise to hypoxia (Table 4). In this case the finding of a normal chest radiograph makes some of these causes less probable.

History of the presenting problem

In practical terms the main issue is to distinguish between a genuinely new condition and the recent identification of something that is gradually progressive. With the chest radiograph reported as normal the main differential diagnoses in this case are shown in Table 5 and the history should pursue these possibilities.

Is the problem really acute?

Try to identify whether—with hindsight—the patient has had respiratory symptoms previously, perhaps on exercise. Has the patient had to stop doing anything or slow down recently?

If the problem seems to be long standing:

• Are there any respiratory or cardiac clues to the diagnosis?

Table 5 Differential diagnosis of hypoxia with a 'normal' chest radiograph.

	Long-standing problem	New condition
Likely diagnoses	Airways disease Interstitial lung disease Obstructive sleep apnoea	Pulmonary embolus Pneumonic process without chest radiograph changes, e.g. atypical pneumonia, miliary tuberculosis, *Pneumocystic carinii* pneumonia
Rare	Restrictive lung disease Upper airway obstruction Neuromuscular disease Cardiac shunts Pulmonary arteriovenous malformation Hepatopulmonary syndrome	Extrinsic alveolitis

- Are there features of untreated asthma, e.g. nocturnal cough, diurnal variation or atopy?
- Are there features of sleep disordered breathing? If this is severe enough to cause daytime hypoxia, then it should be associated with excessive daytime somnolence
- Is there anything to suggest a cardiac problem, e.g. report of a heart murmur?
- Is the patient at risk of interstitial lung disease? (See Section 1.4, p. 160.)

Always remember thromboembolic disease, which may not be associated with chest pain when chronic.

Consider other risks

What acute conditions is the patient at risk of?
- Pulmonary embolism may be suggested by recognized risk factors for thromboembolic disease. (See Section 1.5, p. 163.)
- The risk of atypical pneumonia is increased by exposure to air-conditioning systems (*Legionella*) or birds (*Chlamydia*).
- Miliary TB should be carefully considered in those at high risk, e.g. patients from particular ethnic groups.
- *Pneumocystis carinii* pneumonia (PCP) may present with isolated hypoxia and questioning about risk factors for human immunodeficiency virus (HIV) may be required. This needs tact and discretion and should be left to the end of the history and examination (see *General clinical issues*, Section 2).

Examination

Full general, respiratory and cardiac examinations are required (see Sections 1.1, p. 153 and 1.2, p. 155), but in this case pay particular attention to the following aspects.

General

- Does the patient have a fever or look toxic? These would favour an acute pneumonic process.
- Does the patient look as though he or she has lost weight? In this case weight loss might suggest miliary TB, or *Pneumocystis* as a complication of acquired immune deficiency syndrome (AIDS).
- Are there any other features to suggest AIDS, e.g. oral candidiasis?
- Is the patient likely to have obstructive sleep apnoea (OSA), e.g. obese, thick neck?
- Is the patient clubbed, which might suggest interstitial lung disease or a congenital cardiac shunt in this context?

Respiratory and cardiac

- Are there features of airways disease? Are there crackles in the chest, which might suggest interstitial lung disease in this context?
- Are there cardiac features to suggest pulmonary embolism (see Section 1.5, p. 163)? Are there any cardiac murmurs?

The measurement of PEF, and ideally spirometry, should form part of the clinical assessment—airways disease is common and should not be overlooked.

Neuromuscular

Is there evidence of neuropathy or myopathy? In particular, does the diaphragm move normally?

Approach to investigations and management

Investigations

Chest radiograph

Review the chest radiograph carefully. Take it back to the radiologist for further scrutiny with additional clinical information.
- Is the cardiac silhouette really normal?
- Is there subtle evidence of airspace shadowing (Fig. 9)? This would suggest interstitial lung disease or a pneumonic process.
- Are both hemidiaphragms clearly visible? Check that you are not missing left lower lobe consolidation, which is easy to neglect.
- Are both costophrenic angles clearly visible? A small pleural effusion might be caused by a pneumonic process or to thromboembolism. Sampling of pleural fluid could be diagnostic. (See Section 1.10, p. 176.)

Fig. 9 Radiograph of a 29-year-old homosexual man with a history of dyspnoea and weight loss. Diagnostic possibilities include *Pneumocystis carinii* pneumonia.

Arterial blood gases

An increased $PaCO_2$ (or the demonstration, by calculation, of a normal arterial–alveolar (a–A) oxygen gradient) would suggest true alveolar hypoventilation. Comparison of arterial blood gases measured on room air and 100% oxygen allows calculation of the anatomical shunt, which in normal subjects is less than 5%.

Peak flow, spirometry and lung function

These measurements should be abnormal if there is occult airways disease of sufficient severity to cause hypoxia. In interstitial lung disease there will be a restrictive defect. Upper airway obstruction is an unlikely diagnosis in this case, but would be revealed by the flow–volume loop. (See Section 1.14, p. 184.)

Blood tests

Routine full blood count, biochemistry and inflammatory markers are indicated because of the non-specific nature of symptoms in this case. Serum ACE and calcium are indicated if sarcoid is possible. Atypical pneumonia titres or avian precipitins would be indicated if the history is appropriate.

It may be appropriate, after discussion, to test this patient for HIV (see *General clinical issues*, Section 2 and *Infectious diseases*, Section 1.24).

Computed tomography scan of thorax

This is likely to be a very helpful investigation, but the way in which the study is performed will depend on what is considered to be the most likely diagnosis. Discussion with the radiologist is required: not just an order form stating 'hypoxia—cause?'.
• For suspected thromboembolic disease a spiral protocol is used.
• For suspected interstitial lung disease a high-resolution scan gives the best images and is preferred. Significant pulmonary fibrosis may be invisible on a plain radiograph but seen on CT.

Further investigation for thromboembolism

If the clinical suspicion of thromboembolism is high, then specific tests as discussed in Section 1.5, p. 163, would be appropriate.

BRONCHOSCOPY

Analysis of bronchial lavage fluid is indicated to diagnose PCP and miliary TB. If there is CT evidence of interstitial lung disease transbronchial biopsy is likely to be required; open lung biopsy may be preferred in selected patients.

ECHOCARDIOGRAPHY

A contrast echo is the first choice investigation if an anatomic shunt is identified (estimation of pulmonary artery pressure is a useful piece of extra data from this study). If there is no cardiac shunt then a CT scan will usually identify a pulmonary AVM.

The most useful investigation in respiratory medicine is the old radiograph. This adage normally applies when trying to decide the nature of a solitary pulmonary nodule. However, the principle can be applied prospectively; for patients who you feel uneasy about but are unable to diagnose, it can be helpful to recall them to clinic and repeat their radiograph.

Management

Clearly the management in this case is of the underlying condition. If the underlying condition is untreatable, oxygen should be considered for palliation of symptoms.

Lennox AF, Nicolaides AN. Rapid D-dimer testing as an adjunct to clinical findings in excluding pulmonary embolism. *Thorax* 1999; 54(S2): S33–S36.
The PIOPED investigators. Value of the ventilation–perfusion scan in acute pulmonary embolism. Results of the prospective investigation of pulmonary embolism diagnosis (PIOPED). *JAMA* 1990; 263: 2753–2759.

1.7 Nocturnal cough

Case history

A 45-year-old woman, who has been a life-long non-smoker, is referred with a 6-month history of an annoying dry nocturnal cough. She has no previous history of respiratory problems.

Clinical approach

A chronic persistent cough can be defined as a cough that lasts more than 3 weeks. Causes can be divided according to whether the cough is productive or non-productive (Table 6).

Overall the most common cause of cough is smoking, and the most likely pathology is asthma, COPD or hyperreactive airways, possibly precipitated some time before by an upper respiratory tract infection. In smokers it is always crucial to rule out an underlying malignancy

Table 6 Differential diagnosis of a chronic cough.

Type of cough		Example
Productive	Common	Smoking, COPD/chronic bronchitis, asthma, bronchiectasis
	Consider	Tumour, tuberculosis, pulmonary emboli, congestive heart failure
	Other	Inhaled foreign body
Non-productive	Common	Smoking, asthma, postnasal drip, oesophageal reflux, ACE inhibitors
	Consider	Inflammatory lung disease, e.g. sarcoidosis, connective tissue disease, congestive heart failure, tumour
	Other	Middle ear disease, psychogenic

ACE, angiotensin-converting enzyme; COPD, chronic obstructive pulmonary disease.

such as a lung or throat neoplasm. However, this patient is a non-smoker and there are a number of important causes of chronic cough that are often overlooked:
• postnasal drip
• gastro-oesophageal reflux
• ear and throat problems.

History of the presenting problem

After the patient has told her story, address the following issues with direct questions if they have not already been covered.

Asthma

• When did the problem start? Was it related to a viral illness?
• Have you ever been wheezy, particularly during coughs and colds?
• Do you ever wake up feeling breathless or wheezy in the middle of the night?
• Is there a family history of atopy, i.e. asthma, hayfever, eczema?
• What is your job?

Postnasal drip

There may be a history of hayfever or simply a very runny nose. If asked, some patients can describe a dripping sensation at the back of their throat or swallowing lots of catarrh.

Oesophageal reflux

Many patients with oesophageal reflux will have no symptoms, but check for history of peptic ulceration, indigestion or heart burn.

Cardiac disease

Patients may cough with cardiac failure, or secondary to their medication, especially ACE inhibitors. Are there any risk factors or symptoms of thromoembolic disease? (See Section 1.5, p. 163.)

Inflammatory lung disease

Sarcoidosis or lung manifestations of autoimmune rheumatic disease can simply present with a chronic cough. Look for other manifestations such as joint problems.

Ear and throat disease

Middle ear disease can lead to a cough. Ask about alternations in voice, as underlying vocal cord polyp or malignancy are possible (see *Oncology*, Section 2.6). Ask about sinusitis.

Relevant past history

Asthma

Is there any personal or family history that helps support the diagnosis? For example 'I was always chesty as a child.' 'All my cousins have asthma and my nephew's just been given an inhaler.'

Are there underlying or precipitating factors? For example, allergies—food, pets, eczema and hayfever. Has the patient ever smoked? Do the symptoms get worse in pubs or clubs, or other smoky atmospheres?

Bronchiectasis

If the cough is productive, ask about childhood illness such as pneumonia, TB and diphtheria that would predispose to bronchiectasis.

Examination

Full general, respiratory and cardiac examinations are required (see Sections 1.1, p. 153 and 1.2, p. 155), but examination is unremarkable in many cases presenting with cough as the only symptom. Even so, it is important to look carefully for clues, particularly of the more unusual causes, e.g. autoimmune rheumatic disease, where something such as evidence of small joint disease could be crucial in making the diagnosis.

Respiratory and cardiac

Examine particularly for wheeze and stridor, and for problems in the nose and throat. Use a torch to look for

(a)   (b)

Fig. 11 The same patient shown (a) from the front, dressed, and (b) closer up, from behind and undressed. Kyphoscoliosis can be missed on superficial examination.

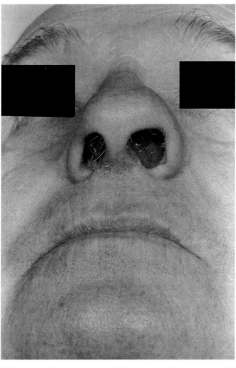

Fig. 12 This patient has snoring and obstructive sleep apnoea. Simple examination shows a polyp which, if treated may improve symptoms.

• Daytime arterial blood gases—the demonstration of daytime hypercapnia will influence the urgency and, possibly, mode of treatment
• Repeat full blood count—to confirm polycythaemia
• Thyroid function tests—hypothyroidism can precipitate weight gain and (rarely) OSA
• Chest radiograph—to exclude lung disease; look also for cardiomegaly

• ECG—may reveal left ventricular hypertrophy or right heart strain
• Spirometry, lung volumes, lying and standing vital capacity or mouth pressures
• Formal ENT evaluation.

Sleep orientated

Overnight oximetry is a useful screening investigation that may be done at home. The diagnosis of polycythaemia secondary to nocturnal hypoxia must be reviewed if the patient reports that she sleeps and there is no desaturation. The absence of nocturnal desaturation would require the assumption of an alternative cause of hypersomnolence (e.g. narcolepsy) occurring with an alternative cause of polycythaemia. However, note that a normal overnight SaO_2 does not exclude the diagnosis of OSA in patients with appropriate symptoms but without polycythaemia.

If the patient has an overnight SaO_2 trace suggestive of OSA, and examination or investigation does not reveal chronic respiratory failure (CRF; or risk factors for CRF), then it is reasonable to manage the patient as having OSA.

If the patient has nocturnal desaturation and risk factors for CRF (e.g. obesity and tobacco-related lung disease) then a more accurate assessment is required. This may involve a limited respiratory sleep study with transcutaneous carbon dioxide monitoring. Full polysomnography with carbon dioxide monitoring is used in some centres. These tests are required because the mode of ventilatory support is determined by the precise diagnosis.

After the institution of mechanical ventilatory support a repeat study is useful to confirm the adequacy of treatment.

 If a patient has daytime sleepiness secondary to OSA that is sufficiently severe to require nasal continuous positive airway pressure (CPAP) ventilatory assistance, they must inform both the DVLA and their motor insurer of the diagnosis.

Management

See Section 2.12, p. 231.

 Chesson AL, Ferber RA, Fry JM *et al.* The indications for polysomnography and related procedures. *Sleep* 1997; 20: 423–487.
Gugger M. Comparison of ResMed Autoset (version 3.03) with polysomnography in the diagnosis of the sleep apnoea/hypopoea syndrome. *Eur Resp J* 1997; 10: 587–591.

1.9 Haemoptysis and weight loss

Case history

A 35-year-old man, who came as a political refugee to the UK 5 years ago, presents with haemoptysis and weight loss. He has been previously fit and well. His chest radiograph is shown in Fig. 13.

Clinical approach

The presentation is vague about the patient's ethnic background and says nothing of his travel history, details of which are critical in this case. Apart from TB, much the most likely diagnosis, other causes of haemoptysis in a young patient are shown in Table 9.

History of the presenting problem

Communication may be difficult: unless the man has good command of English it is unlikely that you will be able to obtain a thorough history without the benefit of an interpreter.

The first thing to do is to establish if haemoptysis is the problem. How long has the patient been coughing up blood? Is the patient sure that the blood is in the phlegm and not in vomit or coming from the throat?

Haemoptysis caused by tuberculosis

A detailed personal, social, family and travel history is required, with particular emphasis on the following:

Fig. 13 Chest radiograph of this patient; note the bilateral apical changes, consistent with *Mycobacterium tuberculosis* infection, as well as the cavity on the periphery of the right upper lobe.

Table 9 Causes of haemoptysis in a young person.

Classification	Examples
Common	Infection, e.g. pyogenic bacteria or MTB
Consider	Bronchiectasis, pulmonary emboli
Rare	Tumour (benign or malignant), Goodpasture's or other vasculitis

MTB, *Mycobacterium tuberculosis.*

• Has the patient been treated for TB in the past? If so, was the patient given antituberculous medication, and how many drugs? Few people remember the names of the tablets: ask for descriptions of them—combination preparations that have distinctive colours and shapes are often used, e.g. Rifater, Rifinah.
• Have family members or close household contacts ever been treated for TB? Many patients deny this, particularly before a diagnosis has been made, because of the stigmas surrounding the disease.
• Where was the patient born? In which countries has the patient lived before coming to the UK? What sort of places has the patient lived in—refugee camps, hostels? The incidence of single-drug- and multidrug-resistant TB varies from region to region and this should be taken into consideration in any subsequent treatment. Remember also that some areas of Western Africa have much higher rates of HIV infection than, say, Bangladesh.

• Where is the patient living now? How many people are living in the patient's home? Many immigrants live in overcrowded housing: from the point of view of contact tracing and subsequent screening it is important to know who the patient's close contacts are.
• Has the patient lost any weight? How is the patient's appetite? Has the patient had any fevers or drenching night sweats? Has the patient needed to change the bedclothes? Weight loss, anorexia, fevers and sweats would all be expected in TB, and their absence would cast doubt on the diagnosis.

Other

• Bronchiectasis—is the patient producing any sputum? How much? Teaspoonfuls or cupfuls? Ask about childhood respiratory infections, including TB and whooping cough, which would predispose to this condition. (See Section 1.3, p. 158)
• Pulmonary emboli—is the patient at risk? (See Section 1.5, p. 163)
• Goodpasture's—exceedingly unlikely in this case, but is there a history of occupational exposure to solvents, paints or petrol?

Examination

Full general, respiratory and cardiac examinations are needed (see Sections 1.1, p. 153 and 1.2, p. 155), but particular attention to the following is required:
• Does the patient look unwell and cachetic? Does the patient appear hot and feverish?
• Is there lymphadenopathy, which would support the diagnosis of TB?
• Is there clubbing and inspiratory crackles that do not clear on coughing, which would support the diagnosis of bronchiectasis?
• What are the signs in the chest? In particular, are there pleural effusions that could be tapped and the pleura biopsied?
• Are there cardiac or pulmonary signs to suggest pulmonary emboli? (See Section 1.5, p. 163.)

Approach to investigations and management

Investigations of haemoptysis

• Chest radiograph—immediate
• Sputum examination for AFB
• Bronchoscopy—within a week if diagnosis not made.

Fig. 14 Chest radiograph of another patient presenting with haemoptysis and later found to have tuberculosis; he had coughed so much that he had a left-sided pneumothorax, which had led to right mediastinal shift. This resolved spontaneously with conservative treatment. His tuberculosis was treated with quadruple therapy.

Investigations

Chest radiograph

This may help narrow down the diagnostic possibilities, but do not forget that TB can mimic many other pathologies, such as lung cancer, other bacterial infections and pneumonitis. Do not forget to look for pleural thickening and evidence of calcification, also for the unexpected (Fig. 14).

Sputum examination

Urgent (same day) examination for MCS and AFB. Send for cytology as well.

Bronchoscopy

Bronchial biopsies, if taken, must be sent both for histology (in formalin) and microbiology (in normal saline). It is good practice for bronchial lavage to be performed and sent for cytology (for malignant cells) and microbiology and virology. Silver staining is not indicated unless there are other reasons to suggest PCP.

Management

Will be according to diagnosis:
• TB: see *Infectious diseases*, Section 2.6
• Bronchiectasis: see Section 2.4, p. 197
• Pulmonary emboli: see *Cardiology*, Section 2.18 and *Haematology and oncology*, Section 3.6.

175

1.10 Pleural effusion and fever

Case history

A 43-year-old woman is admitted to the hospital with fever for the last 7–8 days. Her chest radiograph shows a pleural effusion on the right side (Fig. 15).

Clinical approach

Here the main symptom is fever, suggesting an underlying inflammatory or infective process. The history is short, indicating an acute problem. A pleural effusion on chest radiograph suggests the lungs as the primary site of pathology, but there are other causes of effusion, e.g. cardiac failure, but they are unlikely in this case.

Fever and pleural effusion

Pneumonia with an effusion and empyema are the likeliest diagnoses, but consider:
- TB
- Connective tissue disorder (rheumatoid arthritis/SLE)
- Malignancy (primary bronchial/secondary)
- Mesothelioma
- Pulmonary emboli
- Familial Mediterranean fever (seen in Jewish and Arabic people; recurrent attacks of fever, arthritis, and pleurisy. Prevented by colchicine).

History of the presenting problem

It is important to determine whether the problem really is new or, with hindsight, whether other features were present beforehand. Fever and pleural effusion developing acutely in a previously healthy person are most likely to be caused by an infective pathology. Has there been recent cough and purulent phlegm? Ask about the following if they do not emerge spontaneously in the history:
- Is there any pleuritic chest pain? (bacterial pneumonia/pulmonary embolism).
- Has the patient coughed up blood? (bacterial pneumonia/TB/malignancy).
- Has the patient lost any weight? (tuberculosis/malignancy).
- Has the patient travelled abroad recently? (infection/pulmonary embolism).
- Is the patient a smoker? (bronchial carcinoma).
- Is there any history of night sweats and evening rise of temperature? (TB).
- Has the patient been in contact with anyone with TB?
- Has there been a rash? (may suggest mycoplasma).
- Does the patient suffer from any joint pains in the hands? (rheumatoid arthritis/SLE).

Relevant past history

- Any history of joint pains? (rheumatoid arthritis/SLE).
- Any history of malignancy? (breast, ovarian, lymphoma).

Social and occupational history

- Does the patient smoke?
- Any exposure to asbestos? (benign effusions/mesothelioma).
- A nurse/doctor or other health worker may unwittingly have been in contact with TB.

Examination

Full general, respiratory and cardiac examinations are needed (see Sections 1.1, p. 153 and 1.2, p. 155), but particular attention to the following is required.

General

Look for cachexia, lymphadenopathy (malignancy, TB), jaundice (hepatic metastasis), sputum pot, rash of SLE, rheumatoid hands and nodules. Examine the breasts for any mass (with chaperone if appropriate).

Respiratory

The signs of a pleural effusion (reduced expansion, reduced breath/absent breath sounds and stony dullness) will be present if the effusion is big enough, but these do not help the differential diagnosis.

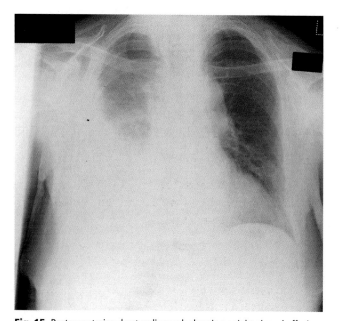

Fig. 15 Posteroanterior chest radiograph showing a right pleural effusion.

Approach to investigations and management

Investigations

Blood tests

Check full blood count, ESR, CRP, rheumatoid factor, antinuclear antibodies, calcium level and liver function tests.

Sputum

For microscopy and culture (specifically including for TB), and for cytology.

Pleural fluid

Examining the pleural fluid is critical.
- If there is associated pneumonia: is the fluid parapneumonic or is it an empyema? If it is opaque/turbid and with a foul smell, then it is clearly an empyema. In cases that are less clear-cut the pleural fluid pH is probably the single most useful test, with empyema strongly suggested by a pH <7.22.
- If there is no associated pneumonia: is the fluid a transudate or an exudate? The two are distinguished by Light's criteria (see below); causes of transudates and exudates are shown in Table 10.
- Send for microscopy and culture: both anaerobic and aerobic, and for TB.
- Send for cytology.
- Measure protein, lactate dehydrogenase (LDH) and pH.

 My colleagues and I demonstrated that with the use of simultaneously obtained serum and pleural fluid protein and lactic acid dehydrogenase (LDH) values, 99% of pleural effusions could be correctly classified as either transudates or exudates. Exudative pleural effusions meet at least one of the following criteria, whereas transudative pleural effusions meet none:
1 Pleural fluid protein divided by serum protein greater than 0.5
2 Pleural fluid LDH divided by serum LDH greater than 0.6
3 Pleural fluid LDH greater than two-thirds the upper limit of normal for the LDH.
(Light's criteria for classification of pleural effusions [1].)

 For suspected malignant effusions it can be helpful to send a large volume and have this spun in the laboratory to magnify the cellular portion.

Table 10 Causes of pleural effusions.

Classification	Example
Transudates	Congestive cardiac failure, cirrhosis, nephrotic syndrome, myxoedema, peritoneal dialysis
Exudates	Malignancy, infectious (bacterial, tuberculosis, fungal, parasitic, viral), pulmonary emboli, collagen vascular (rheumatoid, SLE, Sjögren's syndrome, Wegener's, Churg–Strauss), gastrointestinal (pancreatic disease, subphrenic abscess, oesophageal perforation), yellow-nail syndrome, haemothorax, chylothorax, drug-induced (amiodarone, dantrolene, methotrexate, practolol, nitrofurantoin)

SLE, systemic lupus eythematosus.

Pleural biopsy

Pleural biopsy should be performed in those with an exudative pleural effusion to exclude malignancy. It is reasonable to attempt this with an Abrams' needle, but it is important to remember that because this is a blind (unguided) procedure a negative result does not exclude any diagnosis.

Ultrasound of the chest

In cases of loculated effusion, it is best to aspirate the effusion under ultrasound guidance.

Computed tomographic scan of chest

This investigation quantifies the pleural fluid collection, but also examines the lung parenchyma and may identify unsuspected tumours or solid pleural disease.

Management

The treatment of the effusion depends on the cause, but three cases require special consideration:
- parapneumonic effusions
- empyema
- malignant pleural effusions.

Parapneumonic effusions

Parapneumonic effusions that resolve with appropriate antibiotics are called uncomplicated parapneumonic effusions and do not require tube drainage.

Empyema

- The patient should receive appropriate doses of parenteral antibiotics.
- A chest drain is required: delay in draining an empyema

is associated with an increase in mortality. Use at least a 28 F size drain so that it will not become obstructed with fibrin.

The presence of pleural fluid loculations can prevent complete drainage by mechanical means alone. Intrapleural streptokinase and urokinase have been used to destroy the fibrin membranes that separate the locules and facilitate drainage. Streptokinase (250 000 units) or urokinase (100 000 units) dissolved in 30–60 mL of normal saline is given intrapleurally via the drain, which is then clamped for 1–2 h. On release of the clamp, a successful response is heralded by an increase in the amount of fluid drained and improvement in the chest radiograph. Fibrinolytics can be given daily for 14 days: they do not have any effect on the systemic bleeding parameters.

In patients who remain ill and with inadequate drainage despite intrapleural fibrinolytics, decortication should be considered. This is a major surgical procedure: all fibrous tissue is removed and pus evacuated.

Malignant pleural effusions

Patients with large pleural effusions caused by untreatable malignancies can be very dyspnoiec. This should be treated (unless the patient's life expectancy is very short indeed) with pleurodesis, either locally via a chest drain or by a thoracoscopic approach. In the editor's experience reaccumulation rates are significantly lower after thoracosopic procedures and this approach is preferred unless the patient is expected to die within 1 month.

The indications for inserting a chest drain into a parapneumonic effusion/empyema are:
- pus in pleural cavity (empyema)
- organisms visible in pleural fluid on microscopy
- positive pleural fluid culture
- pleural fluid pH <7.20
- serial reduction in pleural fluid pH, glucose and increase in LDH.

Bouros D, Schiza S, Panagou P, Drositis J, Siafakas N. Role of streptokinase in the treatment of acute loculated parapneumonic pleural effusions and empyema. *Thorax* 1994; 49: 852–855.

Heffner JE. Diagnosis and management of thoracic empyemas. *Curr Opin Pulm Med* 1996; 2(3): 198–205.

Heffner JE, Brown LK, Barbieri C, DeLeo JM. Pleural fluid chemical analysis in parapneumonic effusion. *Am J Respir Crit Care Med* 1995; 151: 1700–1708.

Light RW. *Pleural Diseases* (2nd edn). New York: Lea and Febiger.

1 Light RW, MacGregor MI, Luchsinger PC, Ball WC. Pleural effusions: the diagnostic separation of transudates and exudates. *Ann Intern Med* 1972; 77: 507–513.

1.11 Lung cancer with asbestos exposure

Case history

A 53-year-old taxi driver presents with a chest radiograph that shows evidence of right-sided pleural thickening associated with a moderate pleural effusion. He has previously worked in numerous labouring jobs, including as a lagger.

Clinical approach

Your main concern is that this patient has asbestos-related lung disease and that this could be mesothelioma, although asbestos also causes other pathology (Table 11). It is important to take a detailed occupational history.

How to take an occupational history

- The easiest way of recording employment is by asking the patient what he or she did immediately after leaving school and then recording positions chronologically; people tend to remember their jobs most easily this way.
- Do not forget holiday jobs from school or casual employment (Steve McQueen, the American actor, worked with asbestos for 6 months before he became famous, and he died of asbestos-related lung disease).
- Did anyone in the patient's family work in an asbestos factory and bring the dust home on their clothes?
- On a more short-term basis, particularly if you are worried about the patient's current employment, say in relation to occupational asthma—do the symptoms worsen during the working week and improve at the weekend and during the holidays?

History of the presenting problem

Underlying pathology caused by asbestos exposure

In taking the occupational history, do not forget to ask the following:
- If the patient remembers working with asbestos, how long was this for? How close was the contact and for what length of the working day? For example, was the patient working in the holds of ships unloading bags of asbestos? Were the patient's clothes covered in asbestos dust?

Table 11 Possible asbestos-related lung disease.

Classification	Example
Common	Pleural plaques, pleural thickening
Consider	Asbestos-related fibrosis (asbestosis), lung cancer, mesothelioma

- Did the patient wear protective clothing or masks? Were these provided by the employers?
- Record the names of the companies that they worked for (may be helpful for later reference).

Smoking history

This is necessary because, if there is both asbestos and tobacco exposure, then—for legal purposes—it is desirable to quantify both.

> **!** Take an accurate smoking history and record in the notes when and if the patient has stopped smoking. If patients claim for compensation at a later date, this information will be required.

Symptoms

Persistent pain or rapid progression of symptoms are poor predictive features.
- Has the patient had any chest pain? If so, how long does it last? Does it keep them awake at night?
- Has the patient been short of breath at rest or on exercise?
- Has it been more difficult of late for the patient to lie down without feeling breathless?

Relevant past history

It is important to ascertain whether there have been any previous episodes of chest problems. Did the patient suffer from chest problems as a child? Many previous chest pathologies can leave pleural thickening.

> **Causes of pleural thickening**
> - Asbestos exposure
> - Trauma
> - Previous chest infection/empyema
> - Previous haemothorax
> - Old TB.

Examination

Full general, respiratory and cardiac examinations are needed (see Sections 1.1, p. 153 and 1.2, p. 155), but particular attention to the following is required:
- Does the patient look in good health or obviously unwell?
- Is the patient cachectic and pale?
- Is there clubbing?
- Is there lymphadenopathy?
- What are the signs in the chest?

Approach to investigations and management

> **Investigations of asbestos-related disease**
> - Chest radiograph—posteroanterior and lateral
> - High-resolution computed tomography of the chest
> - Pleural biopsy and aspiration and/or thoracoscopy
> - Open lung biospy.

Investigations

Chest radiograph

In this case, the patient presented with a chest film. In general, look carefully for any pleural thickening—it is easy to miss (Figs 16 and 17a). Is there any calcification, particularly over the diaphragm? Do not forget to look for areas of fibrosis.

Computed tomography scan of chest

This is invaluable when assessing the extent of disease, whether there is pleural thickening, fibrosis or malignancy (Fig. 17b). If appropriate, a CT scan may be followed by a CT-guided biopsy. In cases of bronchogenic cancer and asbestos exposure the presence of fibrosis supports the argument that the patient was exposed to significant quantities of asbestos.

Pleural biopsy and aspiration

> A pleural biopsy with an Abrams' needle can only be carried out in the presence of a moderate to large pleural effusion, otherwise you will puncture the lung and give the patient a pneumothorax.

Fig. 16 Chest radiograph showing obvious left-sided pleural thickening caused by asbestos exposure. (Courtesy of Dr R. Rudd.)

(a)

(b)

Fig. 17 (a) Chest radiograph of a patient with mesothelioma leading to right-sided pleural thickening, which has produced a volume loss and mediastinal shift. (b) Computed tomography scan of the same patient with mesothelioma showing the extent of disease invasion into the right hemithorax.

 Make sure that you send pleural biopsy samples to microbiology, for microscopy and culture (including TB), as well as to histology. The diagnosis may not be malignancy, or there may be dual pathology.

Thoracoscopy

This is generally only available in specialist centres, where it can be performed by chest physicians and/or cardiothoracic surgeons. As with pleural biopsy, the presence of an abnormal amount of pleural fluid is necessary for the procedure to be carried out safely.

Management

The management is dependent on the final diagnosis:
- asbestosis: see Section 2.6.1, p. 202
- mesothelioma: see Section 2.9.2, p. 224
- lung cancer: see Section 2.9.1, p. 220.

1.12 Lobar collapse in non-smoker

Case history

A 55-year-old woman is referred with a 10-day history of productive cough, gradually increasing shortness of breath, and fever. Her symptoms have failed to resolve on oral antibiotics and her chest radiograph shows right upper lobe collapse (Fig. 18), but the same clinical approach would apply to collapse of any lobe (see Fig. 19).

Fig. 18 Posteroanterior chest radiograph showing right upper lobe collapse. Note the tenting of the right hemidiaphragm and the raised right hilum. (Courtesy of Dr I. Vlahos.)

Clinical approach

If there is also consolidation your initial concern must be to treat the acute condition, which is likely to be a lobar pneumonia. The patient should be admitted to hospital, given oxygen (if blood gases reveal hypoxia) and appropriate antibiotics. Sputum and blood cultures should be sent for MCS.

However, collapse alone or collapse/consolidation which is slow to clear (say more than 6 weeks from the start of symptoms) requires investigation because of the possibility that there is an obstructing lesion.

History of the presenting problem

Cause of lobar collapse

A full respiratory history is essential. Be precise.
- When did the shortness of breath start? Was it before the illness that precipitated the patient's admission? If so, how long?
- How did the shortness of breath start? Was it gradual or sudden?
- Has the patient had any associated pains in the chest?
- Is there any history of haemoptysis?
- How long has the patient had the fever? What about night sweats?
- Is inhalation of a foreign body a possibility?

Bacterial infection

Patients with chronic chest problems are particularly prone to infection. In younger, non-smoking patients who are otherwise well, infection may be precipitated by colds or 'flu.

Lung cancer

Consider lung cancer in a middle-aged smoker, particularly if there is any recent history of weight loss and/or anorexia. Be aware, however, that patients with lung cancer do not have to have these symptoms, and can be asymptomatic.

Foreign body

Infants, children and patients with learning difficulties or dementia are particularly at risk. Ask for a history of choking on a peanut, losing a dental filling, or of trauma while eating food.

(a)

(b)

Fig. 19 (a) Posteroanterior chest radiograph and (b) lateral chest radiograph of a left upper lobe collapse. Note the veil-like opacity of the left side. (Courtesy of Dr I. Vlahos.)

Table 12 Differential diagnosis of lobar collapse.

Classification	Example
Common	Infection, i.e. bacteria, tuberculosis
Must consider	Carcinoma of the lung, foreign body
Other causes	Other tumour, e.g. carcinoid, benign adenoma, pulmonary infarct

181

Other

'Odd' symptoms such as flushing, sweats or diarrhoea may be associated with carcinoid. Bronchial adenomas frequently produce haemoptysis.

Relevant past history

Has the patient any other history to support your diagnosis?
• Is the patient a current, ex- or never-smoker?
• Has the patient ever had asthma, bronchitis or any other respiratory problems?
• Is there a personal or family history of TB?

Examination

Full general, respiratory and cardiac examinations are needed (see Sections 1.1, p. 153 and 1.2, p. 155), but particular attention to the following is required:
• Does the patient look in good health or obviously unwell?
• What is the patient's breathing like now? Comfortable or laboured?
• Is the patient cachectic and pale?
• Is there clubbing?
• Is there lymphadenopathy?
• What are the signs in the chest? Is there any evidence of consolidation (bronchial breathing)?

Approach to investigations and management

Investigations of lobar collapse

• Bronchoscopy—in anyone with persistent shadowing
• Computed tomography scan of the chest—useful in many cases.

Investigations

Bronchoscopy

This may be performed as an inpatient if symptoms are slow to resolve, or as an outpatient if persistent shadowing is seen on the chest radiograph. If an endobronchial lesion is seen, it should be biopsied and sent for histology. Bronchial washings should also be sent for cytology (even if nothing was seen) and microscopy.

 Do not forget to request specifically testing for AFB if TB is in the differential diagnosis: it is not performed routinely.

Computed tomography scan of chest

In some centres a CT scan of the chest will be performed before bronchoscopy. This has the advantage of giving the physician performing bronchoscopy a better idea of the anatomical layout of the problem and where to concentrate on taking samples, although if there is lobar collapse this is not a problem. However, a scan should certainly be requested when lung cancer is likely, and this should also include cuts of the liver and adrenals to help stage any potential tumour.

Management

• Chest infection: see *Infectious diseases*, Section 1.4
• Lung cancer: see Section 2.9.1, p. 220
• Foreign body: bronchoscopic removal if possible
• Pulmonary infarct/emboli: see Section 1.5, p. 165
• TB: see *Infectious diseases*, Section 2.6.1.

Foreign bodies

These may be seen at flexible bronchoscopy, but may be difficult to remove. If so, the patient should be given broad-spectrum antibiotics and referred immediately for rigid bronchoscopy in a specialist centre. Long-term exclusion of bronchi can lead to bronchiectasis, associated with chronic cough and repeated chest infections.

1.13 Breathlessness with a normal radiograph

Case history

A 44-year-old woman presents with a 2-year history of exertional dyspnoea. Her chest radiograph is reported as being within normal limits. Her lung function shows:
• FEV_1 83% of predicted
• vital capacity (VC) 79% predicted
• FEV_1/VC ratio 78%
• DL_{CO} 73% predicted
• PaO_2 9.6 kPa
• $PaCO_2$ 4.1 kPa.

Clinical approach

The spirometry effectively rules out obstructive lung disease. Hyperventilation (and its causes) and anaemia are excluded as primary diagnoses by the finding of hypoxia. The differential probably lies between diffuse parenchymal lung disease or a problem of the pulmonary vasculature.

History of the presenting problem

In diffuse parenchymal lung disease the patient may have a dry cough, but there may be no specific features. It will clearly be worth enquiring about systemic or iatrogenic disorders associated with lung disease (see Section 1.4, p. 160). Specific employment histories or recreational interests may also suggest diffuse parenchymal lung disease (see Section 1.11, p. 178, for details of how to take an occupational history).

A history of asthma or rhinitis may suggest the rare possibility of Churg–Strauss syndrome.

Regarding diseases of the pulmonary vasculature: in pulmonary embolus there may be a history of pleuritic chest pain or haemoptysis, but a small proportion of patients present with chronic dyspnoea alone. Ask about risk factors for pulmonary embolism (see Section 1.5, p. 163). This patient could also have primary pulmonary hypertension: hence enquire about appetite suppressants.

Examination

Full general, respiratory and cardiac examinations are needed (see Sections 1.1, p. 153 and 1.2, p. 155), but particular attention to the following is required:
- Skin and joints—may be involved in patients with diffuse parenchymal lung disease (especially sarcoid)
- Clubbing—may feature in diffuse parenchymal lung disease
- Pulse—may be atrial fibrillation in pulmonary embolism
- Cyanosis—unlikely if the PaO_2 remains 9.6 kPa
- JVP—there may be grossly elevated venous pressure or tricuspid regurgitation in chronic pulmonary embolism or primary pulmonary hypertension
- Palpable right ventricular heave—may be present in chronic pulmonary embolism or primary pulmonary hypertension
- Heart sounds—may be a loud P2 in chronic pulmonary embolism or primary pulmonary hypertension
- Auscultation—may be fine inspiratory crackles in diffuse parenchymal lung disease or pleural rubs in pulmonary embolism
- Ankle oedema—may be present in chronic pulmonary embolism or primary pulmonary hypertension.

Approach to investigations and management

Investigations

The priority is to decide whether the patient is suffering from diffuse parenchymal lung disease or a problem of the pulmonary vasculature, and the findings on clinical examination will usually indicate which of these is most likely. The investigation of specific causes follows identification of the diagnostic type, e.g. avian precipitins are measured after the diagnosis of alveolitis is made. The following investigations will each be indicated in some cases: in any particular case start with the ones most likely to give the diagnosis.

Blood tests

It is usual to measure the full blood count, inflammatory markers (CRP and ESR) and simple biochemistry (renal and liver function). A calcium and serum ACE are measured where sarcoid is a possibility.

Electrocardiogram

This may show right heart strain in pulmonary embolism or primary pulmonary hypertension.

Pulmonary function tests

In the case described some lung function tests are given, but measurement of lung volumes by body plethysmography can be useful: fibrotic lung disease should show a reduction in total lung capacity.

High-resolution computed tomography scanning

The relative efficiency of high-resolution CT scanning and chest radiography for detecting diffuse parenchymal lung disease are 94 and 80%, respectively. High-resolution CT findings can predict the histological diagnosis in 82–93% of cases. (See Section 1.4, p. 162.)

Ventilation–perfusion scanning, helical computed tomography or lower leg ultrasound

For more details on the work-up of suspected pulmonary embolism, see Section 1.5, p. 165.

Echocardiography

This is a sensitive technique for detecting primary pulmonary hypertension. However, in view of the gravity of the diagnosis, direct measurement of pulmonary arterial pressure is usually performed both to confirm the diagnosis and to assess whether the patient responds to vasodilators (see *Cardiology*, Sections 1.10, 2.12 and 2.18). Echocardiography can also detect cardiac defects that can be occult causes of secondary pulmonary hypertension.

In primary pulmonary hypertension the patient should be formally assessed to see whether they respond to vasodilating agents. If not, the prognosis is very poor and transplantation or long-term prostacyclin infusion should be considered.

A quarter of cases of hoarseness lasting for more than 2–3 weeks result from cervical or thoracic neoplasm. Bronchoscopy or laryngoscopy is mandatory.

History of the presenting problem

From the patient's story you will need to clarify the following:
- How long have the symptoms been present? Which came first—the voice change, the stridor or the tiredness?
- Is the patient also dyspnoeic?
- Although this patient is obese, has she lost any weight?
- Has the patient any history of cough or haemoptysis?
- Is there any history of dysphagia? This might be due to an underlying mediastinal tumour pressing on the oesophagus.
- Has the patient always been tired? Tiredness is a non-specific symptom, but along with a change in voice and obesity could point to hypothyroidism. Further support for this diagnosis would be obtained if the patient has gained weight recently or been constipated. (See *Endocrinology*, Sections 1.14 and 2.3.1.)
- Has the patient noticed any lymphadenopathy or fever? (suggests lymphoma).
- Are there any signs of superior vena cava obstruction? Swelling of the face and arms, dilated chest wall veins, or raised venous pressure would indicate intrathoracic disease pressing upon the superior vena cava.
- Are there any features of myasthenia gravis? (diplopia or dysphagia).

Management

Depends on diagnosis.

See *Cardiology*, Sections 1.10, 2.12 and 2.18.

British Thoracic Society. Suspected acute pulmonary embolism: a practical approach. *Thorax* 1999; 52 (Suppl. 4): S1–S24.

British Thoracic Society. The diagnosis, assessment and treatment of diffuse parenchymal lung disease in adults. *Thorax* 1999; 54 (Suppl. 1): S1–S30.

Gardner WN. The pathophysiology of hyperventilation. *Chest* 1996; 109: 516–534.

Peacock AJ. Primary pulmonary hypertension. *Thorax* 1999; 54: 1107–1118.

Rich S, Dantzker DR, Ayres SM *et al*. Primary pulmonary hypertension. *Ann Intern Med* 1987; 107: 216–223.

1.14 Upper airway obstruction

Case history

A 56-year-old woman presents with a 5-day history of stridor. She is obese and complains of recent hoarseness of her voice. She also complains of being tired all the time.

Clinical approach

- Wheeze indicates intrathoracic airflow obstruction, and is loudest on expiration.
- Stridor indicates extrathoracic airflow obstruction, and is loudest on inspiration.

This middle-aged patient has stridor, which is a musical sound best heard on inspiration as compared with wheeze, which is heard on expiration. It is caused by the turbulence of air passing through a narrow glottis or trachea, and indicates extrathoracic obstruction. The narrowing of the airway may be intrinsic or extrinsic, and it should be investigated urgently as it may be due to an underlying malignancy.

This patient also complains of a change in her voice and this demands urgent investigation.

Causes of stridor
- Intrinsic narrowing of airway: tumour, stenosis or foreign body
- Extrinsic compression of airway: any neck or mediastinal mass
- Mediastinal fibrosis.

Relevant past history

Check the following:
- Has the patient ever had any thyroid disorder/surgery?
- Stridor can be due to tracheal stenosis secondary to intubation: has the patient ever been intubated, had an operation, or been on a breathing machine?
- Has the patient ever suffered from a lymphoma?
- Does the patient smoke or has she smoked in the past?

Examination

Full general, respiratory and cardiac examinations are needed (see Sections 1.1, p. 153 and 1.2, p. 155), but particular attention to the following is required.

General

- Look for any features of hypothyroidism. (See *Endocrinology*, Sections 1.14 and 2.3.1.)
- Is the thyroid visible or palpable?
- Is there clubbing?
- Look carefully for cervical and axillary lymphadenopathy. Check the abdomen and inguinal regions if you find nodes.
- Is there superior vena cava obstruction? (See *Oncology*, Section 1.8.)

Respiratory

Does she indeed have stridor? Ask her to cough and then take a deep breath with her mouth open—this exaggerates stridor. If there is tight obstruction there may be paradoxical indrawing of the upper thorax during inspiration.

Check for normal symmetrical movement of the chest and mediastinal shift.

Approach to investigations and management

Investigations

Blood tests

Thyroid function tests, full blood count, serum calcium, renal and liver function tests, acetylcholine receptor antibodies if suspicion of myasthenia.

Flow–volume loops

These can be helpful if the picture is not acute. An example of upper airway obstruction is shown in Fig. 20.

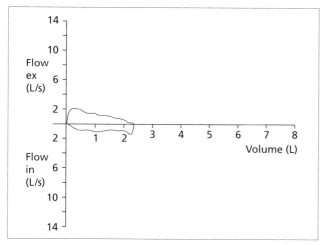

Fig. 20 Flow–volume loop of a patient complaining of exertional dyspnoea. Diagnosis: tracheal stenosis.

Bronchoscopy or laryngoscopy

Mandatory in undiagnosed upper airway obstruction. If the patient is unwell it is prudent to have anaesthetic assistance for this examination.

Tensilon test

This is indicated in suspected myasthenia gravis with underlying thymoma. (See *Neurology*, Section 2.2.5.)

Chest radiograph

This may show mediastinal mass (including thymoma) or lymphadenopathy.

Computed tomography

This is only helpful if intrathoracic disease is identified, or for the staging of localized head and neck disease.

Radionuclide scanning

Thyroid scans can be used to look for retrosternal goitre. Mediastinal thyroid tissue can be of two origins: usually cervical goitre, which extends substernally and brings its blood supply from the neck; more rarely primary intrathoracic goitre, which has its own blood supply (helpful to plan surgery).

Management

As always, the treatment is of the problem diagnosed.
- Laser therapy or stenting can be used for postintubation stenosis.
- If the problem is at the level of the vocal cords, then tracheostomy can be helpful if the problem itself cannot be treated.
- If there is tracheal stenosis that cannot be treated, then the use of a helium–oxygen mixture (which has a low resistance to flow) may provide palliation.

1.15 Difficult decisions

Case history

A 73-year-old man with COPD is admitted with an acute hypercapnic exacerbation. He has previously been confined to his home because of exertional dyspnoea despite the use of domiciliary oxygen and nebulized bronchodilators. He fails to improve with conventional therapy and non-

2 Diseases and treatments

2.1 Upper airway

2.1.1 OBSTRUCTIVE SLEEP APNOEA

Aetiology

OSA results from pharyngeal collapse during sleep, with a consequent abolition or reduction of inspiratory airflow. This process is associated with arousals from sleep and, in turn, daytime sleepiness [1].

The major predisposing factor is obesity but, independent of this, the syndrome is more common in men, perhaps because of gender differences in fat deposition. Other predisposing/exacerbating factors include:
- craniofacial abnormalities
- alcohol and sedative use
- hypothyroidism
- acromegaly
- nasal congestion.

Epidemiology

One to five per cent of adult men have the sleep apnoea syndrome, but the prevalence of OSA is a function of the prevalence of obesity. However, it should be emphasized that not all patients with OSA are sleepy and that some sleepy patients do not have OSA [2].

Clinical presentation

Common
- Snoring
- Excessive daytime somnolence
- Restless or unrefreshing sleep
- Report of witnessed apnoeas from bed partner.

Uncommon
- Nocturnal choking sensation
- Nocturia
- Reduced libido
- Morning headache.

Rare
- Insomnia
- Nocturnal cough
- Gastro-oesophageal reflux
- Polycythaemia.

 Not all patients who are sleepy have OSA. Do not forget to ask questions pertinent to other causes of hypersomnolence and check that the sleep opportunity is adequate.

Physical signs

The patient should have a full respiratory and cardiovascular examination with particular emphasis on:
- general appearance—features of hypothyroidism or acromegaly?
- the upper airway—can the patient breathe through the nose? Is there tonsillar enlargement? Is there retrognathia?
- collar size—when adjusted for height, neck circumference is predictive of OSA (for example a 17-inch collar size in a man 1.78 m tall would give a positive predictive value of >66% of OSA [3])
- evidence of hypertension or cardiac failure
- evidence of coexistent lung disease.

Investigations

Confirming the diagnosis

Some form of overnight study is required. The gold standard test is full polysomnography. The advantage of this test is that it confirms electroencephalographically that the patient is asleep and also identifies other diagnoses (e.g. narcolepsy–cataplexy or periodic limb movement) that might contribute to daytime somnolence.

However, polysomnography is expensive and many patients can be diagnosed using a limited respiratory sleep study or simple oximetry (Fig. 22). It is important to understand the limitations of the diagnostic study employed if the patient subsequently fails to respond to therapy.

Staging the disease

ECG, chest radiograph, FBC—where appropriate consider arterial blood gases, echocardiography, thyroid function tests.

Fig. 22 Traces from a respiratory sleep study in a patient with sleep apnoea. The oximetry trace (a) shows frequent desaturation associated with snoring (b) and obstructive apnoeas (c). The apnoea–hypopnoea index was calculated to be 76/h.

Differential diagnosis

Excessive daytime somnolence

- Inadequate sleep opportunity
- Narcolepsy
- Periodic limb movement
- Idiopathic hypersomnolence.

Disturbed sleep

Chronic respiratory failure due to lung, neuromuscular or other disease.

Treatment

 The first principle of treating any sleep disorder is to establish good sleep habits (known as 'sleep hygiene').

General

- The patient's sleep habits ('hygiene') should be reviewed. The patient should have an adequate sleep opportunity and an appropriate sleeping environment; use of a patient information leaflet may be helpful.
- Where appropriate weight loss should be encouraged.
- The need for treatment is determined by symptoms (usually excessive daytime somnolence) or end-organ complication (e.g. polycythaemia).
- Patients in the UK should advise the DVLA and their motor insurer of their diagnosis.

Dental devices

These devices vary in design but are usually custom made for each patient (Fig. 23). Although they are substantially less effective in edentuluous patients this is not an absolute contraindication. They work by holding the tongue and mandible forward, enlarging the retroglossal space.

Fig. 23 Example of a mandibular advancement device.

Nasal continuous positive airways pressure

This therapy involves the application of positive pressure via a tightly fitting nasal mask which acts as a pneumatic splint to hold the airway open. This therapy has been shown in randomized trials to reduce daytime somnollence [1].

It is usual to perform a titration study to determine the optimal nasal CPAP level and, in many centres, a further study to confirm efficacy of treatment. Compliance with therapy is a function of support offered to patients [4]: it is therefore the view of the College that nasal CPAP services are centralized in specialist centres. Bilevel ventilatory support is sometimes used for OSA patients who require a high level of nasal CPAP.

Surgery

- Surgery to alleviate nasal obstruction may reduce nasal symptoms but is of limited value for OSA.
- Uvulopalatoplasty (UVPP) is sometimes recommended, but current opinion is that subsequent therapy with nasal CPAP is made more difficult by prior UVPP.
- Tracheotomy is the final option for patients with life-threatening OSA who are intolerant of nasal CPAP and other measures.

Complications

Common

- Road traffic accidents; patients with an apnoea/hypopnoea index >10/h have an odds ratio >6 for motor vehicle accidents [5]
- Hypertension [6]
- Snoring (with possible social/marital problems)
- Sexual dysfunction
- Polycythaemia
- Occasional nasal bridge ulceration from mask.

Prognosis

No controlled data on morbidity exist, but in one study 3.3% of 1211 patients with OSA died during a median follow-up of 22 months [4]. Twenty per cent of patients started on CPAP do not continue with treatment.

Prevention

Reducing the weight of the general population would reduce the incidence of OSA.

1 Bennett LS. Adult obstructive sleep apnoea syndrome. *J R Coll Physicians Lond* 1999; 33: 439–444.
2 Davies RJO, Stradling JR. The epidemiology of sleep apnoea. *Thorax* 1996; 51 (Suppl. 2): S65–S70.
3 Davies RJO, Ali NJ, Stradling JR. Neck circumference and other clinical features in the diagnosis of obstructive sleep apnoea syndrome. *Thorax* 1992; 47: 101–105.
4 McArdle N, Devereux G, Heidarnejad H, Engleman HM, Mackay TW, Douglas NJ. Long-term use of CPAP therapy for sleep apnea/hypopnoea syndrome. *Am J Respir Crit Care Med* 1999; 159: 1108–1114.
5 Teran-Santos J, Jiminez-Gomez A, Cordero-Guevara J and the cooperative group Burgos-Santander. The association between sleep apnea and the risk of traffic accidents. *N Engl J Med* 1999; 340: 847–851.
6 Nieto FJ, Young TB, Lind BK *et al.* Association of sleep-disordered breathing, sleep apnea, and hypertension in a large community-based study. Sleep Heart Health Study. *JAMA* 2000; 283: 1829–1836.

2.2 Atopy and asthma

2.2.1 ALLERGIC RHINITIS

Aetiology

Allergic rhinitis can be seasonal (hayfever) or perennial, with around 10% of the population suffering from symptoms. Hayfever is found in up to 20% of young people over the summer months and is often caused by tree and grass pollen and mould spores [1]. Perennial causes include the faeces of the house-dust mite, domestic pets or occupational exposure to dust, fumes and aerosols [2]. It is therefore important to take an occupational history.

Clinical presentation

Patients present with sneezing, itching, watery rhinorrhoea and nasal obstruction.

Physical signs

Look for nasal polyps that can both cause and exacerbate rhinitis.

Investigations

The majority of patients are treated with success empirically; for patients refractory to therapy consider the differential diagnosis (below) and consider occupational history, skin-prick testing, full blood count and eosinophil count.

Differential diagnosis

Other non-allergic causes of rhinitis include infection, nasal polyps, foreign bodies or anatomical variants, nasal tumours, granulomatous diseases, vasomotor (secondary to 'over-the-counter' medication), idiopathic.

Treatment

- Allergen avoidance—not always possible.
- Topical (nasal) steroids—often very effective. Side effects are local irritation and nose bleeds. Check for compliance and technique if there is a failure to improve.
- Oral antihistamines—warn about sedative side effects of some preparations and interactions with other drugs, i.e. terfenadine with erythromycin results in prolonged QT interval.
- Cromoglycates—no major side effects, but require frequent use. Eye drops are particularly effective in allergic conjuctivitis.
- Immunotherapy—desensitization is sometimes possible in selected patients. The technique must be performed in specialist centres.

1 Furham SR. Summer hay fever. In: Durham SR, ed. *ABC of Allergies.* London: BMJ Books, 1998: 16–18.
2 Mackay IS, Durham SR. Perennial rhinitis. In Durham SR, ed. *ABC of Allergies.* London: BMJ Books, 1998: 19–22.

2.2.2 ASTHMA

Aetiology

Asthma is defined as reversible airway obstruction associated with airway inflammation and bronchial hyper-responsiveness [1]. The hyperresponsiveness of the airways is caused by a variety of local stimuli including histamine, leukotrienes and prostaglandins. This produces the reversible airflow obstruction that leads to the characteristic symptoms of shortness of breath, chest tightness and wheeze. Risk factors include:
- a genetic predisposition
- a family or personal history of atopy
- maternal smoking, ethnicity
- socioeconomic status
- male sex.

The role of other factors such as diet and pollution (black smoke, fine particulate matter, ozone and sulphates) remains controversial. While not directly linked to an increased prevalence of the disease, they certainly exacerbate asthmatic symptoms, with increased asthma mortality in areas of high industrial pollution. Other precipitants of asthma attacks include house-dust mites, pollens, moulds, fungi, cat and dog dander, aspirin and non-steroidal anti-inflammatory drugs (NSAIDs) in sensitive patients (approximately 5%), and occupational exposure [2].

Epidemiology

The prevalence of asthma continues to rise worldwide, particularly in developed countries. Approximately 10% of the adult population in the UK have asthma and, despite effective medication, there are still approximately 1600 deaths from the disease each year (these figures do not include COPD).

This continued morbidity and mortality highlights the importance of education of both patients and their doctors, with an emphasis on adequate treatment regimens, good compliance, even with maintenance regimens, and rapid access to medical help when deterioration occurs.

 Patients are at particular risk of dying from asthma if they:
- are taking more than three classes of drugs
- have required hospital admission in the last year
- have psychosocial problems (compliance?)
- have ever had life-threatening asthma.

Clinical presentations

- Severe acute attacks—acute breathlessness and wheeze; hypoxia and/or carbon dioxide retention can lead to stupor and/or confusion

- Chronic asthma—shortness of breath, wheeze, chronic cough, particularly at night when associated with disturbed sleep pattern. Symptoms may be produced by exposure to cold air or exercise.

 An isolated dry cough is perhaps the most overlooked symptom of mild asthma (especially in children). Particularly after colds and 'flu, patients may be left with an annoying dry cough and are frequently referred to specialists for further investigation. Bronchial hyperresponsiveness is often the cause and responds to a course of low-dose inhaled steroids. It is difficult to label such individuals as truly asthmatic (a controversial issue amongst respiratory physicians), although subsequent lung function tests may be helpful. However, patients should be warned that their symptoms may return with a subsequent cold or chest infection.

Physical signs

Life-threatening asthma

- Peak flow <33% of predicted or personal best
- Silent chest
- Cyanosis
- Altered level of consciousness; confusion; coma
- Exhaustion; inability to speak
- Hypotension or bradycardia.

Severe acute attack

- Peak flow <50% of predicted or personal best
- Tachycardia
- Increased respiratory rate: >25 breaths/min
- Cannot complete sentences in one breath
- Use of accessory muscles of respiration, intercostal recession (especially children)
- Increased pulse rate: >110 beats/min.

Moderate

- Peak flow 50–70% of predicted or personal best
- Wheeze
- Dyspnoea
- Chest tightness.

 The British Guidelines on Asthma Management [3] are invaluable, but remember, the patient in front of you is an individual. If you are worried in any way about someone with asthma, especially at night—admit him or her. This is particularly so for those who have an attack that has been going on for some time, if they live alone, do not have a telephone or would find it difficult to return to the hospital. Do not feel pressurized by the patient, nursing staff or the hospital's bed state to send them home.

Investigations

Measure arterial blood gases if patient presents with life-threatening signs, or Sao_2 <94%.
  Blood gas markers for life-threatening asthma are:
- Normal or high $Paco_2$ (≥5–6 kPa/36–45 mmHg)
- Low pH
- Severe hypoxia in spite of oxygen treatment (Pao_2 <8 kPa/60 mmHg).

Chest radiograph

In outpatients, a chest radiograph helps exclude other causes of wheeze, such as infiltrates resulting from eosinophilia or fibrosis. For patients presenting acutely a pneumothorax should be excluded and evidence of infection looked for.

Peak flow

This can be used diagnostically to look for morning dips. Motivated chronic asthmatics can also monitor their progress at home. In patients who clearly do not take measurements on a daily basis, make sure they know their best peak flow and encourage them to at least monitor when they get coughs and cold.

All patients should be given a management plan based on deterioration of their peak flow: credit-card-sized self-management plans are produced by the National Asthma Campaign (Fig. 24).

Lung function tests

These should be performed pre- and postbronchodilator (e.g. salbutamol). They are not helpful acutely, but important as a diagnostic tool to look for evidence of reversibility and to monitor chronic asthmatics.

Allergy testing

Skin-prick tests can help identify allergens that may precipitate asthma attacks, although in practice many of these are not easily avoided.

Differential diagnosis

This includes COPD, congestive heart failure, upper airway obstruction, i.e. foreign body, tumour; pneumothorax, bronchiectasis, pulmonary eosinophilia, Wegener's granulomatosis, Churg–Strauss syndrome.

Treatment

The stepwise approach to the treatment of chronic asthma

(a)

(b)

Fig. 24 Credit-card-sized self-management plan produced by the National Asthma Campaign: (a) front; (b) back. These cards are available free on request from their offices. (With permission of the National Asthma Campaign.)

remains the gold standard (Table 13). For all steps above step 1, inhaled steroids are advocated for controlling airway inflammation and therefore chronic asthma.

The management can be divided into:
- 'relievers' (short-acting β agonists)
- 'preventers' (inhaled steroids)
- 'controllers' (long-acting β agonists and leukotriene receptor antagonists).

It is important to explain to patients that the preventers and controllers must be taken regularly, while the relievers are helpful for acute symptomatic relief. Oral preparations include oral steroids, aminophylline, and the leukotriene receptor antagonists.

In acute severe asthma (Table 14), the patient should not be left sitting in a side room in accident and emergency (A&E). He or she should be in the resuscitation room and monitored for cardiac rhythm and oxygen saturation. The most senior member of the medical team in the hospital (usually the Medical Registrar) should be informed of the patient's condition and urgent anaesthetic and intensive care review should be requested if the patient does not improve rapidly or if the presenting symptoms appear life threatening. Anaesthetists would rather be called to a sick patient than one who has suffered a respiratory arrest.

Table 13 British asthma guidelines for the stepwise management of chronic asthma in adults and school children. (From *Thorax* 1997; 52 (Suppl. 1) S11, Chart 1. With permission of the BMJ Publishing Group.)

Step	Management	Discussion
Step 1	Occasional use of relief bronchodilators	Inhaled short-acting β antagonists 'as required' for symptom relief are acceptable. If they are needed more than once daily move to Step 2. Before altering a treatment step ensure that the patient is having the treatment and has a good inhaler technique. Address any fears
Step 2	Regular inhaled anti-inflammatory agents	Inhaled short-acting β agonists as required, plus beclometasone or budesonide increased to 100–400 µg twice daily or fluticasone 50–200 µg twice daily. Alternatively, use cromoglycate or nedocromil sodium, but if control is not achieved start inhaled steroids
Step 3	High-dose inhaled steroids or low-dose inhaled steroids plus long-acting inhaled β antagonist bronchodilator	Inhaled short-acting β agonists as required, plus either beclometasone or budesonide increased to 800–2000 µg daily or fluticasone 400–1000 µg daily via a large volume spacer; or beclometasone or budesonide increased to 100–400 µg twice daily or fluticasone 50–200 µg twice daily plus salmeterol 50 µg twice daily. In the very small number of patients who experience side effects with high-dose inhaled steroids, either the long-acting inhaled β-agonist option is used, or a sustained release theophylline may be added to Step 2 medication. Cromoglycate or nedocromil may also be tried
Step 4	High-dose inhaled steroid and regular bronchodilators	Inhaled short-acting β agonists as required with inhaled beclometasone or budesonide increased to 800–2000 µg daily or fluticasone 400–1000 µg daily via a large-volume spacer; plus a sequential therapeutic trial of one or more of: • Inhaled long-acting β agonists • Sustained release theophylline • Inhaled ipratropium or oxitropium • Long-acting β-agonist tablets • High-dose inhaled bronchodilators • Cromoglycate or nedocromil
Step 5	Addition of regular steroid tablets	Inhaled short-acting β agonists as required with inhaled beclometasone or budesonide increased to 800–2000 µg daily or fluticasone 400–1000 µg daily via a large-volume spacer and one or more of the long-acting bronchodilators; plus regular prednisolone tablets in a single daily dose
Stepping down		Review treatment every 3–6 months. If control is achieved a stepwise reduction in treatment may be possible. In patients whose treatment was recently started at Step 4 or 5 or included steroid tablets for gaining control of asthma this reduction may take place after a short interval. In other patients with chronic asthma a 3–6-month period of stability should be shown before slow stepwise reduction is undertaken

Newer treatments for asthma

The leukotriene receptor antagonists are the most recent drugs to be added to the therapeutic armamentarium for asthma [4]. They include montelukast and zafirlukast and work by reducing the production of leukotrienes which cause bronchoconstriction, mucus hypersecretion and airway oedema. They may have an anti-inflammatory action (↓ eosinophils). Side effects include abdominal discomfort, diarrhoea and headaches. Their position in the stepwise treatment of asthma has yet to be decided; they may be useful in chronic asthmatics not controlled on inhaled steroids (step 3), as well as exercise-induced and aspirin-sensitive asthma. They have no place in the treatment of acute severe asthma.

1 Rees J, Kanabar D, eds. *ABC of Asthma* (4th edn). London: BMJ Publications, 2000.
2 Jarad NA. Occupational asthma. *J R Coll Physicians Lond* 1999; 33: 537–540.
3 The British Thoracic Society, the National Asthma Campaign, the Royal College of Physicians of London, in association with the General Practitioner in Asthma Group, the British Association of Accident and Emergency Medicine, the British Paediatric Society and the Royal College of Paediatric and Child Health. The British guidelines on asthma management 1995 review and position statement. *Thorax* 1997; 52: Supplement 1.
4 Lipworth BJ. Leukotriene-receptor antagonists. *Lancet* 1999; 353: 57–62.

Stage	Guidelines
1. Immediate treatment	Oxygen 40–60% (CO_2 retention is not usually aggravated by oxygen therapy in asthma) Salbutamol 5 mg or terbutaline 10 mg via an oxygen-driven nebulizer Prednisolone tablets 30–60 mg or intravenous hydrocortisone 200 mg or both if very ill No sedatives of any kind Chest radiograph to exclude pneumothorax *If life-threatening features are present* Add ipratropium 0.5 mg to the nebulized β agonist Give intravenous aminophylline 250 mg over 20 min or salbutamol or terbutaline 250 μg over 10 min. Do not give bolus aminophylline to patients already taking oral theophyllines
2. Subsequent management	*If patient is improving continue* 40–60% oxygen Prednisolone 30–60 mg daily or intravenous hydrocortisone 200 mg 6 hourly Nebulized β agonist 4 hourly *If patient is not improving after 15–30 min* Continue oxygen and steroids Give nebulized β agonist more frequently, up to every 15–30 min Add ipratropium 0.5 mg to nebulizer and repeat 6 hourly until patient is improving *If patient is still not improving give* Aminophylline infusion (small patient 750 mg/24 h, large patient 1500 mg/24 h); monitor blood concentrations if it is continued for over 24 h Salbutamol or terbutaline infusion as an alternative to aminophylline
3. Monitoring treatment	Repeat measurement of PEF 15–30 min after starting treatment Oximetry: maintain Sao_2 >92% Repeat blood gas measurements within 2 h of starting treatment if: Initial Pao_2 <8 kPa (60 mmHg) unless subsequent Sao_2 >92%, or $Paco_2$ normal or raised, or Patient deteriorates Chart PEF before and after giving nebulized or inhaled β agonist and at least four times daily throughout hospital stay
4. When discharged from hospital, patients should have	Been on discharge medication for 24 h and have had inhaler technique checked and recorded PEF >75% of predicted or best and PEF diurnal variability <25% unless discharge is agreed with respiratory physician Treatment with oral and inhaled steroids in addition to bronchodilators Own PEF meter and written self management plan GP follow-up arranged within 1 week Follow-up appointment in respiratory clinic within 4 weeks

PEF, peak expiratory flow.

Table 14 British Thoracic Society guidelines for the management of acute severe asthma in adults. (From *Thorax* 1997; 52 (Suppl. 1): S12, Chart 2. With permission of the BMJ Publishing Group.)

2.3 Chronic obstructive pulmonary disease

Aetiology

The major aetiologic factor is tobacco consumption. Also consider α_1-antitrypsin deficiency (exacerbated by smoking). Smokers vary in their susceptibility to COPD; only 15% developing clinically relevant disease [1]. Coal miners have increased risk.

Pathophysiology

The hallmark of COPD is expiratory flow limitation; this results in a reduced FEV_1 and other characteristic lung function abnormalities (see below). However, the disease is slowly progressive and the picture therefore depends on the severity of the disease at the time of assessment [2].

Epidemiology

Prevalence is approximately 6% in men and 3% in women, being determined by smoking rates.

Clinical presentation

Because the severity of COPD necessarily passes from mild to severe, patients who present with severe disease are those that have not been identified at an earlier stage.
• Common—recurrent respiratory infections, morning cough, exertional dyspnoea
• Uncommon—picked up because of sleep disordered breathing or need for other medical intervention (e.g. elective surgery); these patients may have tolerated the common symptoms above
• Rare—cor pulmonale, ventilatory failure.

Physical signs

May be none in early disease.
• Common—hyperinflation, wheeze, coarse crackles
• Uncommon (unless disease advanced)—cyanosis, weight loss, cor pulmonale (oedema and raised JVP). Hoover's sign refers to the paradoxical inward movement of the lower lateral rib cage during inspiration.

Investigations

Spirometric tests

Depending on severity there will be a reduction in FEV_1 that is disproportionate to the fall in VC, leading to a FEV_1/VC ratio of <70%. A normal FEV_1 effectively excludes COPD but a normal peak flow can occur in mild disease. Residual volume (RV), functional residual capacity (FRC) and total lung capacity (TLC) are elevated in COPD but these measurements are not routinely made in primary care; similarly the flow–volume loop shows characteristic scalloping of the expiratory limb (Fig. 25 and see Section 3.6.2).

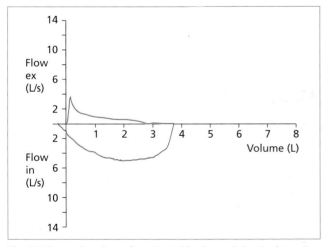

Fig. 25 Flow–volume loop of a patient with advanced chronic obstructive pulmonary disease (COPD). In this case expiratory flow limitation is severe, and marked scalloping of the curve is observed virtually throughout expiration.

Dynamic hyperinflation as a mechanism of dyspnoea in COPD

As COPD patients are flow limited during expiration, end-expiratory lung volume (EELV) has to increase when the demand placed on the respiratory system is increased (as during exercise). For a patient with severe COPD the increase in EELV could be as much as a litre.

Bronchodilator challenge

Perform this when the patient is stable. Look for improvement in FEV_1, a positive result requiring >10% and >200 mL increase. Patients can experience symptomatic relief despite a 'negative' study; if benefit needs to be documented it can be helpful to measure exercise capacity (for example by the shuttle walk test [3]).

Steroid challenge

Indicated in disease of more than moderate severity. Give prednisolone 30 mg once a day for 2 weeks; a positive result must be >10% and >200 mL increase in FEV_1.

Steroids have multiple side effects. Think which of these you are going to warn the patient about. If you are anxious that a patient is going to be susceptible to a particular side effect you may wish to give high-dose inhaled steroids instead (e.g. beclamethasone 1000 µg twice a day for 6 weeks via a spacer).

Chest radiograph

This can exclude alternative pathology. Look for bullae in advanced disease and hyperinflation (low flat diaphragms, increased number of ribs visible). An example is shown in Fig. 26.

Arterial blood gases

If SaO_2 is 92% or less, patients may benefit from domiciliary oxygen and should have their arterial/earlobe gas measured on room air. Guidelines for the administration of domiciliary oxygen are found in Section 2.12.1, p. 231.

Differential diagnosis

Because the symptoms of COPD are relatively non-specific, virtually any cardiac or pulmonary condition could feature in the differential. From a practical point of view it is important to ensure that other causes of airflow limitation, especially asthma, are not overlooked.

Fig. 26 Chest radiograph of a patient with emphysema. Note the low, flat diaphragms and hyperinflation. Few lung markings are seen at the bases indicating the possibility of bulbous disease.

Treatment

Emergency

See *Emergency medicine*, Section 1.10.

Stable patients

All patients with COPD should stop smoking; this is the single most important determinant of outcome. Nicotine replacement used in conjunction with a smoking cessation clinic can increase quit rates. 'Flu vaccination is recommended.

 Tell patients to stop smoking when you see them for other reasons. Doctors' advice is a potent stimulus to quit.

Treatment options for COPD are stratified by stage as shown in Table 15. On-going studies examining the role of inhaled steroids in COPD may influence management in the future [4].

In patients with very advanced disease, specialist assessment is indicated if preliminary investigations suggest that lung volume reduction surgery (LVRS), transplantation or non-invasive ventilatory support is indicated.

• LVRS is a new therapy that is most effective in patients with heterogeneous lung disease predominantly involving the upper lobes. It is currently offered only at a few centres in the UK.

• Non-invasive ventilatory support is indicated (see Section 2.12.3, p. 234) in patients with daytime hypercapnia and symptoms attributable to this, particularly if they have recurrent admissions.

• Lung transplantation (see Section 2.13, p. 236) is an option for some patients.

Complications

• Common—infection (bacterial and viral), steroid side effects
• Uncommon—cor pulmonale, pneumothorax, ventilatory failure, polycythaemia, heart failure
• Rare—pulmonary hypertension, peripheral neuropathy.

Prognosis

In general is inversely related to age and postbronchodilator FEV_1 such that:
• age <60 and FEV_1 >50% predicted → 90% 3-year survival
• age >60 and FEV_1 >50% predicted → 80% 3-year survival
• age >60 and FEV_1 <50% predicted → 75% 3-year survival.

Table 15 The spectrum of chronic obstructive pulmonary disease (COPD).

Symptoms	FEV_1 (representative) (% predicted)	Management options (to consider)
Healthy	100%	Stop smoking
Smoker's cough	75%	Antibiotics for infection, inhaled bronchodilators
Exertional dyspnoea Some signs, sputum	50%	Combination BDs Steroid reversibility 'Flu vaccination Pulmonary rehabilitation
Dyspnoea on minimal exertion or rest Wheeze, cyanosis Hyperinflation	25%	Nebulized BDs Assess for domiciliary O_2 Assess for lung volume reduction surgery

BDs, bronchodilators.

The 5-year survival in patients admitted with a hypercapnic exacerbation is 28% [5].

is the end result of various pathologic processes [1–3], as listed in Table 16.

1 British Thoracic Society. BTS Guidelines for the management of chronic obstructive pulmonary disease. *Thorax* 1997; 52: S1–S28.
2 Burrows B, Earle RH. Course and prognosis of chronic obstructive lung disease. A prospective study of 200 patients. *N Engl J Med* 1969; 280: 397–404.
3 Singh SJ, Morgan MDL, Scott S, Walters D, Hardman AE. Development of a shuttle walking test of disability in patients with chronic airways obstruction. *Thorax* 1992; 47: 1019–1024.
4 Burge, PS. EUROSCOP, ISOLDE and the Copenhagen City Lung Study. *Thorax* 1999; 54: 287–288.
5 Warren PM, Flenley DC, Millar JS, Avery A. Respiratory failure revisited: acute excerbations of chronic bronchitis between 1961 and 68 and 1970–76. *Lancet* 1980; i: 467–471.

2.4 Bronchiectasis

Aetiology

Bronchiectasis is the term used to describe abnormal irreversible dilatation of the bronchi because of the destruction of the muscular and elastic components of their wall. It was first described by Laennec in 1819 and

Pathology

The primary problem in bronchiectasis is subnormal respiratory defences against infections. This may be caused by:
• immunoglobulin deficiency
• impaired mucociliary clearance
• bronchial obstruction.

As a result the airway contains excess mucus and this results in bronchial infection, with recruitment of neutrophils and monocytes into the lungs. Proteolytic enzymes such as elastase and cytokines are released into the lung and result in the destruction of the elastic and muscular components of the bronchial wall. Recurrent episodes of this type finally result in bronchiectasis.

Clinical presentation

Symptoms

• Patients mildly affected may present with symptoms (Table 17) only during exacerbation.
• Severely affected patients may have some or all the symptoms continuously and may develop cor pulmonale.

Signs

See Table 18.

Table 16 Conditions associated with bronchiectasis.

Classification	Examples
Postinfectious	Tuberculosis, measles, whooping cough, bronchiolitis in infancy caused by respiratory syncytial virus, bacterial pneumonia
Bronchial obstruction	Foreign body, adenoma, enlarged external lymph nodes, middle lobe syndrome
Allergic bronchopulmonary aspergillosis	—
Impaired host defence	Hypogammaglobulinaemia, Kartagener's, Young's syndrome, primary ciliary dyskinesia (syndrome characterized by bronchiectasis, situs inversus and recurrent sinusitis)
Cystic fibrosis	—
Rare conditions	Rheumatoid arthritis (3.1% of patients), Sjögren's syndrome, relapsing polychondritis, systemic lupus erythematosus, Marfan's syndrome, ulcerative colitis, Crohn's disease, sarcoidosis, yellow-nail syndrome (lymphoedema, yellow nails and pleural effusions), toxic gas inhalation (ammonia), gastric aspiration, tracheobronchomegaly (Mounier–Kuhn syndrome), congenital cartilage deficiency (Williams—Campbell syndrome), bronchopulmonary sequestration, α_1-antitrypsin deficiency

Table 17 Symptoms of bronchiectasis.

Common
Cough
Sputum production
   Mild: <10 mL/24 h
   Moderate: 10–150 mL/24 h
   Severe: >150 mL/24 h
Dyspnoea
Haemoptysis
Fever and pleuritic chest pain during infective exacerbation

Uncommon
Sinusitis in 30%
Halitosis

Rare
Discoloured nails in yellow-nail syndrome
Infertility in Young's syndrome
Male infertility (in cystic fibrosis)
Profuse recurrent haemoptysis without purulent sputum (bronchiectasis haemorrhagica sicca)
Other features of associated conditions

Table 18 Signs of bronchiectasis.

Common
Wheeze
Crackles
Nasal polyps or sinusitis
Clubbing in 10% of patients

Uncommon
Peripheral oedema in cor pulmonale
Cyanosis in hypoxaemia

Rare (i.e. syndrome specific)
Examples include rheumatoid hands, butterfly rash, Marfanoid features

Investigations

Investigations in bronchiectasis are carried out to diagnose its presence and extent, and also to find an underlying aetiology (Figs 27 and 28, Table 19).

Treatment

Options include the following:
- Postural drainage—this should be performed at least twice daily. It helps prevent chest infections by removing secretions.
- Antibiotics—helpful during infective exacerbation. They are best used by basing choice on previous sputum culture result.
- Bronchodilators—β_2 agonists, anticholinergics and theophyllines in cases with airway obstruction.
- Oxygen/non-invasive ventilation (NIV)—the guidelines used in practice are based on data obtained from patients with COPD (qv, see Sections 2.12.1 and 2.12.3). Patients with bronchiectasis can be difficult to ventilate successfully using NIV, although this should not preclude its use for palliative purposes or as a bridge to transplantation.

Fig. 27 Plain chest radiograph of a woman with bronchiectasis. Abnormalities are most prominent in the right lower zone.

Fig. 28 Computed tomography scan of a patient with gross bilateral bronchiectasis. Many of the bronchi have a classic 'signet ring' appearance generated by an enlarged bronchus and a neighbouring vessel.

- Diuretics (with care) in the presence of cor pulmonale.
- Surgery—resection of a lobe in genuinely localized bronchiectasis or in life-threatening haemoptysis. Lung transplantation is an option (see Section 2.13, p. 236).

Specific treatments

- Regular immunoglobulin infusion in agammaglobulinaemia
- Prednisolone in allergic bronchopulmonary aspergillosis.

Complications

The complications of bronchiectasis are:
- recurrent pneumonia
- empyema and lung abscess
- pneumothorax

Table 19 Investigations in bronchiectasis.

Test type	Description	Possible finding
Generic	Chest radiograph	May be normal Tram lines, linear radioluciences (cylindrical bronchiectasis) Toothpaste lines: thick parallel markings (varicose bronchiectasis) Cysts (cystic bronchiectasis) May show features of rheumatoid arthritis, sarcoidosis, and pleural effusion in yellow-nail syndrome etc.
	High-resolution computed tomography scan	Is the investigation of choice. It is non-invasive and has a sensitivity of 84% and specificity of 82% in detecting bronchiectasis
	Lung function tests	Obstructive pattern without hyperinflation
	Arterial blood gases	In advanced disease may show hypoxia and/or hypercapnia
	Sputum cultures	May grow *Staphylococcus aureus*, *Pseudomonas aeruginosa* as well as more common respiratory pathogens
Specific (for certain diseases)	Serum immunoglobulins	May show IgG/IgG subclass/IgA deficiency
	Sweat sodium concentration	Increased in cystic fibrosis
	Eosinophils/IgE	Increased in ABPA
	ANCA/autoantibodies	If connective tissue disease is suspected
	ACE/calcium	If sarcoid is suspected

ABPA, allergic bronchopulmonary aspergillosis; ACE, angiotensin-converting enzyme; ANCA, antinuclear cytoplasmic antibodies.

- cor pulmonale
- massive haemoptysis
- brain abscess
- amyloidosis.

Prognosis

- Dismal prognosis in the preantibiotic era with patients dying from infections
- Death now mainly as a result of cor pulmonale.

Prevention

- Administration of vaccines against measles, pertussis, influenza, TB
- Prompt removal of foreign bodies and obstructing lesions
- Antibiotics in bronchopulmonary infections.

See *Rheumatology and clinical immunology*, Sections 1.1 and 2.1.1.
1 Cohen M, Sahn SA. Bronchiectasis in systemic diseases. *Chest* 1999; 116: 1063–1074.
2 Stockley RA. Bronchiectasis. *Medicine* 1999; 27 (10): 113–116.
3 Luce JM. Bronchiectasis. In: Murray, Nadel, eds. *Textbook of Respiratory Medicine* (2nd edn). W B Saunders, 1994: 1398–1417.

2.5 Cystic fibrosis

Aetiology

Cystic fibrosis (CF) is an autosomal recessive disease caused by a defect in the gene encoding an epithelial cell transmembrane protein termed the cystic fibrosis transmembrane conductance regulator (CFTR). The gene is located on the long arm of chromosome 7 and the most common mutation in the UK is ΔF508. The function of this protein is to serve as a chloride channel and also as a regulator of an epithelial sodium channel; however, the exact mechanism by which defects in CFTR-mediated ion transport cause the phenotype of cystic fibrosis (CF) is unknown [1].

The lungs of CF patients are thought not to be infected at birth, but endobronchial bacterial colonization occurs within the first months of life and usually progresses to colonization with *Pseudomonas aeruginosa*. Lung destruction follows with the development of an obstructive respiratory defect and eventually respiratory failure.

Table 20 Presentations of cystic fibrosis.

Classification	Example
Respiratory disease (40%)	Frequent infections; recurrent bronchitis/bronchiolitis
Malabsorption (30%)	Failure to thrive, rectal prolapse, intussusception, fatty diarrhoea
Meconium ileus (20%)	
Rare	Infertility (men), cirrhosis or portal hypertension, nasal polyps, adult bronchiectasis

Epidemiology

Prevalence in Europeans is 1 in 2500; it is rare in Afro-Caribbeans (1 in 17 000) and very rare in Orientals (1 in 90 000).

Clinical presentation

Presentations of CF are shown in Table 20. The average age of newly diagnosed patients is 4.8 years, but may be up to 65 years. Diabetes occurs in 6% of adults.

 Consider CF as a potential diagnosis in adult patients with recurrent purulent chest infections.

Physical signs

These will depend on the presentation and stage of disease.

An adult patient with CF is likely to be clubbed with signs of hyperinflation. Crackles and/or wheeze may be audible. In advanced disease there may also be cyanosis or respiratory distress. The patient may appear undernourished (see below); hepatosplenomegaly may be present.

Investigations

The diagnosis of CF is based on one or more clinical features consistent with the CF phenotype (see above) plus one of:
• two CF gene mutations
• a positive sweat test
• abnormal nasal potential differences.

Gene mutations

In excess of 800 mutations are recognized: most UK laboratories only screen for 12 of these, covering an estimated 93% of the UK patients. Thus, it is possible for a patient to have CF without routine genotyping identifying a mutation. Conversely the finding of one mutation does not diagnose CF because the carrier frequency of the single gene is 1 in 25.

Sweat test

This should be performed at least twice.

Nasal potential differences

Although this can be useful for patients with a borderline sweat test, this test should not be considered diagnostic in isolation outside specialist centres.

 Investigations relevant to the management of an acutely unwell CF patient would depend on clinical presentation. In specialist CF centres all patients would undergo annual review. As well as symptomatic enquiry and a physical examination this would include, from a physician's perspective:
• chest radiograph (Fig. 29)
• full lung function tests
• full blood count (FBC), urea and electrolytes, calcium, liver function tests
• sputum microbiology
• ECG.

Fig. 29 Chest radiograph of an adult patient with cystic fibrosis. Hyperinflation and cystic change (most obvious in the right upper lobe) is evident. A Portacath is seen over the left lung field.

Differential diagnosis

This is the differential diagnosis of the presenting symptom.

Treatment

The best care of the CF patient requires multidisciplinary team working between a physician, nurse, social worker, physiotherapist, nutritionist, general practitioner and a genetic counsellor [2]. In CF centres all patients undergo annual review which allows assessment by this multidisciplinary team as well as the physician (see above).

Respiratory system

Respiratory symptoms should be managed aggressively with the aim being to defend pulmonary function.
• Standard therapy comprises antibiotics (both for acute infection and in colonized patients) and physiotherapy.
• Sputum clearance may be enhanced in some patients by the administration of nebulized recombinant deoxyribonuclease ('DNase').
• Bronchodilators and anti-inflammatory drugs are often helpful also.

Gastrointestinal disease

Ninety per cent of CF patients have pancreatic insufficiency and benefit from replacement of enzymes and fat-soluble vitamins. Professional dietetic assessment is indicated for all patients.

There is no specific therapy for CF liver disease, but supportive management is as for other causes of cirrhosis/portal hypertension.

Transplantation

In advanced disease lung transplantation (see Section 2.13, p. 235) offers the best chance of survival [3]. For patients awaiting a transplant, non-invasive positive pressure ventilation can be a useful bridge; endotracheal ventilation of patients with advanced CF is almost always unsuccessful.

Broadly speaking, patients may be considered suitable for transplantation if the FEV_1 is <30% predicted or, if rapidly declining, greater than this. Other features favouring transplantation are the development of ventilatory failure and increasing hospitalizations. Because cadaveric organs are in short supply there is increasing interest in living donor bilateral lobar lung transplantation.

 In advanced CF, respiratory failure as a result of overwhelming infection is a common cause of death. Endotracheal ventilation does not alter the outcome in this situation and hence this treatment is not usually offered.

Complications

Of pulmonary disease

The more severe complications occur in more advanced disease:
• sinusitis and nasal polyps
• bacterial respiratory infection
• pneumothorax
• haemoptysis
• aspergillosis
• respiratory failure and pulmonary hypertension.

Of gastrointestinal disease

CF adults may have abdominal pain, but the cause is seldom appendicitis or other surgically remediable problems. Although surgical advice should be sought where appropriate, most experts prefer to have a high threshold for abdominal surgery. Other complications include:
• Obstruction
• Malabsorption
• Glucose intolerance/diabetes
• Cirrhosis and portal hypertension.

Other/iatrogenic

The total list of possible complications of CF is enormous but includes:
• infertility in men
• pregnancy—represents a hazard if the FEV_1 is <40–50% predicted or if there is pulmonary hypertension
• ototoxicity from repeated aminoglycosides
• Portacath complications.

Prognosis

The median survival of newborns with CF is now estimated to be about 40 years; this compares with 14 years in 1969. The 5-year survival after transplantation is around 50%.

Prevention

For parents who are CF gene carriers (e.g. because a sibling with CF is already identified), prenatal diagnosis is possible. The risks of chorionic villous sampling are roughly equal to those of amniocentesis but with the advantage of giving an earlier result.

Therapy aimed at preventing the phenotypic expression of CF by gene replacement is not yet a practical clinical option [1–4].

See *Cell biology,* Section 1.
See *Gastroenterology,* Sections 1.10 and 2.4.
1 Stern M., Alton E. The pathogenesis of cystic fibrosis and progress towards gene therapy. *J R Coll Physicians Lond* 1999; 33: 434–439.
2 Varlotta L. Management and care of the newly diagnosed patient with cystic fibrosis. *Curr Opin Pulm Med* 1998; 4: 311–318.
3 Shapiro B, Veerarghaven S., Barbers RG. Lung transplantation for cystic fibrosis: an update and practical considerations for referring candidates. *Curr Opin Pulm Med* 1999; 5: 365–370.
4 Rosenstein BJ, Zeitlin PJ. Cystic fibrosis. *Lancet* 1998; 351: 277–282.

2.6 Occupational lung disease

2.6.1 ASBESTOSIS AND THE PNEUMOCONIOSES

 Prevention is better than cure.

Aetiology and pathology

The pneumoconioses are occupational lung diseases caused by inhalation of a variety of industrial dusts. Strictly speaking, asbestosis is a subtype of the pneumoconioses but, because of its relative prevalence, tends to be considered separately. Likewise, coal worker's pneumoconiosis (CWP) merits its own discussion [1–6].

CWP aside, the pneumoconioses can be divided into two subgroups (Table 21):
• benign forms—tend to be asymptomatic. Recognized by the chest radiograph appearances that they produce: small, round opacities caused by perivascular collections of dust
• fibrotic forms—produce, as the name suggests, pulmonary fibrosis associated with a restrictive lung defect. They may cause symptoms and sometimes progress to respiratory failure.

Table 21 Industrial substances whose dusts cause pneumoconiosis.

Disease type	Causative agent (disease name)
Benign disease	Iron (siderosis)
	Tin (stannosis)
	Barium (bariosis)
	Antimony
Fibrotic disease	Asbestos
	Silica (silicosis)
	Beryllium (berylliosis)
	Aluminium ores (Shaver's disease or aluminosis)

Asbestosis

The interstitial fibrosis produced by asbestos exposure is dose related, with length and level of exposure relating directly to the development and severity of symptoms. The fibrosis tends to be in the lower lobes and is frequently associated with pleural thickening and the appearance of pleural plaques on chest radiograph. Asbestos exposure can also lead to mesothelioma and lung cancer, particularly adenocarcinoma.

Coal worker's pneumoconiosis

CWP is seen in workers exposed to coal dust and accounts for 90% of claims for industrial compensation. The condition is generally divided into:
• simple CWP—based on the chest radiograph appearances of small, round opacities that represent small fibrous nodules in the lung, predominantly in the upper lobes
• complicated CWP (massive progressive fibrosis, MPF)—a patient is said to have advanced to MPF when these fibrous lesions have reached more that 3 cm in diameter. Histologically, these larger lesions commonly undergo necrosis and cavitation.

CWP associated with rheumatoid arthritis is known as Caplan's syndrome.

Clinical presentation

This may include:
• breathlessness
• cough
• jet black sputum production (CWP only).

Physical signs

Few in early disease; later:
• decreased chest expansion
• inspiratory crackles
• wheeze (CWP)
• clubbing (asbestosis, but not silicosis; rarely in CWP).

Investigations

Chest radiograph

The International Labour Office has produced a method of classification for the radiographic changes seen in pneumoconiosis. These classifications are largely based on the size and number of opacities seen on the chest radiograph and are used by medical panels when discussing compensation claims.
• For benign pneumoconiosis, small, round opacities are diagnostic of the disease.

(a)

(b)

(c)

(d)

Fig. 30 (a) Chest radiograph of a patient with previous asbestos exposure with extensive pleural plaques. (Courtesy of Dr J. Moore-Gillon.) (b) Chest radiograph showing widespread pulmonary fibrosis secondary to asbestos exposure. (Courtesy of Dr R. Rudd.) (c) Chest radiograph showing the progressive massive fibrosis of coal worker's pneumoconiosis in a coal miner. (Courtesy of Dr R. Rudd.) (d) Computed tomography scan of the thorax; note the posterior changes, with pleural thickening and the adjacent early changes of asbestosis. (Courtesy of Dr J. Moore-Gillon.)

• Asbestos can produce a number of changes, including pleural thickening, pleural (holly leaf) plaques, fibrosis and evidence of tumours (Fig. 30a,b).
• Silicosis produces classical eggshell calcification around the hilar lymph nodes, as well as peripheral nodules.
• For CWP, see above (Fig. 30c).

Lung function tests

These show a restrictive picture with decreased FVC, TLC, RV and gas transfer.

High-resolution computed tomography scan

Prone and supine films will help reveal the extent of the disease, and is particularly helpful when extensive pleural disease masks the lung parenchyma (Fig. 30d).

Treatment

A priority is avoidance of further dust exposure. The workplace should, if necessary, consider review of protective equipment used by other employees. The benign pneumoconioses require no other treatment.

Fibrotic disease is normally considered resistant to therapy, excepting berylliosis, where high-dose prednisolone can produce a clinical improvement. Occasionally, courses of steroids are tried in patients with asbestosis who are showing rapid deterioration of their lung function. Treatment of CWP is largely supportive.

Complications

These may include:
- respiratory failure
- right heart failure
- TB in silicosis.

1 Waldron HA. *Lecture Notes on Occupational Medicine* (4th edn). Oxford: Blackwell Scientific Publications, 1990.
2 Jarad NA. Asbestos-related disease. *J R Coll Physicians Lond* 1999; 33: 537–540.
3 Morgan WKC, Gee JBL. Asbestos-related disease. In: Morgan WKC, Seaton A, eds. *Occupational Lung Diseases* (3rd edn). Philadelphia: W.B. Saunders, 1995.
4 Morgan WKC and Gee JBL. Coal worker's pneumoconiosis, and other pneumoconiosis. In: Morgan WKC and Seaton, eds. *Occupational Lung Diseases* (3rd edn). Philadelphia: W.B. Saunders, 1995.
5 Rudd RM. Asbestos-related disease. In: Brewis RAL, Corrin B, Geddes DM, Gibson GJ, eds. *Respiratory Medicine* (2nd edn). London: W.B. Saunders, 1998: 545–569.
6 Morgan WKC, Elmes P, McConnochie. Pneumoconiosis. In: Brewis RAL, Corrin B, Geddes DM, Gibson GJ, eds. *Respiratory Medicine* (2nd edn). London: W.B. Saunders, 1998: 570–604.

2.7 Diffuse parenchymal (interstitial) lung disease

2.7.1 CRYPTOGENIC FIBROSING ALVEOLITIS

Aetiology

Not known (by definition). More common in cigarette smokers. Speculation regarding viral or occupational aetiology. Rarely familial.

Pathophysiology

Cryptogenic fibrosing alveolitis (CFA) involves lung injury; immunological and inflammatory response; and fibrogenesis. There is evidence that the fibrogenic response becomes autonomous. Transgenic animals over-expressing transforming growth factor β develop progressive fibrosing lung disease indistinguishable histologically from CFA.

Pathology

The typical appearance is of 'usual interstitial pneumonia', where there is a patchy distribution of interstitial fibrosis, chronic inflammatory cell infiltrate and enlarged cystic air spaces.

Epidemiology

Usually age >50 years. Affects men slightly more often than women: incidence 5–10 per 100 000; prevalence 15–20 per 100 000.

Clinical presentation

Insidious (at least 3–6 months) onset of otherwise unexplained breathlessness without wheeze. There may be a dry cough, but sputum production is unusual. Haemoptysis is uncommon and suggests malignancy (see below).

Physical signs

Bibasilar fine inspiratory crackles. Clubbing in 75% of cases. In advanced cases there is cyanosis and signs of pulmonary hypertension/right ventricular failure.

Look for non-pulmonary features that would suggest alternative diagnoses, e.g. rash, arthropathy, lymphadenopathy.

Investigations

Pulmonary function studies show evidence of restriction and impaired gas exchange.

Chest radiograph shows small lung fields and reticulo-nodular shadowing, particularly at the bases and lung peripheries, but becoming widespread in advanced cases. Lymphadenopathy is not expected. There may be features of pulmonary hypertension.

High-resolution CT scan reveals bibasilar reticular abnormalities with honeycombing and minimal or no ground glass opacities: the appearances may be virtually pathognomonic.

Transbronchial lung biopsy or bronchiolar lavage do not support another diagnosis, i.e. there are no granulomas on biopsy and no excess lymphocytes on lavage.

Differential diagnosis

CFA is a diagnosis of exclusion. Definition (International Consensus Statement) requires: (i) the presence of a surgical biopsy (transbronchial biopsy specimens are too small to make the diagnosis, but can be useful in excluding other conditions) showing the usual interstitial pneumonia pattern of pathology; (ii) exclusion of known causes of interstitial lung disease such as drug exposures, environmental exposures and rheumatological disease; (iii) restrictive pulmonary function tests and/or impaired gas exchange; and (iv) typical features on chest radiography or high-resolution CT scans. The diagnosis is less certain in the absence of a surgical lung biopsy.

The following must be excluded:
- Diffuse rheumatological lung disease
- Occupational lung disease (asbestosis, hard metal disease)
- Chronic extrinsic allergic alveolitis
- Chronic sarcoidosis
- Various drugs (especially cytotoxics: bleomycin, busulfan, BCNU, methotrexate), inhaled agents and toxins (e.g. paraquat)
- Irradiation.

Treatment

There have been no prospective, placebo-controlled, randomized trials. As first-line treatment, most authorities recommend low-dose prednisolone (10–20 mg/day) with azathioprine (1.5–2.5 mg/kg/day, max 150 mg/day). The length of time for which treatment should be given is not known, but most recommend a minimum of 3–6 months and, if disease stabilizes or improves, continuing for at least 1 year thereafter. Many other agents have been tried, including high-dose corticosteroid (e.g. methylprednisolone 1 g i.v./day for 3 days) and cyclophosphamide for accelerated disease.

In end-stage disease, single lung transplantation is used in selected cases: the alternative is palliative treatment (oxygen, diuretics, opiates).

Complications

- Respiratory failure and cor pulmonale.
- Ten-fold increased risk of lung malignancy.

Prognosis

Median survival is <3 years: 10 years' survival is 5–10%.

The Diffuse Parenchymal Lung Disease Group. The diagnosis, assessment and treatment of diffuse parenchymal lung disease in adults. *Thorax* 1999; 54: Suppl 1.
Mason RJ, Schwarz MI, Hunninghake GW, Musson RA. NHLBI workshop summary. Pharmacological therapy for idiopathic pulmonary fibrosis. Past, present and future. *Am J Resp Crit Care Med* 1999; 160: 1771–1777.
Joint Statement of American Thoracic Society and European Respiratory Society Idiopathic pulmonary fibrosis: diagnosis and treatment. International consensus statement. *Am J Resp Crit Care Med* 2000; 161: 646–664.

2.7.2 BRONCHIOLITIS OBLITERANS AND ORGANIZING PNEUMONIA

There is a great deal of confusion in the literature regarding these and similar terms!
- Bronchiolitis obliterans describes a condition that presents with breathlessness in which there is obliteration of the terminal bronchioles by fixed fibrosis.
- Cryptogenic organizing pneumonia (the term recommended by the American Thoracic Society/European Respiratory Society nomenclature committee) describes a disorder presenting with pneumonia-like features in which intra-alveolar histological changes spread proximally to the terminal bronchiole, which can be obliterated, but with loose fibrous tissue different from that seen in bronchiolitis obliterans.

Bronchiolitis obliterans

Aetiology

May be associated with rheumatological disease, particularly rheumatoid arthritis or Sjögren's syndrome, or after lung transplantation. Less often associated with infection, inhaled gases, drugs, or cryptogenic (cause unknown).

Pathology

Predominantly affects the terminal bronchioles, with significant narrowing and sometimes obliteration of the lumen by a mixture of cellular infiltration and fibrosis.

Clinical presentation

Progressive breathlessness, often with little wheeze. Cough is rarely productive. Haemoptysis does not occur.

Physical signs

Examination of the chest is likely to be unremarkable, excepting for evidence of respiratory failure and cor pulmonale in advanced cases.

Investigations

- Lung function tests show fixed airflow obstruction with increased residual volume. Total gas transfer for carbon monoxide is reduced, but when corrected for alveolar volume is normal.
- Chest radiograph shows large lung fields. There is no evidence of infiltration.
- High-resolution CT scan reveals patchy attenuation ('mosaicism'), which is characteristic.
- Blood tests may suggest rheumatological disease.

Wegener's is low—approximately 10% [3,5]. Alternative possibilities are:
- biopsy of upper airway lesions
- renal biopsy (if evidence of nephritis)
- open lung biopsy.

Other investigations

- Screening blood tests—renal and liver function tests, antinuclear antibodies (ANA), Rh factor, ACE and autoantibodies
- Urine—looking for proteinuria, haematuria and cellular casts as evidence of renal involvement
- Chest radiograph—may show pulmonary infiltrates, nodules, haemorrhage or a combination of these abnormalities (45% of patients)
- High-resolution CT scanning—may be a useful adjunct to diagnosis and for monitoring disease progression.

Differential diagnosis

The differential depends on the nature of the presenting symptom. The more difficult differential can be of eosinophilia. Where there is significant diagnostic doubt, the case for obtaining biopsy material is strengthened.

Treatment

- Wegener's—steroids ± cyclophosphamide ± plasmapharesis. Septrin may have a role for patients with disease confined to the upper airway. Azathioprine is often used to maintain remission
- Churg–Strauss—steroids ± cyclophosphamide ± plasmapharesis.

Complications

- Wegener's—chronic renal insufficiency (42%; a quarter of these will require dialysis), hearing loss (35%), nasal deformities (28%), tracheal stenosis (13%) and visual loss (8%)
- Churg–Strauss—essentially a more benign condition than Wegener's, but myocardial damage and gastrointestinal tract involvement are recognized.

Prognosis

- Wegener's—13% mortality
- Churg–Strauss—11% morbidity in long-term follow-up.

See *Nephrology*, Section 1.9.
See *Rheumatology and clinical immunology*, Sections 1.10, 1.20 and 2.5.
1 Burns A. Pulmonary vasculitis. *Thorax* 1998; 53: 220–227.
2 Stirling RG, Chung KF. Leukotriene antagonists and Churg–Strauss syndrome: the smoking gun. *Thorax* 1999; 54: 865–866.
3 Hoffman GS, Kerr GS, Leavitt RY *et al.* Wegener granulomatosis: an analysis of 158 patients. *Ann Intern Med* 1992; 116: 488–498.
4 Guillevin L, Cohen P, Gayraud M, Lhote F, Jarrousse B., Casassus P. Churg–Strauss syndrome. Clinical study and long-term follow up of 96 patients. *Medicine (Baltimore MD)* 1999; 78: 26–37.
5 Schnabel A, Holl-Ulrich K, Dalhoff K, Reuter M, Gross WL. Efficacy of transbronchial biopsy in pulmonary vasculitides. *Eur Resp J* 1997; 10: 2738–2743.

2.8.4 PULMONARY EOSINOPHILIA

Aetiology/pathology

Pulmonary eosinophilia is the term used for a group of disorders of different aetiology, characterized by peripheral blood eosinophilia and eosinophilic pulmonary infiltrates [1–3]. The causes of pulmonary eosinophilia are:
- allergic bronchopulmonary aspergillosis
- drug-induced pulmonary eosinophilia
- tropical pulmonary eosinophilia
- Löffler's syndrome
- Churg–Strauss syndrome
- hypereosinophilic syndrome
- eosinophilic pneumonia.

Allergic bronchopulmonary aspergillosis

This is mainly caused by *Aspergillus fumigatus*, but may be caused by other *Aspergillus* species and *Candida*. Inhaled spores are deposited in secretions and proliferate resulting in mucus plugging of the airways. There is production of IgE and IgG antibodies and eosinophilic infiltration of the lungs. Proximal bronchiectasis occurs as a result of local immune reaction.

Drug-induced pulmonary eosinophilia

Various drugs can cause pulmonary infiltrates, eosinophilia, fever and pulmonary symptoms such as wheeze and cough:
- aspirin
- methotrexate
- sulphonamides
- captopril
- naproxen
- tetracycline

- carbamazepine
- nitrofurantoin
- tolazamide
- chlorpropamide
- penicillamine
- bleomycin
- chlorpromazine
- penicillin
- gold
- imipramine
- phenytoin
- sulfasalazine.

Tropical pulmonary eosinophilia

The common causes are:
- *Wuchereria bancrofti*
- *Brugia malayi*
- *Ancylostoma duodenale*
- *Strongyloides stercoralis*
- *Toxocara canis.*

Hypereosinophilic syndrome

This is characterized by marked blood eosinophilia and eosinophilic infiltration of the heart, lungs, skin, central nervous system and other organs. It usually affects men in the fourth decade and has a high morbidity and mortality.

Chronic eosinophilic pneumonia

This is characterized by blood eosinophilia with pulmonary eosinophilic infiltration for which there is no obvious cause.

Epidemiology

- Allergic bronchopulmonary aspergillosis—the most common cause of eosinophilia. Occurs worldwide and at any age
- Drug-induced pulmonary eosinophilia—dependent on local patterns of drug use
- Tropical pulmonary eosinophilia—commonly seen in Asia, Africa and South America
- Chronic eosinophilic pneumonia—mainly affects middle-aged women with a history of asthma.

Clinical presentation

- Allergic bronchopulmonary aspergillosis—most patients present with asthma. Ten per cent have night sweats, fever or malaise.
- Drug-induced pulmonary eosinophilia—Cough, dyspnoea and fever may start within hours of taking the drug.

- Tropical pulmonary eosinophilia—most patients are young adults and present with cough, mainly nocturnal. Breathlessness, chest pain, fever, weight loss and anorexia may occur. If untreated, symptoms may persist or remit spontaneously and recur later.
- Hypereosinophilic syndrome—patients present with fever, anorexia and weight loss along with symptoms secondary to the organ affected. In 60% of cases the heart is affected with arrythmias and heart failure. In 50% of cases the lungs are involved and the patient complains of cough.
- Chronic eosinophilic pneumonia—patients present with cough, dyspnoea, fever and weight loss.

Physical signs

- Allergic bronchopulmonary aspergillosis—there may be signs of consolidation or simply wheeze
- Drug-induced pulmonary eosinophilia—wheeze and respiratory distress
- Tropical pulmonary eosinophilia—wheeze
- Hypereosinophilic syndrome—signs of mitral and tricuspid valve incompetence. Pulmonary consolidation and pleural effusions can occur.

Investigations

Allergic bronchopulmonary aspergillosis

- Blood eosinophilia is moderate (500–2000/mm^3).
- All patients show a positive immediate skin-prick test to *A. fumigatus*.
- IgG precipating antibodies to *A. fumigatus* are found in over 90% of patients.
- Total serum IgE is elevated during acute episodes, and serum IgE can be used to monitor treatment.
- Chest radiograph may show segmental or lobar collapse or bronchiectasis. In the acute phase transient pulmonary infiltrates may be seen.

Drug-induced pulmonary eosinophilia

Chest radiograph may show transient pulmonary infiltrates.

Tropical pulmonary eosinophilia

- Blood eosinophilia is high (5000–60 000/mm^3).
- IgE is markedly elevated.
- Antifilarial antibodies are present in high titre.
- Chest radiograph may be normal, but more typically shows diffuse mottling with lesions 1–3 mm in diameter.

Chronic eosinophilic pneumonia

• There is likely to be peripheral eosinophilia, anaemia, raised ESR and elevated IgE.
• Lung function tests show a restrictive or mixed defect.
• Chest radiograph shows peripheral pulmonary densities that have been described as 'photograph negative of pulmonary oedema'.

Treatment

Allergic bronchopulmonary aspergillosis

Treatment is with oral corticosteroids during acute episodes. Response to treatment can be monitored by radiologic clearing, resolution of eosinophilia or serum IgE levels.

Drug-induced pulmonary eosinophilia

Withdrawal of the drug results in resolution of the symptoms, which can be hastened by corticosteroids.

Tropical pulmonary eosinophilia

• Treatment of filarial disease is with diethylcarbamazine, building up to a dosage of 6 mg/kg per day for 3 weeks. Marked delay in treatment is associated with poor clinical response and development of pulmonary fibrosis.
• Mebendazole, albendazole or pyrantel pamoate are used if *Ascaris* or *Necator* are the cause.
• Thiabendazole is the drug of choice for *Strongyloides stercolaris*.

Hypereosinophilic syndrome

Treatment is with corticosteroids. In resistant cases, hydroxycarbamide (hydroxyurea) may be helpful.

Chronic eosinophilic pneumonia

This responds rapidly to corticosteroids, and failure to respond within 48–72 h raises the possibility of alternative diagnosis such as bronchiolitis obliterans and organizing pneumonia (BOOP, see Section 2.7.2). The dosage of corticosteroids is gradually tapered as relapses are common. Most patients regain normal lung function; a few may develop a persistent obstructive defect, and rarely pulmonary fibrosis may occur.

See *Infectious diseases*, Section 1.21.
1 Douglas NJ, Goetzl EJ. Pulmonary eosinophilia and eosinophilic granuloma. In: Murray JF, Nadel JA, eds. *Textbook of Respiratory Medicine* (2nd edn). Philadelphia: W. B. Saunders, 1994: 1913–1932.
2 Muers MF. Eosinophilic lung diseases. *Medicine* 1999; 27: 11; 167–169.
3 Harrison R. The eosinophilic lung diseases. *CME Bull Resp Med* 1998; 1(2): 27–29.

2.8.5 IATROGENIC LUNG DISEASE

Aetiology

A number of respiratory conditions may be precipitated by standard medical therapy [1], either by damage to the lung parenchyma or by disturbing the pulmonary physiology. These effects must be remembered when prescribing such treatments, and highlight the importance of taking a thorough past medical and drug history when interviewing patients. Potential mechanisms include:
• bronchoconstriction
• alveolitis
• radiotherapy.

Bronchoconstriction

Some of the drugs that can produce bronchoconstriction are:
• aspirin and the other NSAIDs
• penicillins
• tetracyclines
• cephalosporins
• cromoglycate
• β blockers
• anticholinesterases
• opiates
• iodine contrast media
• *N*-acetyl-cysteine.

 Remember, drugs do not have to be given systemically to produce problems. Even eye drops such as timolol can produce wheeze and chest tightness, particularly in elderly patients.

Alveolitis

Some of the drugs that can affect the lung parenchyma are listed in Table 23. Some of these effects are potentially reversible on withdrawal of the treatment, while others may produce irreversible damage.

Table 23 Drugs that can affect the lung parenchyma.

Drug type	Drug name
Cardiac	Amiodarone
	Procainamide
	Quinidine
Antibiotics	Nitrofurantoin
	Sulphonamides
	Penicillins
Anti-inflammatory	Sulfasalazine
	Penicillamine
	Gold
Cytotoxics	Bleomycin
	Mitomycin
	Busulfan
	Chlorambucil
	Cyclophosphamide
	Methotrexate
	Carmustine

Radiotherapy

Radiation, prescribed with a view to eradicating tumour cells, also damages healthy tissues. When given to the thorax for the treatment of lymphoma, breast or lung cancer, it can produce a pneumonitis in the underlying lung. The risk of damage is proportional to the dose of radiotherapy.

Clinical presentation

The clinical presentation will be determined by the nature of the underlying pathophysiology. In general:
• bronchoconstriction presents with wheezing after drug administration
• pneumonitis or alveolitis is likely to have a slower onset with exertional dyspnoea and fine inspiratory crackles being prominent.

Investigations

In bronchoconstriction, monitoring peak flow is worthwhile to see if this improves after a couple of days. It is then worth requesting lung function testing pre- and post-bronchodilator to see if mild asthma or COPD has been unmasked.

In alveolitis there should be radiological changes visible on plain chest radiograph or high-resolution CT (Fig. 32), as well as appropriate changes in pulmonary function tests—reduced lung volumes with a reduced K_{CO}.

Radiotherapy produces more localized fibrosis that may progress to cause lung contraction. The edge is often sharply defined (Fig. 33).

Ensure that patients with radiation fibrosis are told that they have an abnormal chest radiograph, especially if the changes are persistent. This can save them unnecessary investigations in the future.

Treatment

For all suspected drug side effects it is necessary to stop the offending medication and replace with another class of drug if necessary.

Patients with bronchoconstriction may also require a bronchodilator, at least in the short term until their symptoms improve, as well as a short course of corticosteroids.

In alveolitis some patients will respond to steroid therapy; in others the damage will be irreversible, but nonprogressive. Serial K_{CO} measurements are recommended by some authorities for patients taking amiodarone and other agents particularly associated with alveolitis.

1 Seaton A, Seaton D, Leitch AG. Drug-induced lung disease, oxygen toxicity and related syndromes. In: *Crofton and Douglas's Respiratory Disease*. Blackwell Scientific Publications, 1985.

2.8.6 SMOKE INHALATION

Aetiology

This term includes inhalation of a wide array of substances. In addition to the effects of toxic substances there is thermal injury to the respiratory tract, limited to the upper airways and resulting in laryngeal oedema. In fires, heat decomposition and pyrolysis causes the release of an enormous number of toxins such as carbon monoxide, cyanide, oxidants and products of preformed chemicals, which result in cytotoxic anoxia.

Studies of fire fighters and victims of fires have shown that smoke inhalation results in acute airflow obstruction and a non-specific increase in airway responsiveness after smoke inhalation.

Clinical presentation

Presentation depends on the severity of exposure, and ranges from mild airway obstruction to coma with extensive thermal injury and laryngeal oedema. In cases of severe exposure, pulmonary oedema and adult respiratory distress syndrome (ARDS) may develop immediately or following a latent period of 3–30 h. Patients may also present with symptoms of carbon monoxide poisoning (headache, confusion, clumsiness).

It is desirable to find out whether any chemicals or toxic gases were involved in the incident.

(a)

(b)

(c)

(d)

Fig. 32 (a) Chest radiograph of a man with ischaemic heart disease showing an implantable cardioverter defibrillator and pulmonary shadowing; he was thought to have heart failure. Computed tomography scans of the same patient (b) supine and (c) prone, taken the next day. The pulmonary shadowing does not change in position and therefore is more consistent with fibrosis secondary to amiodarone. (d) Computed tomography scan of the same patient 2 years later showing complete resolution of the fibrosis; the amiodarone had been stopped soon after the results of first scan and he was given a 6-month course of oral steroids.

 Smoke inhalation

- May include inhalation of various chemical fumes.
- Patients may be asymptomatic or gravely ill.
- It is essential to find out whether toxic chemicals were involved.
- Beware of thermal burns and possibility of laryngeal oedema. (An experienced anaesthetist should be present.)
- Smoke inhalation kills more fire victims than thermal injury.

Physical signs

Assess airway, breathing and circulation and resuscitate if necessary; otherwise look for:

- tachypnoea
- cyanosis
- thermal burns
- listen for crackles (pulmonary oedema) and wheeze
- cherry red skin, visual field defects and papilloedema of carbon monoxide poisoning.

Investigations

- Arterial blood gases—look for PaO_2, $PaCO_2$ and presence of acidosis
- Lactate level (lactic acidosis)
- Renal function (myoglobinuria secondary to muscle necrosis in carbon monoxide poisoning)

Fig. 33 Chest radiograph of a woman who had received mantel radiation for Hodgkin's lymphoma 30 years previously. The left upper lobe shows extensive tethering and fibrosis. She was referred to the chest physicians on the basis of this radiograph for bronchoscopy, with no reference to previous films. The changes had been present for many years.

• Carboxyhaemoglobin and methaemoglobin to assess the severity of inhalation
• Chest radiograph—look for pulmonary oedema and lung infiltrates
• Cardiac rhythm (arrhythmias in carbon monoxide poisoning)
• Oxygen saturation—monitor continuously.

 Carboxyhaemoglobin is detected by pulse oximeters; therefore Sao_2 may not be an accurate reflection of oxygenation in carbon monoxide poisoning.

Treatment

Depending on exposure:
• care of thermal injury
• high-flow oxygen to correct hypoxia
• nebulized bronchodilators to relieve airway obstruction
• intravenous fluids to correct any dehydration
• hyperbaric oxygen in case of carbon monoxide levels over 40% or over 25% with seizures or arrhythmias
• intubation and ventilation if needed. Prophylactic intubation is required in severe cases
• treatment of pulmonary oedema, which can be caused by arrhythmia.

Complications

Depending on severity:
• renal failure secondary to myoglobinuria caused by rhabdomyolysis
• pulmonary oedema
• ARDS
• bronchiolitis obliterans—this usually develops 2–8 weeks after exposure, even in patients who were asymptomatic at initial presentation. It is characterized by non-productive cough and dyspnoea. It is more likely to develop in patients exposed to less soluble gases such as nitrogen dioxide and phosgene. This gradually progresses to respiratory failure.
• Increased airway responsiveness with repeated episodes of smoke inhalation (seen in fire fighters).

Prevention

Prevention will depend upon safeguard against fires in both residential buildings and chemical work places.

 Blanc PD, Schwartz DA. Acute pulmonary responses to toxic exposures. In: Murray JF, Nadel JA, eds. *Textbook of Respiratory Medicine* (2nd edn). Philadelphia: W.B. Saunders, 1994: 2056–2057.
Speizer FE. Environmental lung diseases. *Harrison's Principles of Internal Medicine* (12th edn). McGraw-Hill: 1061–1062.

2.8.7 SICKLE CELL DISEASE AND THE LUNG

Aetiology

The two major pulmonary problems that occur in sickle cell disease are:
• infection, leading to pneumonia
• veno-occulsion resulting in pulmonary emboli and infarction.
Together they make up the 'acute chest syndrome' [1].

Epidemiology

Infection is more common in children, although the risk of pneumococcal pneumonia has been reduced by the use of antibiotic prophylaxis. Adolescents and adults are more at risk of pulmonary emboli and infarction, which can lead to pulmonary hypertension and cor pulmonale.

Clinical presentation

Any 'Sickler' presenting with fever, pleuritic chest pain and shortness of breath should be carefully assessed and admitted for observation.

Aggression and/or confusion should not be mistaken for a psychotic or 'drugged-up' individual; the patient may well be hypoxic and septic.

Physical signs

These are fever, dyspnoea, crackles in lung fields, confusion, evidence of consolidation or opacities on chest radiograph.

Investigations

Emergency

For acutely ill patients obtain:
• full blood count—severe anaemia may require transfusion or exchange tranfusion
• urea and electrolytes—make sure the patient is not dehydrated
• chest radiograph—looking for pulmonary shadowing, consolidation and opacities (Fig. 34)
• arterial blood gases—looking for hypoxia; acidosis is a marker of the severity of the illness
• ECG.

Short term

Aimed at identifying reversible disease:
• ventilation–perfusion (V/Q) scan or spiral CT—look for emboli and infarction
• sputum for MCS
• echocardiographic assessment of pulmonary hypertension.

Fig. 34 Chest radiograph of a patient with sickle cell disease; there is right middle and lower lobe collapse and consolidation caused by pneumonia. Also note the cardiomegaly and small spleen. Less obvious are the surgical clips from a previous cholecystectomy. (Courtesy of Dr I. Vlahos.)

Long term

Lung function tests—note that sickle cell patients often have reduced indices even when in relative good health.

Treatment

Emergency

Try to reassure the patient, while:
• administering broad-spectrum intravenous antibiotics and fluids
• administering high-flow oxygen, humidified if possible
• giving adequate analgesia
• anticoagulating as for pulmonary emboli if veno-occlusion is suspected.

Hypoxia in sickle disease is often ascribed to co-administration of analgesics and/or sedatives. This could be a dangerous assumption and you can check it by measurement of $Pa\text{CO}_2$. Reduction of respiratory drive should not affect the a–A gradient.

Short to long term

Close co-operation between haematologist and respiratory physician is helpful. Prophylactic antibiotics will help reduce episodes of infection. The patient may require life-long anticoagulation.

Complications

Repeated pulmonary emboli and infarction may lead to pulmonary hypertension, cor pulmonale and right heart failure in relatively young patients.

See *Haematology*, Section 1.2.
1 Sergeant GR. Pulmonary system. In: *Sickle Cell Disease*. Oxford: Oxford University Press, 1992, 150–167.

2.8.8 HUMAN IMMUNODEFICIENCY VIRUS AND THE LUNG

Aetiology/epidemiology

Lung pathology is common in patients with HIV infection and particularly in those with low CD4 counts. Like the immunocompetent, they are prone to the common viral and bacterial infections; but they are also at risk of atypical infections such as PCP [1–3]. PCP was a common cause of death in AIDS patients until the introduction of septrin prophylaxis in those with CD4 counts <200. It now tends to be seen as a first presentation of the disease in previously undiagnosed HIV.

Tuberculosis is a major cause of mortality and morbidity in HIV patients, particularly in developing countries, and non-tuberculous mycobacteria including *Mycobacterium avium intercellulare* (CD4 <100), *M. kansasii* and *M. chelonea* are also seen. Multidrug-resistant TB started to become a substantial problem in the early 1990s, with between 80 and 100% mortality. The relative numbers of patients infected with multi-drug resistant TB in Western countries remains small, but the plight of the developing world is uncertain.

Cytomegalovirus (CMV) pulmonary infection rarely occurs alone; if it is found, its presence does not affect the outcome of other lung infections. Fungal infections, e.g. *Cryptococcus neoformans*, tend to be seen as part of a disseminated syndrome.

Tumours such as Kaposi's sarcoma (KS) commonly occur in the lung as well as the skin, although lymphoma tends to arise in extrapulmonary sites in HIV patients.

Clinical presentation

The management of HIV patients with pulmonary symptoms can be difficult. Do not forget that acute shortness of breath can be caused by bacterial pneumonia, asthma or pulmonary emboli, just as in the immunocompetent. However, patients with HIV more commonly present with a history of gradually increasing breathlessness, fever, mild to moderate sputum production or just dry cough, and occasionally haemoptysis.

Physical signs

- How unwell is the patient? Are they hypoxic?
- Look for clubbing.
- Look closely in the mouth and on the skin for KS as well as other stigmata or evidence of immunodeficiency.
- Note any intercostal recession.
- Listen for crackles and wheezing.

Investigations

Chest radiograph

This may be virtually diagnostic (Fig. 35); but on the other hand it may appear normal, especially in early PCP and KS.

 Do not allow a false sense of security if the chest radiograph appears normal.

Oxygen saturation

Before and after exercise. Low postexercise oxygen saturation is almost diagnostic of PCP.

Fig. 35 Chest radiograph of a young man who presented with progressive shortness of breath, dry cough and a fever; note the classic bilateral perihilar appearance of the interstitial shadowing that is highly suggestive of *Pneumocystis carnii* pneumonia, which was later proved on bronchoscopic lavage to be the diagnosis. (Courtesy of Dr I. Vlahos.)

Arterial blood gases

Hypoxia demands explanation even if the chest radiograph seems normal.

Bronchoscopy

Because of the wide range of respiratory pathology seen in the immunosuppressed, bronchoscopy is required in this group of patients if there are new respiratory symptoms and the diagnosis is not obvious. Make sure that samples are sent for the regular investigations, but in particular:
- cytology to look for PCP
- microscopy to look for AFB
- virology to look for CMV.

Intrapulmonary KS is unusual without cutaneous KS, but not impossible.

 Sedation in HIV disease

Some newer antiretroviral agents, notably indinavir, efavirenz, nelfinavir, ritonavir and saquinavir, may greatly slow metabolism of hypnotic agents by interaction with cytochrome p450. Check what your patient is taking, or he or she may stay sleepy for several hours or longer.

Computed tomography scan of chest

Useful when other investigations are negative or disease is slow to resolve. Not essential in all patients but can be useful in unexplained hypoxia or fever (may see lymph nodes).

Treatment

Pneumocystis pneumonia

- High-dose intravenous septrin, oxygen and steroids (if PaO_2 <9.3). Do not forget to monitor bloods including FBC and liver function tests carefully. Second-line treatment in those unable to tolerate septrin is pentamidine or dapsone and trimethoprim.
- Because of the improved overall prognosis of HIV patients, full supportive care (including intubation and mechanical ventilation) is usually recommended if indicated on physiological grounds.

In severe PCP large bullae may form. Pneumothorax could explain a sudden deterioration.

Kaposi's sarcoma

KS may improve in patients with a high viral load who are started on antiviral drugs. Otherwise, refer to an oncologist for intravenous chemotherapy.

Tuberculosis

The frequency of atypical presentations is increased but management is along conventional lines. Interactions with new-generation antivirals are a problem; specialist advice is required [4]. See *Infectious diseases*, Sections 1.39 and 2.6.

Do not forget that drug regimens are different for atypical mycobacteria and multidrug-resistant TB.

See *Infectious diseases*, Sections 1.26 and 2.11.
1 Miller R. AIDS and the lung. In: Adler MW, ed. *ABC of AIDS*. London: BMJ Publishing group, 1999: 26–33.
2 Miller R. Respiratory manifestations of AIDS. In: Mindel A, Miller R, eds. *AIDS, A Pocket Handbook of Diagnosis and Management* (2nd edn). Arnold, 1995.
3 Breen R, Johnson M. Respiratory infections in patients with HIV. *J R Coll Physicians Lond* 1999; 33(5): 430–433.
4 Pozniak AL, Miller R, Ormerod LP. The treatment of TB in HIV-infected persons. *AIDS* 1999; 13(4): 435–445.

2.9 Malignancy

2.9.1 LUNG CANCER

Aetiology/pathology

Smoking remains the chief cause, although other aetiological factors include asbestos, arsenic and some heavy metals. Various histological types are recognized (Table 24).

Epidemiology

Bronchial carcinoma is undoubtedly one of the leading causes of mortality in the UK with around 35 000 deaths per year [1–3]. It is more common in men, although the incidence in women continues to increase (male : female $\approx 2 : 1$).

Clinical presentation

Common

Any abrupt change in respiratory symptoms in a past or current smoker merits investigation:
- cough
- haemoptysis
- shortness of breath (may represent an effusion or lobar collapse)
- chest pain.

Uncommon

Rarer presentations reflect the vagaries of anatomy or distribution of metastases:
- wheeze or stridor
- dysphagia as a result of oesophageal compression by enlarged mediastinal nodes
- nerve involvement, e.g. hoarseness secondary to recurrent laryngeal nerve palsy
- Horner's syndrome
- neuralgic pain as a result of tumour spread, e.g. Pancoast's, rib involvement

Table 24 Common histological cell types of lung cancer.

Histological classification	Types
Non-small-cell lung cancer	Squamous cell Adenocarcinoma Large cell
Small cell lung cancer	Synonym: oat cell

Table 25 Non-metastatic manifestations of lung cancer.

Syndrome	Mechanism
Cushing's syndrome	Ectopic adrenocorticotrophic hormone
SIADH	Ectopic antidiuretic hormone
Hypercalcaemia	Parathyroid hormone-like peptide
Hypertrophic pulmonary osteoarthropathy	Unknown
Eaton–Lambert syndrome	Unknown

SIADH, syndrome of inappropriate antidiuretic hormone secretion.

- loss of power and/or numbness in a limb or confusion resulting from brain metastasis
- facial swelling caused by superior vena caval obstruction
- confusion secondary to hypercalcaemia
- confusion secondary to hyponatraemia caused by syndrome of inappropriate antidiuretic hormone (SIADH) secretion
- cushingoid features and/or increased pigmentation (ectopic adrenocorticotrophic hormone secretion).

 Non-metastatic manifestations of lung cancer (Table 25).

Physical signs

Examination is often made with the benefit of a chest radiograph.

Common

Look for:
- clubbing
- tobacco-stained fingers
- cachexia
- pallor.

Uncommon

- Lymphadenopathy—feel carefully, including behind the sternomastoids
- Evidence of consolidation or pleural effusion on percussion and auscultation
- Liver edge secondary to metastases
- Bone pain caused by metastases
- Facial swelling and collateral venous circulation.

Rare

- Stridor secondary to tracheal or main bronchus involvement
- Horner's syndrome
- Pigmentation
- Skin metastases.

Fig. 36 Chest radiograph of a 56-year-old man presenting with cough, haemoptysis and weight loss. Note the large left hilar mass. Bronchoscopic biopsy revealed a large-cell carcinoma.

Fig. 37 Chest radiograph of a man with widespread nodular shadowing caused by diffuse adenocarcinoma of the lung.

Investigations

Chest radiograph

Posteroanterior and lateral views help to localize the lesion, especially for the bronchoscopist (Figs 36 and 37).

Bronchoscopy

If there is a visible lesion:
- biopsy for histology
- washings and brushing to cytology
- washings to microbiology for MCS and AFB (remember that infection can mimic carcinoma).

The surgeon will want to know the endobronchial anatomy.

(a)

(b)

Fig. 38 This woman presented with incoordination in her left arm associated with mild loss of sensation. (a) Magnetic resonance imaging of her brain revealed a pontine lesion and (b) chest radiograph revealed left upper lobe mass associated with right paratracheal lymphadenopathy. She had a diagnosis of squamous cell carcinoma of the lung and was given palliative radiotherapy to the brain.

Computed tomography scan

For staging the tumour the scan needs to include the thorax, liver and adrenals to look for metastases, as well as the brain if there is evidence of neurological involvement (Fig. 38).

Percutaneous biopsy under computed tomography guidance

This is useful when bronchoscopy does not establish the diagnosis. The patient should be warned that there is a 10% chance of pneumothorax; they must be fit enough to tolerate such a complication.

Mediastinoscopy

Mediastinal nodes shown to be enlarged on CT/magnetic resonance imaging (MRI) are biopsied. This helps differentiate hyperplastic lymphadenopathy from tumour invasion. This can alter tumour staging and therefore operability. In some centres the nodes are sampled and analysed under frozen section before proceeding.

Positron emission tomography scans

These are becoming a useful tool in identifying tumour involvement of mediastinal nodes as well as other local spread.

Sputum cytology

This is mainly useful in patients who would not tolerate a bronchoscopy.

Blood tests

These are not diagnostic but can identify complications:
* FBC—anaemia may indicate the progression of disease and/or bone marrow involvement
* Urea and electrolytes—↓ Na may indicate SIADH; ↑ urea dehydration
* Liver function tests—if deranged may indicate metastatic disease.

Differential diagnosis

This is of the presenting problem but could include:
* infection—consolidation from a pneumonia, TB
* lung abscess
* bronchial adenoma.

Complications

The vigour with which complications are treated will depend on the patient's general performance status and local expertise (Table 26).

Table 26 Complications associated with lung cancer.

Problem	Treatment
Dyspnoea	DXT, endobronchial DXT, laser or cryotherapy, stenting, opiates
Bone metastases	DXT, non-steroidal analgesics. Prophylactic surgery is recommended if a lesion is found in a non-fractured weight-bearing bone
Brain metastases	Palliative DXT, steroids Excision occasionally recommended for single metastasis
SVC obstruction	DXT, stenting
Haemoptysis	DXT, laser bronchoscopy
Electrolyte abnormality	Correct as appropriate (see *Endocrinology*, Sections 1.1 and 1.2)

DXT, Deep X-ray therapy; SVC, superior vena cava.

Treatment

Emergency

- Radiotherapy (DXT) for superior vena caval (SVC) obstruction or tracheal/bronchial obstruction (see *Oncology*, Section 1.8)
- Laser bronchoscopy or stenting of tracheal or main bronchial obstruction—requires swift referral to specialist centre
- Pain control—early referral to Macmillan/palliative care team.

Short term

Surgery

The most important step is to decide whether the patient is a candidate for surgery or not. Age should not be a barrier for referral. Those with solitary peripheral lesions should always be referred. In general, patients presenting with central lesions, metastases or small-cell lung cancer (SCLC) are not candidates for thoracotomy. If in any doubt, always make a swift referral to your local cardio-thoracic surgeon, as in most cases resection is the only treatment likely to be curative. Make sure the patient comes back to see you immediately if they are turned down for surgery.

Non-surgical treatment

RADIOTHERAPY

High-dose DXT with curative intent may be given to patients with non-small cell lung cancer (NSCLC) without metastases who decline surgery. Patients with extrathoracic spread are generally given a palliative dose to control local symptoms as high-dose DXT has not been shown to alter prognosis but can lead to considerable morbidity.

Prophylatic cranial DXT in SCLC has been shown to improve prognosis; however, postoperative DXT following resection does not improve prognosis [4].

CHEMOTHERAPY

Oral and/or intravenous treatment is given with DXT in small-cell disease. Trials continue to evaluate its usefulness in NSCLC and before or after lung resection.

Pain and symptom control

It is essential to introduce patients and family to support teams as soon as is appropriate.

Prognosis

Overall 5-year survival is 5.5%.

Prevention

Smoking cessation

 Tomorrow, tomorrow, tomorrow … No, today.

Never underestimate your ability to counsel patients about smoking cessation—your words may just be the crucial encouragement the patient needs [5]. Particularly if you have never smoked, do not appear distant and virtuous; imagine your worst habit, even if it is not life threatening, and how difficult it would be to give up.

Recent government-sponsored initiatives in the UK may lead to increased availability of clinics to help people quit smoking. It is worth knowing what is available in your area so that you can readily advise. Although most nicotine replacement therapies (NRT) are not available on NHS hospital formularies, have an idea of what is available and encourage patients to see their general practitioners for further advice. Preparations include nicotine patches, gum, vaporizer (inhalator), sublingual tablets and nasal spray.

 Encourage patients to quit, help them set a date on which to stop and refer them to a specialist smokers' clinic if appropriate. Record your advice in their notes and general practitioner letter, and take the opportunity to ask how they are getting on if you see them again in clinic.

See *Pain Relief and Palliative Care*, Sections 2.9 and 2.10.
See *Oncology*, Section 2.9.

1 Brown JS, Spiro SG. Update on lung cancer and mesothelioma. *J R Coll Physicians Lond* 1999; 33(6): 506–512.
2 Seaton A, Seaton D, Leitch AG. Cancer in the lung. In: Seaton A, Seaton D, Leitch AG, eds. *Crofton and Douglas's Respiratory Disease*. Oxford: Blackwell Science, 1995.
3 Spiro SG. Bronchial tumours. In: Brewis RAL, Corrin B, Geddes DM, Gibson GJ, eds. *Respiratory Medicine* (2nd edn). London: W.B. Saunders, 1995: 924–961.
4 Jett JR. Is there a role for adjuvant therapy for resected non-small cell lung cancer? *Thorax* 1999; 54 (Suppl. 2): S37–S41.
5 McEwen A, West R. How to intervene against smoking. *J R Coll Physicians Lond* 1999; 33: 513–515.

2.9.2 MESOTHELIOMA

Aetiology

Asbestos fibre has been used extensively for its fire-resistant properties in the building industry, in shipbuilding and for brake and clutch lines in cars. It was mined in countries as far apart as the former USSR, Canada and South Africa, and transported to countries such as the UK by boat. The crocidolite form of asbestos is now known to be particularly hazardous in causing the associated lung diseases [1–4].

Asbestos fibres are inhaled and become lodged in the alveoli where they are incompletely phagocytosed by macrophages. The resulting inflammatory reaction leads to local tissue damage and fibrosis, and is thought to increase susceptibility to malignant change.

Epidemiology

The effects of asbestos tend to occur 20–40 years after the initial exposure. Therefore, as asbestos controls only became law in the late 1970s, it is predicted that we will continue seeing cases well into the 21st century.

Clinical presentation

- Shortness of breath (often caused by pleural effusion)
- Weight loss
- Chest wall pain.

Physical signs

Evidence of a pleural effusion and/or pleural thickening with:
- decreased expansion on the affected side
- decreased breath sounds on the affected side.

A careful occupational history is required from anyone presenting in this way (See Section 1.11).

Investigations

Despite vigorous investigation it is sometimes not possible to obtain diagnostic histology confirming mesothelioma in life. Special stains can help and it may be worth discussing this with the pathologist. See Section 1.11, p. 178.
- Pleural biopsy and aspiration
- Thoracoscopy and biopsy
- CT scan of the chest (Fig. 39).

Differential diagnosis

- Lung cancer—there is a symbiotic relationship between asbestos and smoking, with lung cancer being five times more common in smokers exposed to asbestos than smokers who have no exposure
- Sarcoma
- Benign pleural thickening.

Treatment

Emergency

- Drain associated pleural effusions if the patient is very short of breath.
- Only consider pleurodesis once you have a tissue diagnosis.

 Both pleural biopsy and thoracoscopy must be performed in the presence of a pleural effusion.

Short term

- Radical surgery, involving rib and lung resection, is attempted in a very few patients with limited disease.
- Pain can be a major problem and difficult to control, even with opiates; involve the experts, i.e. the palliative care (Macmillan) team early. Local DXT may sometime help. Cervical cordotomy can help intractable unilateral pain.
- Surgical or medical pleurodesis can help prevent recurrent pleural effusions.
- Drain sites should be irradiated to prevent recurrence; mesothelioma is notorious for seeding along tracks.

Long term

Trials with γ-interferon are underway.

(a)

(b)

(c)

Fig. 39 (a) Chest radiograph of a man with left-sided mesothelioma; (b) computed tomography scan of the thorax shows extensive mesothelioma extending from apex, and (c) from the pleura into the thoracic cavity at the level of the left upper lobe. (Courtesy of Dr J. Moore-Gillon.)

Complications

- Repeated pleural effusions
- Severe pain.

Prognosis

Poor, with limited response to therapy. Median survival 12–18 months.

Prevention

There will continue to be a rise in the number of cases until at least 2015 as the rules controlling the use and handling of asbestos were only enforced in the late 1970s. The 20–40 years' latency from exposure to symptoms means that patients who were youngsters then will continue to present for some time.

Compensation claims

Patients with mesothelioma, asbestosis, diffuse pleural thickening and lung cancer associated with asbestosis are entitled to state compensation and receive a disability pension. Patients may also be able to make a claim against previous employers for any asbestos-related condition, including pleural plaques, and may receive compensation if the employers have been negligent in exposing them to asbestos.

If a patient wishes to pursue this course of action, the law generally allows them only 3 years in which to commence legal action after the date on which they first knew they had an asbestos-related condition. It is good practice to record that you advised the patient of this point when you diagnose an asbestos-related condition.

Similar procedures for both state benefits and claims against employers may be followed for coal worker's pneumoconiosis (CWP) and occupational asthma and a small number of other industrial lung diseases.

Disease associations

• Non-pleural mesothelioma tumours may occur as primary disease on the pericardium, usually presenting as constrictive pericarditis. Diagnosis is normally made by pericardial biopsy.

• Peritoneal mesothelioma causes vague symptoms of tiredness, lethargy and loss of appetite, followed by abdominal distension caused by ascites. Diagnosis may be made by laparoscopic omental biopsy.

See *Oncology*, Section 2.9.
1 Brown JS, Spiro SG. Update on lung cancer and mesothelioma. *J R Coll Physicians Lond* 1999; 33: 506–512.
2 Edge JR. Mesothelioma. *British Journal of Hospital Medicine* 1983; 29: 521–536.
3 Morgan WKC, Gee JBL. Asbestos-related disease. In: Morgan WKC, Seaton A, eds. *Occupational Lung Diseases* (3rd edn). W. B. Saunders, 1995.
4 Rudd RM. Asbestos-related disease. In: Brewis RAL, Corrin B, Geddes DM, Gibson GJ, eds. *Respiratory Medicine* (2nd edn). W.B. Saunders, 1995: 545–569.

2.9.3 MEDIASTINAL TUMOURS

Aetiology

The mediastinum is the part of the thorax lying between the two pleural sacs and contains the heart and various other thoracic viscera. It is a site where masses of different pathology are not uncommon: they can occur at any age and may be solid or cystic [1–3].

Based on a lateral chest radiograph, the mediastinum can be divided into three compartments (Fig. 40). Table 27 shows the normal constituents of the three compartments of the mediastinum as well as the tumours and cysts that may occur in each compartment.

Clinical presentation

Fifty per cent of all mediastinal masses are asymptomatic and 90% of these are benign. The likelihood of malignancy is higher in infants and children than in adults. The signs and symptoms of mediastinal masses depend upon the compression and invasion of nearby intrathoracic structures (Table 28). Mediastinal tumours may also be associated with various endocrine syndromes: myasthenia gravis with thymoma being particularly noteworthy (See *Neurology*, Section 2.2.5).

Investigations

The diagnostic approach to mediastinal masses can be divided into:
• imaging techniques
• techniques for obtaining tissue samples.

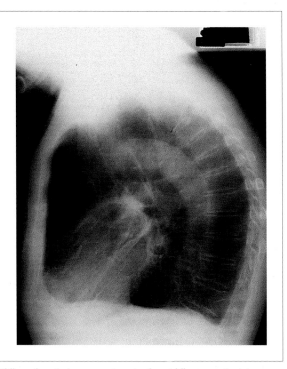

Fig. 40 Lateral chest radiograph showing division of the mediastinum into anterior, middle and posterior compartments, the middle compartment containing the heart and great vessels.

Table 27 Normal constituents of the mediastinum and tumours arising from them.

Compartment	Location	Normal contents	Examples of mediastinal mass
Anterior	Superior and anterior to the heart shadow	Thymus gland (remnant), internal mammary arterier and veins, lymph nodes, fat	Thymoma, lymphoma, retrosternal thyroid and parathyroid mass, fibroma, lipoma, teratoma, seminoma, choriocarcinoma
Middle	Posterior and inferior to the anterior compartment	Heart, pericardium, great vessels, trachea, major bronchi, phrenic nerves	Aortic arch aneurysm, pericardial cysts, left ventricular aneurysm, vascular lesions
Posterior	Lies within the margins of the thoracic vertebrae	Oesophagus, thoracic duct, descending thoracic aorta, azygos and hemiazygos veins, sympathetic chain	Oesophageal tumours, neurogenic tumours (neurofibroma, neurilemoma, neurosarcoma, ganglioneuroma, neuroblastoma, chemodectoma, phaeochromocytoma), diaphragmatic hernia, rare tumours (Adkin's tumour, Descending aortic aneurysm chordoma, mediastinal sarcoma

SVC, superior vena cava; TB, tuberculosis.

Table 28 Clinical presentation of mediastinal tumours.

Structure involved	Signs and symptoms
Trachea and main bronchus	Stridor, cough, dyspnoea, recurrent chest infections
Phrenic nerve	Diaphragmatic paralysis
Oesophagus	Dysphagia
Sympathetic trunk	Horner's syndrome
Superior vena cava	Non-pulsatile distension of neck veins, cyanosis and swelling of the face, neck and upper arm, dilated veins on chest wall
Pericardium	Pericardial effusion, pericarditis
Left recurrent laryngeal nerve	Left vocal cord palsy with hoarse voice

Imaging techniques

Chest radiograph

Most mediastinal tumours are discovered incidentally by posteroanterior or lateral chest radiographs.

Computed tomography

This helps evaluate the origin of a mediastinal mass and can also diagnose certain lesions confidently, e.g. teratoma.

Magnetic resonance imaging

This can offer superior definition to CT scanning and may be preferred prior to surgery.

Radionuclide scanning

These techniques can be used for specific lesions such as:
- radioiodine scanning for ectopic thyroid tissue

- uptake of thallium (^{201}Tl) by Hodgkin's lymphoma
- radioactive gold may be useful in localizing extra-medullary haematopoiesis.

Techniques for obtaining mediastinal tissue

- Mediastinoscopy
- Mediastinotomy.

Treatment

The treatment of a mediastinal mass would depend on the nature and location of the lesion.

1 Pierson DJ. Disorders of the pleura, mediastinum and diaphragm. In: *Harrison's Principles of Internal Medicine* (12th edn). McGraw-Hill: 1111–1116.
2 Pierson DJ. Tumours and cysts of the mediastinum. In: Murray JF, Nadel JA, eds. *Textbook of Respiratory Medicine* (2nd edn). W.B. Saunders: 2278–2290.
3 Benjamin SP, McCormack LJ, Effler DB, Groves LK. Primary tumours of the mediastinum. *Chest* 1972; 62: 297–303.

2.10 Disorders of the chest wall and diaphragm

Aetiology

A variety of chest wall disorders can lead to nocturnal hypoventilation and chronic respiratory failure, which occurs when the load placed on the respiratory muscle pump exceeds the pump's capacity. Abnormalities are initially present at night when the patient is often supine (increasing load) and drive is physiologically reduced, especially in rapid eye movement (REM) sleep.

The most common disorders are:

- post-tuberculous sequelae
- scoliosis
- kyphosis
- fibrothorax
- ankylosing spondylitis.

Post-tuberculous sequelae

Prior to the advent of combination chemotherapy, thoracoplasty was used as a treatment for pulmonary TB. Other therapies previously used (e.g. artificial pneumothoraces, phrenic nerve crush and plombage) may exacerbate load–capacity imbalance, but seldom cause ventilatory failure on their own. In the 1950s 30 000 thoracoplasties were performed in the UK.

Scoliosis

- Scoliosis is classified as congenital if there are associated spinal abnormalities (such as a hemivertebra).
- Scoliosis may also occur in association with neurological disease, notably poliomyelitis, muscular dystrophies, spinal muscular atrophy and syringomyelia.
- Most often no cause is found, when scoliosis is then termed idiopathic.

Kyphosis

When it occurs early in life (e.g. tuberculous osteomyelitis) kyphosis may cause CRF, but kyphosis alone in later life (e.g. resulting from osteoporosis or malignancy) seldom causes respiratory failure.

Fibrothorax

In fibrothorax stiffness of the thorax occurs because of pleural disease, especially after haemothorax, tuberculous empyema or asbestos exposure.

Ankylosing spondylitis

This is an unusual cause of CRF unless there is another pathology of which COPD would be the most likely.

Epidemiology

In a Swedish registry study of patients receiving home oxygen or ventilation [1] the annual demand was calculated at 3 per 10^6 population. Eighty-seven per cent of the patients had scoliosis, and half of these were as a result of previous polio.

Clinical presentation

Scoliotic patients should be regularly reviewed once their VC is less than 1.5 L.

 A minor change may precipitate respiratory failure. Consider infection or prescription of sedative drugs.

- Common—exertional dyspnoea, orthopnoea. Symptoms of nocturnal ventilatory failure (morning headache, daytime somnolence, mood or personality change)
- Uncommon—acute respiratory failure, cor pulmonale.

Physical signs

The patient should have a full respiratory, cardiac and skeletal examination looking particularly for:

- cyanosis
- carbon dioxide retention flap, dilated veins, papilloedema
- skeletal/rib-cage deformity
- presence of scars suggestive of phrenic nerve crush
- elevated JVP (may suggest pulmonary hypertension or cor pulmonale)
- respiratory signs
- ankle swelling.

Investigations

- FBC—may show polycythaemia
- arterial blood gases—may demonstrate daytime hypercapnia
- ECG—in case of rhythm disturbance and RVH
- Pulmonary function—these disorders are usually associated with a restrictive defect. Measurement of lung volumes is desirable
- Imaging—a chest radiograph is usual, although it can be almost uninterpretable in severe scoliosis. Spinal radiographs can be examined to determine the Cobb angle (Fig. 41). Angles less than 70° are seldom associated with respiratory failure unless a dual pathology exists
- Overnight transcutaneous O_2/CO_2 study—to detect incipient respiratory failure. An example of a patient with nocturnal respiratory failure despite initial normal gas tensions is shown in Fig. 42
- Echocardiography—is used to assess pulmonary artery pressure.

Differential diagnosis

There is no plausible differential diagnosis to the condition of scoliosis. Instead the clinical evaluation should seek to determine whether the magnitude of symptoms is

Fig. 41 Radiograph of a scoliotic patient. The Cobb angle is calculated by drawing lines parallel to the sections of spine above and below the curve. In a normal subject with a straight spine the angle is 0°, but in this case it is 66°.

appropriate for the degree of skeletal disease. If not, a second diagnosis should be sought.

Treatment

For patients who are still growing, early treatment (see below) can prevent worsening of curvature. Screening of school-age children is therefore important, as is regular review of children found to have a scoliosis.

Spinal stabilization

For children with an increasing curvature, treatment options include:

• external fixation (e.g. with a trunk brace)
• internal surgical stabilization by vertebral fusion or insertion of rods.
Although there are arguments for and against both procedures, the role of surgery is becoming increasingly important. Surgery may also be considered in adults but the main aim here is the palliation of pain.

Oxygen

Controlled oxygen therapy is indicated if the PaO_2 is <7.3 kPa. In most cases this will be combined with nocturnal nasal inspiratory pressure support (see below). Portable oxygen systems may palliate exertional dyspnoea.

Domiciliary ventilatory support

For patients with symptoms of CRF, home mechanical ventilation is effective [2]. The most commonly used technique is inspiratory pressure support delivered via a nasal mask.

Complications

See also Section 2.11, p. 230.

Common

• Musculoskeletal (relating to spinal deformity) and joint related
• Respiratory tract infection
• Hypertension.

Less common

• Chronic respiratory failure [3]
• Pulmonary artery hypertension.

Fig. 42 Overnight O_2/CO_2 study in a patient with a scoliosis. Three dips in SaO_2 (upper line) are demonstrated with an associated rise in $tcpCO_2$, (lower line) which correspond to REM sleep. Note that this patient has gas tensions in the normal range initially and therefore probably has normal daytime blood gases.

Contraindications

Carbon dioxide retention

Carbon dioxide retention is not an absolute contraindication, but the clinician will need to assess the magnitude of carbon dioxide retention and weigh the risks/symptoms attributable to this against the benefit of improving hypoxia.

Smoking

Smoking in the presence of home oxygen is a fire hazard [3]. For this reason some clinicians do not prescribe oxygen to patients who admit a continued tobacco habit. Others argue that as some patients dishonestly deny continued smoking, this approach is unreasonable.

Practical details

For survival benefit LTOT needs to be used for a minimum of 15 h per day and is therefore best given via an oxygen concentrator. In England and Wales this is prescribed by the patient's general practitioner, but in Scotland this is the responsibility of the local chest physician.

Short-burst oxygen is more conveniently prescribed from a cylinder. Most of the devices for ambulatory oxygen administration are not currently available on prescription in the UK; they are either purchased by the specialist respiratory unit (often with charitable funds) or the patient themselves [4].

Outcome

For patients with COPD, LTOT reduces hospital admission and improves survival [1, 2].

Complications

- As well as smoking, oxygen presents a general fire risk [5]
- Services must be installed to locally determined standards.

1 Nocturnal Oxygen Therapy Trial Group. Continuous or nocturnal oxygen therapy in hypoxaemic chronic obstructive lung disease. *Ann Intern Med* 1980; 93: 391–398.

2 Medical Research Council. Long-term domiciliary oxygen therapy in chronic hypoxic cor pulmonale complicating chronic bronchitis and emphysema. Report of a working party. *Lancet* 1981; i: 681–686.

3 Maxwell DL, McGlashan JA, Andrews S, Gleeson MJ. Hazards of domiciliary oxygen therapy. *Respir Med* 1993; 87: 225–226.

4 Wedzicha JA. Domiciliary oxygen therapy services: clinical guidelines and advice for prescribers. *J R Coll Physicians Lond* 1999; 33: 445–447.

5 West GA, Primeau P. Nonmedical hazards of long-term oxygen therapy. *Respir Care* 1983; 28: 906–912.

2.12.2 CONTINUOUS POSITIVE AIRWAYS PRESSURE

Principle

CPAP describes the application of a constant pressure to the airway; the pressure may be applied to a cuffed endotracheal or tracheostomy tube or via a nasal or facial mask. It is important to appreciate that, by contrast to non-invasive ventilation (see Section 2.12.3, p. 233), no airflow will occur in a patient receiving CPAP in the absence of respiratory muscle activity (Fig. 43).

The increased airway pressure exerts a dilating force on the upper airway (hence its use in OSA, see Section 2.1.1, p. 188) and, if the upper airway is patent, increases EELV (hence its use in respiratory tract infection).

Indications

Acute

- Respiratory tract infection
- Pulmonary oedema (but caution in ischaemic heart disease)
- Postoperatively.

Chronic

- OSA
- Snoring
- Sleep-disordered breathing associated with congestive cardiac failure.

Contraindications

Nil.

Practical details

CPAP may be either high or low flow. High-flow CPAP is driven by piped air with room air entrained using a flow generator; flows in excess of 100 L/min may achieved in this way. Although this apparatus does not provide ventilatory assistance, the high flows mean that the work of breathing is much reduced. This mode is preferred for acute applications.

For domiciliary use, lightweight portable machines are available. Newer machines are able to sense flattening of the inspiratory flow curve and adjust the pressure level accordingly. It is hypothesized that this approach will improve patient adherence in OSA [1].

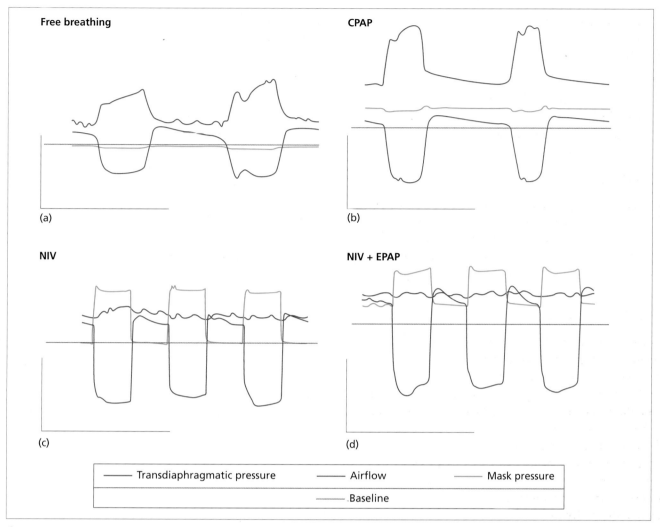

Fig. 43 Continuous positive airway pressure (CPAP) is not the same as non-invasive ventilation (NIV). In both free breathing (a) and CPAP (b) the patient still has to make an effort—shown by the large changes in transdiaphragmatic pressure. For NIV, either without expiratory positive airways pressure (EPAP) (c) or with EPAP (d), the patient's effort is minimal, but the ventilator is imposing a pressure change on the system.

Outcome

Acute

By increasing EELV V/Q matching is improved and, consequently, oxygenation. CPAP may not influence the course of the underlying disease so, for example, a patient developing ARDS may improve initially on CPAP but then subsequently require intubation if lung injury progresses.

Chronic

Although the effect of CPAP, if any, on cardiovascular mortality in OSA remains to be determined, randomized studies show it to be of value in improving daytime wakefulness and quality of life.

Complications

• Local—nasal bridge ulceration (Fig. 44), irritation of the nasal mucosa

Fig. 44 This patient was receiving domiciliary ventilatory support via a nasal mask. Nasal bridge ulceration occurred and he had to switch to an alternative interface to continue his treatment.

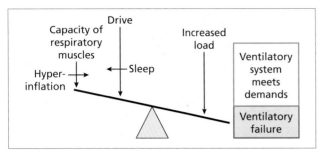

Fig. 45 As with other organ system failure, respiratory failure occurs when the load on the system exceeds capacity; this may occur acutely or chronically. During sleep the drive to the respiratory muscle pump is physiologically reduced and it is for this reason that chronic respiratory failure in its early stages demonstrates only nocturnal abnormalities.

• Systemic—may reduce cardiac preload and consequently afterload.

1 Loube DI. Technologic advances in the treatment of obstructive sleep apnea syndrome. *Chest* 1999; 116: 1426–1433.

2.12.3 NON-INVASIVE VENTILATION

Principle

Respiratory failure results from an imbalance between the capacity of the respiratory muscle pump and the load placed upon it; this imbalance may occur chronically or acutely and for a variety of reasons (see Fig. 45). Unless treatment of the underlying cause is immediately efficacious, mechanical support is required to relieve respiratory failure. This can be given either invasively via an endotracheal tube or non-invasively.

The latter option, termed non-invasive ventilation, may be positive pressure via a nasal/facial mask or negative pressure (as for example with an 'iron lung'). In recent years the clinical uses of non-invasive positive-pressure ventilation (NIPPV) have expanded significantly.

The masks used for CPAP (see Section 2.12.2, p. 232) are also used for NIPPV and this can lead to confusion in the minds of some medical and paramedical staff. The difference between CPAP and NIPPV is not trivial and is that:
• with CPAP a constant pressure is applied to the airway
• in NIPPV a pulse of positive pressure is applied (see Fig. 43). The rate may be controlled by the machine or, more often, the patient is able to trigger the machine by initiating a breath.

If a positive pressure is applied in the expiratory phase (EPAP) in addition to the pulse delivered to support inspiration, then the machine is said to allow bilevel pressure application.

Indications

Acute

Established indications are:
• Acute NIPPV reduces intubation rate in patients with acute decompensated COPD [1]. NIPPV can also facilitate weaning [2].
• Acute respiratory failure can also be treated with NIPPV [3] but this requires the support of a specialized ICU/high-dependency unit (HDU).

 NIV treats respiratory failure. Do not be tempted to try and treat other conditions with it.

Chronic

The main indications are:
• restrictive thoracic disorders
• COPD
• neuromuscular and control of breathing disorders.
The timing of initiation of domiciliary NIV requires specialist assessment which will take into consideration the diagnosis, symptom load and physiological data [4].

Contraindications

Acute

• Patient too obtunded to co-operate
• Patient unable to protect airway
• Claustrophobia or anatomical facial deformity
• Haemodynamic instability.

Chronic

Claustrophobia or anatomical facial deformity.

Practical details

It is important that the operator is familiar with the ventilator to be used. Outside specialist units it is probably preferable to use a single model. For acute indications a full face mask is preferred, but for chronic applications a nasal mask is usually the first choice. Further detail as to how to set up a machine are beyond the scope of this work but may be found elsewhere, together with details on alternative interfaces and methods of ventilatory support such as negative pressure ventilation [5].

When using NIV for the management of acute decompensated COPD it is necessary to decide whether or not the patient is a candidate for endotracheal ventilation

Fig. 46 Algorithm for the management of acute respiratory failure using non-invasive ventilation (NIV). CVP, central venous pressure.

(ETV) if NIV fails (see Section 1.15, p. 185). A suggested algorithm is shown in Fig. 46. If the patient is a candidate for ETV then recent data suggest that patients with a pH <7.30 after bronchodilators are best managed in an HDU/ICU environment by a physician with special expertise in NIV [6].

Outcome

Acute

In a study performed in general wards in the UK with COPD patients with a pH in the range 7.25–7.35 the mortality was 20% with standard therapy and 10% with NIV. This was stratified by pH so that for patients in the range 7.3–7.35 rates were 14.5 and 5%, respectively, and for patients with pH 7.25–7.30 were 29 and 21%, respectively [6].

Chronic

At the Brompton Hospital the 5-year chance of continuing NIV (which relates approximately to survival) was 79% for scoliosis, 94% for previous TB, 100% for past polio, 81% for neuromuscular disease, 43% for COPD. Bronchiectatics had a particularly poor prognosis; median survival 0.7 years [7].

Complications

These include:
- nasal bridge ulceration (see Fig. 44)
- aerophagy.

1 Brochard L, Mancebo J, Wysocki M *et al*. Noninvasive ventilation for acute exacerbations of chronic obstructive pulmonary disease. *N Engl J Med* 1995; 333: 817–822.
2 Nava S, Ambrosino N, Clini E *et al*. Noninvasive mechanical ventilation in the weaning of patients with respiratory failure due to chronic obstructive pulmonary disease. *Ann Intern Med* 1998; 128: 721–728.
3 Antonelli M, Conti G, Rocco M *et al*. A comparison of non-invasive positive pressure ventilation and conventional mechanical ventilation in patients with acute respiratory failure. *N Engl J Med* 1998; 339: 429–435.
4 Clinical indications for non-invasive positive pressure ventilation in chronic respiratory failure due to restrictive lung disease, COPD, and nocturnal hypoventilation—a consensus conference report. *Chest* 1999; 116: 521–534.
5 Simonds AK. *Non-Invasive Respiratory Support*. London: Chapman and Hall, 1996.
6 Plant PK, Owen JL, Elliott MW. Use of non-invasive ventilation (NIV) in acute exacerbations of COPD—Subgroup analysis of a multicentre randomised controlled trial. *Am J Respir Crit Care Med* 1999; 159: A15.
7 Simonds AK, Elliott MW. Outcome of domiciliary nasal intermittent positive pressure ventilation in restrictive and obstructive disorders. *Thorax* 1995; 50: 604–609.

2.13 Lung transplantation

Principle

The aim of transplantation is to replace a poorly functioning organ with a better one [1]. Operative procedures from cadaveric donors are:
- single (approximately 50% of the total)
- double lung transplantations (approximately 25% of the total)
- heart–lung transplantation (approximately 25% of the total).

There has been recent interest in living lobar transplantation [2], but the final position of this approach remains to be decided.

Indications

The general indication is pulmonary disease that is clinically and physiologically severe despite maximal medical therapy. As a rule of thumb the life expectancy of the condition should be less than that of the transplant recipient (see below), i.e. 2–3 years or less. The patient should be adequately nourished with an appropriate psychological state and social support.

In practice the most common diagnoses are, in order:
- COPD (including α_1-antitrypsin deficiency)
- CF
- primary pulmonary hypertension
- idiopathic pulmonary fibrosis
- pulmonary hypertension secondary to congenital cardiac disease.

There are detailed guidelines on the severity of these conditions in relation to the timing of transplantation [3].

Contraindications

Absolute contraindications are:
- unstable clinical condition
- neoplasia
- uncontrolled/untreatable infection; this does not disqualify patients with airway colonization
- significant cardiac dysfunction (unless heart–lung transplantation is considered)
- cigarette usage; drug/alcohol dependency
- serious psychological disorder.

Relative contraindications: because the supply of donor organs does not meet the demand, many units operate age restrictions.
- ventilator-dependent patients have a worse prognosis and many units feel it unethical to offer organs to these patients if non-ventilator-dependent patients also require an organ. This does not apply to patients using non-invasive ventilators.
- previous cardiac surgery, pleurectomy or pleurodesis increase operative difficulty and risk. Prior history of simple pneumothorax (and tube drainage) does not.

Practical details

Preoperative

Ideally the patient should be on as low a dose of corticosteroids as possible. Bridging strategies such as prostacyclin infusions (for primary pulmonary hypertension (PPH)) and non-invasive ventilation are of value.

Operative

Surgical details are beyond the scope of a medical text, but it should be noted that organ retrieval, preservation and assessment are crucial.

Postoperative

Regular follow-up of the patient is key. In particular repeated transbronchial biopsies are required, and the patient must perform daily spirometry.

Complications

The decline in survival is biphasic. In the first 3 months the leading causes of death are infection and primary graft failure. Later, chronic rejection becomes more important and is characterized by bronchiolitis obliterans and, physiologically, airflow obstruction.

Retransplantation is a controversial issue. While this procedure can be life saving in case of failure of the transplanted organ, many centres feel that it is unethical to offer individuals a second organ while other patients die on the transplant list because of a shortage of donor organs.

1 Thulrock EP. Lung transplantation. *Am J Respir Crit Care Med* 1997; 155: 789–818.
2 Dark JH. Lung: living related transplantation. *Br Med Bull* 1997; 53: 892–903.
3 American Society for Transplant Physicians (ASTP)/American Thoracic Society (ATS)/European Respiratory Society (ERS)/International Society for Heart and Lung Transplantation (ISHLT). International guidelines for the selection of lung transplant candidates. *Am J Respir Crit Care Med* 1998; 158: 335–339.

3 Investigations and practical procedures

3.1 Arterial blood gas sampling

Principle

To measure the oxygen and carbon dioxide tensions and acid–base status of arterial blood.

Indications

Arterial blood gas sampling was a research procedure until the mid 1960s. It is now widely performed, either by direct arterial puncture or from indwelling arterial lines. Indications include:
- respiratory failure (type I or II)
- renal failure
- hepatic failure
- cardiac failure
- drug intoxication (aspirin, narcotics)
- endogenous acid overproduction (ketoacidosis or lactic acidosis)
- severe illness, cause unknown.

For interpretation of data, see Section 3.6.1.

Contraindications

May need care in presence of bleeding disorders.

Important information for patients

The procedure should be explained to the patient. The possibility of requiring more than one attempt should be mentioned.

Practical details

Before investigation

The patient should be lying or sitting comfortably and an appropriate site selected. The radial artery of the non-dominant arm is most commonly used, but the brachial or femoral arteries can be used. Make sure you have enough sterile gauze to apply immediate pressure after the procedure.

The investigation

Clean the skin over the wrist with an antiseptic solution.

Palpate the artery between the tips of the forefinger and the middle finger of one hand.

Introduce the needle with the heparinized syringe attached to it between the fingers, at an angle of 45°, and slowly advance the needle along the line of the artery. On puncturing the artery, a small spurt of blood entering the syringe will be seen.

Withdraw 3–4 mL of blood and press a sterile pressure dressing over the site of puncture.

Expel any air bubbles and cap the syringe. The syringe should be labelled and sent to the lab immediately on ice if a blood gas machine is not available at the 'bedside'.

The role of local anaesthesia remains controversial. Although used by some, especially in paediatric practice, skilled operators maintain that it adds unnecessary complexity to the procedure.

After investigation

The pressure dressing should be kept in place for 5 min or until all bleeding stops.

Complications

In practice, complications are rare:
- haematoma
- arterial spasm leading to distal ischaemia
- femoral nerve lies lateral to the femoral artery and can be injured if femoral artery is the chosen site
- median nerve lies medial to the brachial artery and can be injured.

Lightowler JV, Elliott MW. Local anaesthetic infiltration prior to arterial puncture for blood gas analysis: a survey of current practice and a randomised double blind placebo controlled trial. *J R Coll Physicians Lond* 1997; 31 (6): 645–646.

3.2 Aspiration of pleural effusion or pneumothorax

Principle

To aspirate fluid from a pleural effusion or air from a pneumothorax. This can be carried out using a syringe and a cannula, which is less traumatic than a chest drain (see Section 3.4), and should be considered before chest drain insertion in most cases.

Indications

• Pleural effusion—aspiration is preferred where the aim is to collect a diagnostic sample (just a few millilitres) or if the aim is simply to palliate symptoms by removing fluid where the cause is known
• Pneumothorax—aspiration is preferred unless there is respiratory embarrassment or bilateral pneumothoraces.

Contraindications

Gross abnormalities of coagulation clotting require correction. Herpes zoster or local pyoderma imply the need to choose an alternative, healthy skin area.

Important information for patients

The procedure should be explained to the patient and the possibility of developing a pneumothorax should be mentioned.

Practical details

Before procedure

A simple aspiration can be performed without local anaesthesia if the patient is co-operative. In anxious patients, lidocaine should be infiltrated into the skin and the parietal pleura. Except in the case of a diagnostic aspiration of fluid (when a 20-mL syringe and green needle suffice) the equipment required is:
• a wide-bore (grey) venflon
• a three-way tap
• a 50-mL Luer lock syringe.
In the case of an effusion, a jug and a giving set with fluid chamber cut off will also be required.

Pleural effusion technique

The patient should be seated comfortably, either on the edge of a bed resting forward onto one or more pillows on a bedside table, or 'cowboy style' on a chair (back-to-front, facing the chair back, with arms resting on the chair back).

The area of stony dullness corresponding to the radiograph should be identified and one interspace below this marked with a biro, usually in the line of the scapula.

Having cleaned the skin, the venflon is inserted while aspirating with a syringe. Remember to enter the pleural cavity just above the rib to avoid injury to the neurovascular bundle.

When fluid is obtained, advance the cannula while removing the stylet and connect the three-way tap with the 50-mL syringe and the giving set attached.

By aspirating and then expelling into the jug, the effusion is aspirated. The purpose of the giving set is to avoid air inadvertently entering the pleural space.

Not more than 1500 mL of fluid should be aspirated in a single session as re-expansion pulmonary oedema may occur. Discontinue aspiration if the patient experiences cough, dyspnoea or faintness (signs of rapid mediastinal shift).

Pneumothorax technique

In case of a pneumothorax, with the patient in the supine position, aspirate the air from the second intercostal space in the midclavicular line. Discontinue the procedure if more than 2.5 L are aspirated (a large leak will need chest drain), if resistance is felt or if patient coughs excessively.

After procedure

Apply a dressing and request a chest radiograph.

Complications

• Entry into the pleural cavity may precipitate vasovagal syncope (give intravenous atropine)
• Rapid aspiration of effusion can lead to re-expansion pulmonary oedema
• Pneumothorax
• Haemothorax.

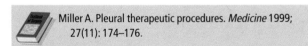
Miller A. Pleural therapeutic procedures. *Medicine* 1999; 27(11): 174–176.

3.3 Pleural biopsy

Principle

Pleural biopsy is used to obtain a sample of the parietal pleura for cytological and microbiological examination.

Indications

All cases of exudative pleural effusion of undetermined cause. Discrete pleural lesions are best biopsied under radiological control because of the difficulty matching the surface landmarks to radiological anatomy.

Contraindications

- Absence of adequate pleural fluid
- Borderline respiratory function—production of a pneumothorax can precipitate respiratory failure
- Empyema—risk of development of multiple subcutaneous abscesses
- Presence of a bleeding diasthesis
- Thrombocytopenia (if platelets <50 000/mm^3, platelets should be transfused before the procedure).

Important information for patients

The procedure should be explained to the patient and the possibility of developing a pneumothorax should be mentioned.

Practical details

Before procedure

Premedication with an opiate or midazolam will help to reduce pain and anxiety.

The patient should be comfortable during the procedure and this is best achieved by having him or her sitting on the edge of the bed or on a stool with arms and head resting on one or more pillows on a bedside table. The operator stands behind the patient.

The site for the biopsy should be selected with care on the basis of a recent chest radiograph and clinical presentation. The best site is in the intercostal space below the spot where the tactile fremitus is lost and the percussion note becomes dull, superior to the rib below and hence avoiding the neurovascular bundle.

The procedure

The procedure can be performed either using the Abrams' needle or the Cope's needle. The Abrams' needle is more common and hence will be described here.

After positioning the patient and cleaning the skin with sterile solution, the skin and underlying tissues are infiltrated with 1% lidocaine. It is essential to anaesthetize the parietal pleura, which is rich in pain receptors. Do this as follows: once you have entered the pleural cavity and are aspirating pleural fluid, withdraw the needle slightly until nothing comes on aspiration. At this stage the needle is in contact with the parietal pleura: infiltrate with lidocaine, and allow 5 min for it to act.

Prepare for the biopsy by using a scalpel to make a small incision (0.5 cm) in the skin and the tissues, dissecting if necessary with forceps.

Introduce the Abrams' needle into the pleural space using constant and firm pressure. Then remove the stylet and, with the inner cannula in the closed position, attach a syringe to the inner cannula.

Rotate the inner cannula anticlockwise in the outer cannula to open the distal notch.

Aspirate pleural fluid and withdraw the needle slowly until it hooks onto the pleura.

Rotate the inner cannula into the closed position and remove the whole needle.

A specimen of the pleura should be found in the tip of the needle. Three specimens are normally obtained at the 3 o'clock, 6 o'clock and 9 o'clock positions.

After procedure

A dressing at the site should be applied and a chest radiograph should be requested.

Complications

Although many complications are possible these are not common in practice:
- vasovagal syncope (give intravenous atropine)
- pneumothorax/haemopneumothorax
- bronchopleural fistula if the viseral pleura is damaged
- bleeding because of damage to the intercostal artery or vein
- visceral damage—spleen, liver, kidney.

3.4 Intercostal tube insertion

Principle

Intercostal tube insertion enables drainage fluid, air, blood or pus from the pleural cavity. It can be life saving, and may have to be performed rapidly and in unusual places. All doctors should be able to perform it.

Indications

- Tension pneumothorax
- Bilateral pneumothorax
- Empyema (use a tube of large diameter 28–32 F)
- Any patient with pneumothorax who is to be ventilated
- Haemothorax
- Any pleural effusion adversely affecting patients breathing (and not relieved by aspiration)
- To drain the pleural cavity dry prior to pleurodesis.

Contraindications

There are no absolute contraindications. However:
• bleeding diastheses should be corrected before chest drain insertion when possible
• it can be difficult to insert a drain if the pleura is thickened.

 Patients with COPD may have large bullae that resemble pneumothoraces. They will not be helped by intercostal tube drainage.

Important information for patients

The procedure should be explained to the patient and the possibility of developing a haemothorax should be mentioned.

Practical details

Before procedure

Premedication with an opiate or midazolam will reduce pain and anxiety; however, bear in mind the respiratory depression that can occur as a result of these drugs.

The patient should be lying supine with the head end of the bed elevated 30–45° and the arm held behind the head. A recent chest radiograph should be reviewed and the site of insertion should be marked. The drain should be inserted in the triangle of safety:
• between the anterior and posterior axillary lines, preferably anterior to the mid-axillary line
• below the axillary vessels
• in the level of or above the nipple (i.e. fifth intercostal space)
• above the rib avoiding the neurovascular bundle.

The procedure

Infiltrate the clean skin and parietal pleura with 2% lidocaine.

Incise the skin in the line of the ribs (2 cm) and dissect soft tissue with artery forceps.

Insert two strong non-absorbable sutures: one simple suture to secure the drain and one vertical mattress suture to close the wound after removal of the drain. A purse string suture results in a circular wound, which heals with a scar and should not be used.

When the pleura is breached, insert the drain with the trocar retracted so that it acts as a rigid directional guide only. Do not use excessive force as you may damage the underlying viscera.

In case of a pneumothorax aim the drain towards the apex. In case of an effusion, aim the drain inferiorly.

Once the drain is inserted, remove the trocar slowly and connect the tube to the underwater seal system.

Secure the drain and apply sterile dressing.

After procedure

• Obtain a chest radiograph to check position of the drain.
• Always maintain the level of water above the bottom of the tube in the underwater seal system.
• The bottle should be kept below the chest level.
• Never clamp the chest drain in case of pneumothorax (risk of developing a tension pneumothorax).
• Check daily if it is draining, bubbling or swinging.

Removal of chest drain

• In case of a pneumothorax, it can be removed once there is no bubbling, minimal swinging with respiration and chest radiograph shows a fully expanded lung.
• In case of a pleural effusion, it can be removed once it is draining less than 30 mL of fluid in 24 h.

The drain should be removed with the patient performing a Valsalva manoeuvre. A chest radiograph should be performed afterwards to check for pneumothorax.

Complications

These can include:
• bronchopleural fistula caused by injury to the lung
• visceral injury (liver, heart, diaphragm, spleen, stomach)
• thoracic duct injury causing chylothorax
• long thoracic nerve damage causing winging of the scapula
• haemothorax.

 American College of Surgeons Committee on Trauma,1993. Light RW. *Pleural diseases* (2nd edn). Lea and Febiger: 311–320.

3.5 Fibreoptic bronchoscopy and transbronchial biopsy

3.5.1 FIBREOPTIC BRONCHOSCOPY

Principle

Fibreoptic bronchoscopy allows inspection of the bronchial tree and the biopsy of abnormal lesions.

Indications

The indications given under the American Thoracic Society Guidelines are:
- diagnostic
- therapeutic.

Diagnostic

- Evaluate lung lesions that appear on chest radiograph
- Assess airway patency
- Investigate unexplained haemoptysis
- Search the origin of suspicious or positive sputum cytology
- Obtain specimen for microbiological examination in suspected infections
- Investigate cause of SVC obstruction, vocal cord palsy, unexplained pleural effusion and paralysis of a hemidiaphragm
- Evaluate a suspected tracheoesophageal fistula
- Evaluate the airways for suspected bronchial tear after thoracic trauma
- Determine the extent of respiratory injury after inhalation of noxious fumes or aspiration of gastric juice.

Therapeutic

These are often performed via an endotracheal tube:
- Remove foreign bodies
- Remove secretions or mucous plugs
- Perform difficult intubations.

3.5.2 TRANSBRONCHIAL BIOPSY

Principle

To obtain diagnostic tissue, usually in cases of suspected diffuse parenchymal lung disease.

Indications

Although the samples obtained are small and sometimes crushed, transbronchial biopsy achieves a high diagnostic yield in diffuse parenchymal lung diseases that have centrilobular accentuation, such as granulomatous and metastatic diseases. These include:
- sarcoidosis—75–89% diagnostic yield
- carcinoma—64–68% diagnostic yield
- infection
- eosinophilic pneumonia
- alveolar proteinosis.

Complications

The risk of developing a pneumothorax is 10%; however, this can be reduced by avoiding the right middle lobe and the lingula and with the use of fluoroscopy.

Sokolowski RW, Burgher LW, Jones FL *et al.* Guidelines for fibreoptic bronchoscopy in adults. *Am Rev Respir Dis* 1987; 136: 1066.
British Thoracic Society. The Diagnosis, assessment and treatment of diffuse parenchymal lung disease in adults. *Thorax* 1999; 54: Supplement 1.

3.6 Interpretation of clinical data

3.6.1 ARTERIAL BLOOD GASES

What is measured

Whenever you take a set of blood gases, make sure that you clearly record the date, time, patient's name and their inspired concentration of oxygen. This is crucial for interpretation and comparison with other results: a Po_2 of 12 kPa is normal if the patient is breathing air but grossly abnormal if they are on 60% oxygen!

Blood gas machines record various data (Table 29), and many also give a value for base excess/deficit. Calculation of base excess/deficit is designed to make it easy to separate metabolic from respiratory causes of pH disturbance. Various algorithms are used in these calculations, the principles being as follows.

Table 29 Measurements made by blood gas machines.

	Normal range	Notes
Po_2	>10.6 kPa (breathing air)	Hypoxia <8 kPa
pH	pH 7.37–7.43	
H^+	37–43 nmol/L	
Pco_2	4.7–6.0 kPa	Respiratory failure: If Po_2 <8 kPa and Pco_2 <6.5 kPa = Type I If Pco_2 >6.5 kPa = Type II
HCO_3^-	22–28 mmol/L	In dealing with problems of respiratory failure or acid–base disturbance, measurement of plasma bicarbonate is often helpful

Table 31 Causes of restrictive and obstructive lung defects.

Type of defect	Spirometric pattern	Examples
Restrictive	Increased FEV_1/FVC ratio	Pulmonary fibrosis, respiratory muscle weakness, obesity, pleural disease, chest wall and skeletal disorders
Obstructive	Decreased FEV_1/FVC ratio	COPD, asthma

COPD, chronic obstructive pulmonary disease; FEV_1, forced expiratory volume in 1 s; FVC, forced vital capacity.

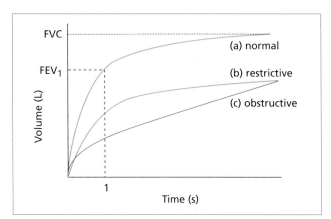

Fig. 49 Spirometry curves for (a) a normal patient; (b) patient with a restrictive lung defect; and (c) patient with an obstructive lung defect. FEV_1, forced expiratory volume after 1 s; FVC, forced vital capacity.

Gas transfer

TL_{CO} and K_{CO} are measurements of gas diffusion across the alveolar membrane. K_{CO} is corrected for lung volume as $K_{CO} = TL_{CO}/Va$, where Va is the alveolar volume available for gas exchange. In the laboratory, carbon monoxide is used to calculate this diffusion capacity, hence the 'CO' after the terms.

If you imagine the alveolar membrane in its healthy state as being thin and permeable, say like a sheet of tissue paper, any pathological process that causes it to become thickened and coarse will slow down the movement of carbon monoxide (or oxygen) from the lung into the blood stream. Conversely, increased levels of blood and therefore haemoglobin, either in the blood stream or in the alveoli, will cause an increase in the uptake of oxygen (Table 32).

Flow–volume loops

These measure the expiratory and inspiratory flow of air (L/s) against actual volume exhaled or inhaled. The upper, expiratory curve starts with the patient at maximum/forced inhalation (TLC) and ends at total/forced expiration (RV).

The curves have characteristic shapes according to the

Table 32 Causes of increased and decreased K_{CO}.

Change in K_{CO}	Mechanism	Examples
Increased	Reduced V_A	Skeletal deformity, pleural disease and respiratory muscle weakness
	Increased capillary blood volume	Left-to-right shunt, lung haemorrhage, polycythaemia
Reduced	Destruction of lung tissue	Emphysema
	Impairment to diffusion by disease	Fibrosing alveolitis
	Reduced blood flow to pulmonary capillaries	Pulmonary vascular disease or hypertension, right-to-left shunt
	Reduced uptake by blood	Anaemia

underlying disease process and whether the pathology is causing intra- or extrathoracic obstruction to the airflow, thus distorting the shape of the curve from the normal. The most important patterns are those of expiratory flow limitation (Fig. 50).

3.6.3 OVERNIGHT OXIMETRY

This relatively cheap and easy test can be used as a baseline investigation to screen for possible sleep apnoea patients who report disturbed sleep and/or daytime somnolence. The patient's SaO_2 is continuously recorded via a finger probe while they rest.

Analysis of the results looks for drops in the saturation and the frequency of these events, which may represent episodes of apnoea. (See Section 1.8, p. 172.) Patients with recurrent hypoxic episodes and/or large dips in their oxygen should be referred for formal assessment by a physician interested in sleep disorders.

3.6.4 CHEST RADIOGRAPH

Stand back at least 1–2 m and take a long hard look. Does anything strike you straight away? If so, fine, but do not ignore the rest. Then proceed systematically as described below.

Heart

• Is the heart size normal or does it look enlarged? Estimate the cardiac width with that of the thorax; the heart should fill less than half the thoracic width.
• Follow the contours of the heart; are there any 'bits' that should not be there? Do they correspond to enlarged ventricles or atria or are they something else?
• Is there anything sitting behind the heart that makes it look distorted, e.g. dilated oesophagus, stomach?

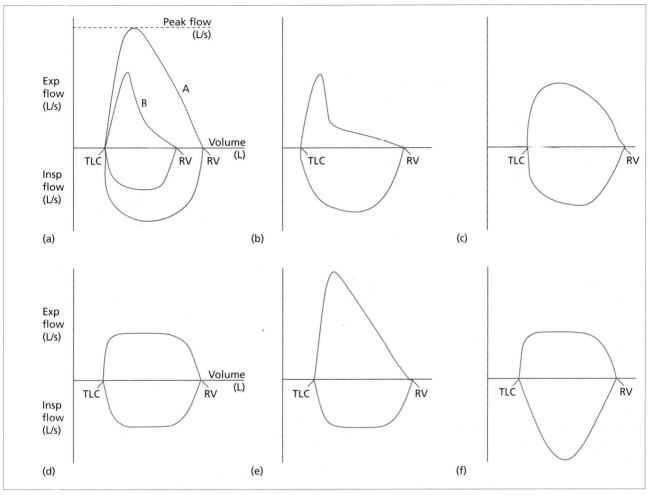

Fig. 50 Flow–volume loops: (a) normal patient (A); and obstructive lung disease (B), e.g. asthma, chronic obstructive pulmonary disease (COPD); (b) emphysema; (c) restrictive lung defect, e.g. pulmonary fibrosis; (d) fixed intra- or extrathoracic obstruction, e.g. tracheal tumour; (e) variable extrathoracic obstruction, e.g. tracheal stenosis outside the thoracic cavity, works like a one-way valve, opening on expiration while collapsing on inspiration; (f) variable intrathoracic obstruction. RV, residual volume; TLC, total lung capacity.

Lungs

• First of all, ignore the lung fields, and take a good look around the edge of the lung at the pleura—is it thickened or calcified? Are there any obvious pleural plaques? These can look surprisingly like retained self-adhesive ECG pads (and vice versa!).

• Now inspect the lung fields. Are all the pulmonary lobes and fissures present, or are they distorted, collapsed or consolidated? If there is an abnormality—where is it, how would you describe it? Shape (oval, round, wedge), size, texture (honeycomb, patchy).

Bones

• Are they of equal density throughout, or do they look 'moth-eaten'? Is there any evidence of cysts or osteolytic changes? Is there any evidence of old or new fractures, e.g. pathological fractures?

• Look carefully along the ribs for fractures or notches. Turning the chest radiograph on its side and studying the ribs often helps detract your attention from everything else.

 If a radiograph seems normal do not forget to double check the bones, the apices and the area behind the heart. Are you missing a small pneumothorax? Is there an extrathoracic abnormality (e.g. a mastectomy)? If in doubt, ask a radiologist!

Figure 51 shows in diagrammatic fashion the radiographic patterns of lobar collapse, and examples of lobar collapse.

3.6.5 COMPUTED TOMOGRAPHY SCAN OF THE THORAX

There are a number of indications for CT scans of the thorax and, as with all investigations, you need to be

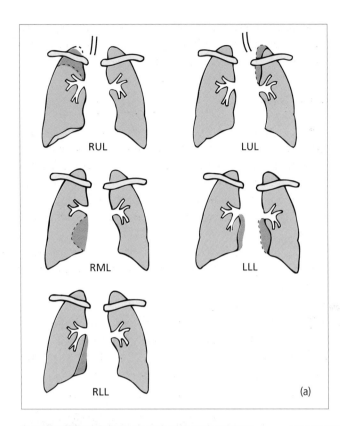

Fig. 51 (a) Diagrammatic representation of the radiographic patterns of lobar collapse. Helpful information may be provided by the position of the trachea, the hilar vascular shadows and the horizontal fissure. (b) Chest radiograph of right upper lobe collapse secondary to *Mycobacterium* infection. Note the tracheal deviation and air bronchogram. Right upper lobe collapse also tends to cause elevation of the horizontal fissure, tenting (but not elevation) of the right diaphragm and a raised right hilum. (c) Potentially difficult radiograph of right middle lobe collapse. The key is the increased opacification obscuring the right cardiac border. (d) Lateral view of the right middle lobe collapse patient in (c) with a wedge of opacity in the region of the middle lobe. (e) Left lower lobe collapse; note the classic presence of 'sail sign', where the collapsed lobe lies behind the heart; also left mediastinal shift, left hilar depression and loss of the left hemidiaphragm. (See Fig. 19, p. 181 for radiographs of left upper lobe collapse, and also Fig. 18, p. 180 for another example of RUL collapse.) LLL, left lower lobe; LUL, left upper lobe; RLL, right lower lobe; RML, right middle lobe; RUL, right upper lobe. (Courtesy of Dr I. Vlahos.)

detailed on the request form as to the reasons for the test in order for the radiologists to give you the best possible service. A variety of techniques are used.

Figure 52 shows the principal mediastinal structures seen on CT scanning of the thorax.

Type of scans

High-resolution scans

Here the lung is imaged at small intervals or sections. These are often invaluable in the diagnosis of parenchymal lung disease and can be diagnostic of certain conditions, thus avoiding further more invasive investigations, e.g. sarcoidosis—beading, and pulmonary fibrosis—honeycombing of the lung.

You should also ask for the radiologist to perform prone and supine films, i.e. scan the patient lying on both back and front. This is to ensure that pulmonary interstitial fluid is not mimicking the changes of fibrosis: fluid will move downwards, while fibrosis remains in the same area of the lung on both views (Fig. 53).

Conventional scans

Staging scans for suspected lung cancer (or other discrete lesions like abcesses) involve the scanner imaging at wider intervals. The images are reproduced in two settings:
• bony or soft-tissue windows—highlight lymph node enlargement, soft-tissue involvement and bony lesions
• lung windows—concentrate on the lung parenchyma, producing images of the tumour as well as the condition of the surrounding lung, i.e. coexisting emphysema, bullae or fibrosis.

Helical computed tomography

Spiral CT is the latest technological improvement in this form of scanning. It is fast and a complete scan can be completed in one breath-hold. They are increasingly useful in the diagnosis of pulmonary emboli when contrast media is used to create a pulmonary angiogram.

Reading a scan

When you assess a CT scan, remember that you are viewing it as though you are standing at the patient's feet looking upwards, so the patient's liver is on the left of the picture and the spleen on the right, etc. Like the chest radiograph, try to follow a system through the scans.
• Follow the main vessels such as the descending and ascending aorta and its arch.
• Look carefully for enlargement of the hilar and para-tracheal lymph nodes and any other soft-tissue changes (Fig. 54).
• Look at the lung windows—study the lung parenchyma and run your eye carefully around the pleura looking for any thickening, plaques and/or adjacent fibrosis.
• Finally, show a radiologist and, for your education, ask them to talk you through the scan.

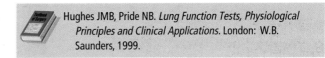

Hughes JMB, Pride NB. *Lung Function Tests, Physiological Principles and Clinical Applications.* London: W.B. Saunders, 1999.

Acknowledgements

The authors and editor would like to thank the following people for their help in the preparation of this module: Professor M. Green, Imperial College of Science Medicine and Technology, Dr J. Moore-Gillon, Department of Respiratory Medicine, Barts and The London NHS Trust, London, Dr L. Kuitert, Department of Respiratory Medicine, Barts and The London NHS Trust, London and Dr I. Vlahos, Academic Department of Radiology, Barts and The London NHS Trust, London.

(a)

(b)

Fig. 53 Computed tomography scan of the thorax (a) supine and (b) prone, of a man with pulmonary fibrosis. Note the different positioning of the patient on the scanning table (at the bottom of both films). The honeycombing appearance of the lungs remains posterior in both views.

Fig. 54 Computed tomography of the thorax; note the mass of lymph nodes that is distorting the normal architecture of the mediastinum. This patient was subsequently diagnosed as having sarcoidosis.

Fig. 52 (*Opposite*) Principal mediastinal structures on computed tomography scanning of the thorax. Remember that you are viewing the sections from below, i.e. the left of the thorax is on the right of the figure. (a and b) Section above the aortic arch. The trachea (T), oesophagus (O), right brachiocephalic vein (RBV), left brachiocephalic vein (LBV), innominate vein (IV), left common carotid artery (LCCA), and left subclavian artery (LSA) are visible. (c and d) Section at the level of the aortic arch (A). The superior vena cava (SVC) is visible. (e and f) Section below aortic arch. Both ascending (AA) and descending (DA) aortas are visible. The trachea (T) is bifurcated and pulmonary arteries (PA) are seen. Note in (f) that the bifurcation of the trachea is present behind the pulmonary arteries, but difficult to see in cross-section. (g and h) Section at the level of the pulmonary veins (PV). Lower lobe intrapulmonary arteries and bronchi are not shown in the diagram. (Computed tomography scans courtesy of Dr I. Vlahos.)

4 Self-assessment

Answers on pp. 265–271.

Question 1
The following are true of mesothelioma (T/F):
A Painless pleural effusion is a common presentation
B Evidence of asbestos exposure is absent in >10% of cases
C Metastasis occurs in <20% of cases
D The right lung is more commonly affected than the left lung
E The mean latency to presentation is in the range 20–29 years.

Question 2
A 50-year-old man presents with a 4-year history of exertional dyspnoea and this radiograph (Fig. 55). He has a past history of atrial fibrillation but is otherwise well. What questions would you ask? What investigations would you suggest?

Fig. 55 Question 2: Chest radiograph.

Question 3
A Snoring
B Short sleeps in day are very refreshing
C Heavy snoring in spouse
D Nocturia
E Crawly sensation in legs in the evening
F Sensation of inability to move limbs while waking
G Motor vehicle accident
H Morning headache
I Short sleeps in day are unrefreshing.

In a patient with unwanted daytime somnolence, which condition do the features listed most suggest. Each answer may be used once, more than once, or not at all.
1 Narcolepsy cataplexy syndrome
2 Obstructive sleep apnoea syndrome
3 Periodic limb movement
4 Chronic (type II) respiratory failure
5 Inadequate sleep opportunity
6 Symptom not discriminating.

Question 4
A 44-year-old woman presents to A&E 4 weeks after a hysterectomy which had been performed for menorrhagia with left-sided pleuritic chest pain. Her chest radiograph is reported as normal and she has a PaO_2 of 9.5 kPa and a $PaCO_2$ of 4.0 kPa. Pending further investigation she is treated with a therepeutic dose of low-molecular-weight heparin for a presumptive diagnosis of pulmonary embolus. Your hospital does not have facilities for pulmonary angiography. Select the optimal management course:

A Do V/Q scan. Continue to treat for pulmonary embolus if high probability of pulmonary embolus. If low or intermediate probability arrange helical computed tomography and only continue to treat for pulmonary embolus if shown on CT.
B Check D-dimer level; continue to treat for pulmonary embolus unless normal.
C Continue to treat for pulmonary embolus without further investigation.
D Arrange helical CT and D-dimer test. Continue to treat for pulmonary embolus unless CT shows an alternative credible diagnosis or unless both CT negative for pulmonary embolus and D-dimer levels within normal range.
E Do V/Q scan. Continue to treat for pulmonary embolus only if high probability of pulmonary embolus.

Question 5
The following statements concerning ethical aspects of mechanical ventilation are correct (T/F):
A The same ethical considerations apply to withholding mechanical ventilation as to withdrawing it
B An adult patient may not elect to have mechanical ventilation withdrawn
C An adult patient who wishes to receive mechanical ventilation should do so irrespective of their diagnosis

D The next of kin (e.g. spouse) may withhold consent to ventilate an adult patient

E The next of kin (e.g. parent) may withhold consent to ventilate a paediatric patient.

Question 6

A 71-year-old woman presents to A&E with a Glasgow Coma Score of 6 having been found collapsed at home. Her neighbours noticed that she has been less active than usual and has stopped shopping at the local supermarket for the last 4 weeks, complaining of increasing shortness of breath and drowsiness. She has a history of tuberculosis, treated 50 years ago and on examination has had a left-sided thoracoplasty. Her blood gases on admission (having had 60% oxygen in the ambulance) are pH 7.2; PO_2 12.1; PCO_2 14.5; HCO_3^- 38.0.

1 The most likely diagnosis is:

A Multiple pulmonary emboli

B Emphysema with O_2 narcosis

C Acute on chronic type II respiratory failure

D Life-threatening asthma

E Metabolic acidosis.

2 What would be your initial management plan?

Question 7

A CT scan of thorax, prone and supine

B Sputum examination

C Lung function tests

D Bronchoscopy

E Overnight oximetry.

For each of the following conditions, select the most specific investigation from the list of options above for determining the diagnosis. Each options may be used once, more than once, or not at all:

1 Loud snoring associated with morning headache

2 Suspected lung cancer

3 Shortness of breath associated with amiodarone

4 *Pneumocystis carinii* pneumonia

5 Asthma.

Question 8

In patients with lung disease secondary to asbestos exposure (T/F):

A Lung fibrosis is largely reversible with steroids

B They are not entitled to compensation payments unless they develop mesothelioma

C Pleural plaques are predominantly apical

D Necrotic cavities are a feature of advanced disease

E When a patient dies of asbestos-related disease, the case should be discussed with the coroner.

Question 9

A man is admitted following his first grand mal fit. He had fallen over at home in his bedroom, jerked a few times, got up and went to the bathroom; fell over again, hit his head and had a grand mal fit lasting 5 min (witnessed by his wife). He also had a 3-week history of shortness of breath: initially this occurred one morning when he tried to climb up the stairs at home and suddenly became acutely short of breath; there was no associated chest pain, no cough or haemoptysis. He had smoked until the onset of dyspnoea.

The patient went to his general practitioner: the chest radiograph showed bilateral hilar enlargement (Fig. 56). Currently, he is mildly short of breath and has some chest tightness. Observations and examination: slightly short of breath at rest; no lymphadenopathy; not cyanosed or pale. Cardiovascular system (CVS): pulse 100; BP 140/80; JVP not raised; heart sounds—ejection systolic murmur loudest over left sternal edge. Respiratory system (RS): trachea central; percussion normal; breathe sounds vesicular.

1 What does his ECG (Fig. 57) show?

2 What is the diagnosis?

3 What would you expect his arterial blood gases to show? Pick one option from the list below:

A An acute respiratory alkalosis secondary to anxiety

B Chronic type 2 respiratory failure

C Normal blood gases

D Hypoxia with a normal pH

E A metabolic acidosis.

Question 10

Cryptogenic fibrosing alveolitis (CFA) (T/F):

A Is more common in men

B Usually affects between the fifth and the sixth decade

C Is normally not accompanied by cough

D Is never familial

E Is characterized by late inspiratory crackles which disappear on bending forward.

Fig. 56 Question 9: Chest radiograph.

Fig. 57 Question 9: Lead ECG of the patient taken at time of admission; look carefully at the axis and chest leads. All the leads were correctly positioned!

Question 11

In pulmonary embolism (T/F):

A A pleural effusion occurs in up to 50% of the patients

B Transudative pleural effusion may occur in pulmonary embolism

C A blood-stained pleural effusion is a contraindication for anticoagulants

D Anticoagulants dissolve the clots

E Thrombolytics can be given within 14 days.

Question 12

A Tracheostomy narrowed by mucous plug in a self-ventilating patient with O_2 10 L/min added

B Hepatopulmonary syndrome

C Acid maltase deficiency

D *Pneumocystis carinii* pneumonia

E Rendu–Osler–Weber syndrome

F Pulmonary embolus

G Acute asthma

H Amiodarone lung

I Lobar pneumonia.

For each of the scenarios given above, match the most likely pathophysiologic mechanism causing hypoxia. Each answer may be used once, more than once, or not at all.

1 Right to left shunt

2 Alveolar hypoventilation

3 Impaired diffusion

4 Reduced inspired oxygen

5 *V/Q* mismatch.

Question 13

A 42-year-old Irish accountant presents with a 3-month history of an annoying dry cough. She has no other symptoms. Her chest radiograph has been reported as normal but you notice that there is some perihilar haziness and fine shadowing in both lower zones (Fig. 58). What is the diagnosis? What two investigations might you perform?

Fig. 58 Question 13: Chest radiograph.

Question 14

A 16-year-old woman presents in outpatients with a 3-month history of nocturnal dry cough; she has had several courses of antibiotics with no change in her symptoms. Her chest radiograph is clear.

What is the most likely diagnosis from the options below?

A *Pneumocystis carinii* pneumonia
B Oesophageal reflux
C Asthma
D Bronchiolitis obliterans
E Emphysema.

What investigation might you organize as an outpatient department? What might you ask her to do at home? How would you treat her?

Question 15

Bronchiectasis (T/F):

A Does not occur in rheumatoid arthritis
B Can be diagnosed by a chest radiograph
C With haemoptysis is an absolute indication for bronchoscopy
D Can result in amyloidosis
E Caused by bronchial obstruction commonly affects the lingula lobe of the left lung.

Question 16

Sarcoidosis (T/F):

A Is more common in females
B Affects the lungs in fewer than 50% of patients
C Can be diagnosed by the Kveim test
D Is associated with elevated serum ACE in all patients
E Is best diagnosed by a transbronchial biopsy if dyspnoea is present.

Question 17

A Methotrexate
B Opiates
C Dapsone
D Montelukast
E Salbutamol.

For each of the drugs listed above, pick the most appropriate statement from the list below. Each option may be used once, more than once, or not at all:

1 Can cause bronchoconstriction at its recommended dose
2 Is given orally in the treatment of moderate exercise-induced asthma
3 Is used with trimethaprin as an adjuvant drug in the treatment of *Pneumocystis carinii* pneumonia
4 Can be used as a prophylaxis treatment of exercise-induced asthma
5 Can cause pulmonary fibrosis at therapeutic doses.

Question 18

A 67-year-old man who is tetraplegic and in ventilatory failure as a result of motor neuron disease is receiving ventilatory support via facemask ventilation. He can only remove the facemask for 2–3 min and requests discontinuation of mechanical ventilation repeatedly over a 2-week period of inpatient assessment. Select the best course of management (it may be assumed in the question that other options for mechanical ventilation have been explored and that the patient is competent and free of psychiatric disease).

A Refuse because this action will result in the patient's death
B Agree but suggest that he carries out this manoeuvre away from hospital premises (e.g. at home)
C Agree but avoid opiates and/or benzodiazepines in case his respiration is compromised
D Agree but give opiates and/or benzodiazepine drugs if he becomes breathless
E Agree and give opiates and/or benzodiazepine drugs prior to stopping mechanical ventilation.

Question 19

In sarcoidosis (T/F):

A Hypercalcemia is best treated with pamidronate
B Haemoptysis is not a common symptom
C Chest radiograph changes determine disease activity
D The third cranial nerve is the most common nerve affected
E Proximal myopathy may be the presenting symptom.

Question 20

A Caring for laboratory animals
B Silk manufacturing worker
C Coal miner
D Cement manufacturing
E Demolition worker
F Air hostess
G Food processing industry
H Cotton manufacturing worker
I Shepherd.

For each lung condition below select the most likely occupational association from the list above. Each answer may be used once, more than once, or not at all.

1 Byssinosis
2 Mesothelioma
3 Pneumoconiosis
4 Asthma.

Question 21

Consider the lung function tests in Table 33.
1 Which description best describes these results?
A Restrictive lung defect
B Obstructive lung defect

Table 33 Question 21: Lung function tests.

	Value	% Predicted
FEV_1	1.64 L	65
VC	1.80 L	55
TLC	3.63 L	61
FRC	2.50 L	75
RV	1.92 L	79
TL_{CO}	2.15 mmol/kPa/min	29
K_{CO}	0.92	71

See text for abbreviation definitions.

C Within normal limits
D Restrictive lung defect with reduced gas transfer.
2 The most likely diagnosis is:
A Scoliosis
B Asthma
C Fibrosing alveolitis
D Sarcoid
E Diaphragm paralysis.

Question 22

According to the UK National Asthma Guidelines, the following observations are true of an adult patient with asthma in the acute severe category rather than the life-threatening category (T/F).
A A tachycardia of greater than 120 beats/min
B PO_2 less that 8.0 kPa, irrespective of treatment with oxygen
C Silent chest
D Peak flow ≤50% predicted or best
E First-line treatment should be nebulized β agonists.

Question 23

Sarcoidosis can (T/F):
A Be associated with polydipsia and polyuria
B Be frequently associated with arthralgia
C Result in massive haemoptysis
D Result in liver granulomas in less than a quarter of the cases
E Result in blindness.

Question 24

Concerning the obstructive sleep apnoea syndrome, the following are true (T/F):
A Hyperthyroidism is a recognized predisposing condition
B Uvulopalatoplasty is indicated in patients with severe disease (e.g. an apnoea/hypopnoea index >30/h)
C The clinician should inform the DVLA at the time the diagnosis is made
D The main reason for treatment is to reduce long-term cardiovascular mortality
E Domiciliary oxygen is indicated if polycythaemia occurs.

Question 25

The following are recognized causes of dyspnoea with a normal radiograph (T/F):
A Use of the oral contraceptive pill
B Left upper lobe collapse
C Primary pulmonary hypertension
D Miliary tuberculosis
E Anaemia.

Question 26

Smoke inhalation (T/F):
A Does not result in airway obstruction
B Can be associated with development of ARDS up to 24 h later
C Can result in visual field defects
D May be complicated by rhabdomyolysis
E May cause bronchiolitis obliterans.

Question 27

A Paracetamol
B *N*-acetyl-cysteine
C Cefuroxime
D Flecainide
E Amiodarone
F Methadone
G Fenfluramine
H Hydralazine
I Gold.
For each respiratory disease below, give the drug from the selection listed above that is most likely to be the cause. Each answer may be used once, more than once, or not at all.
1 Pulmonary eosinophilia
2 Pleural effusion
3 Asthma
4 Alveolitis
5 Pulmonary hypertension.

Question 28

Churg–Strauss syndrome (T/F):
A May result in gastrointestinal bleed
B Is not associated with nasal polyps
C May be accompanied by pleural effusion in fewer than 10% of the patients
D Does not result in renal failure
E Is treated with high-dose corticosteroids.

Question 29

A 65-year-old man is admitted with hypercapnic respiratory failure. The general practitioner's letter says that he attends your hospital's chest clinic and is considered to have severe chronic obstructive pulmonary disease. He does not respond to bronchodilators, controlled oxygen and non-invasive mechanical ventilation. He is too confused for you to have a meaningful conversation but his wife is present. What management issues need immediate consideration and how would you pursue these?

Question 30

Pulmonary eosinophilia (T/F):

A Should be investigated with a transbronchial biopsy

B Is accompanied by a pleural effusion in over 60% of cases

C Is commonly caused by allergic bronchopulmonary aspergillosis

D May result in pulmonary fibrosis due to chronic eosinophilic pneumonia

E Usually occurs in young males.

Question 31

A The patient's wife says he has been becoming increasingly depressed

B Presence of right lower lobe consolidation pattern

C Use of domiciliary oxygen therapy and nebulized bronchodilators

D Drowsy with small pupils

E Pleuritic chest pain

F Data on hospital computer from blood taken 2 months ago show Hb 8.8 g/dL and serum creatinine 400 mmol/L

G History of hernia repair 2 weeks previously

H Use of high-flow oxygen in ambulance

I Has been becoming more forgetful recently.

A 65-year-old man is admitted with hypercapnic respiratory failure. The general practitioner's letter says that he attends your hospital's chest clinic and is considered to have severe chronic obstructive pulmonary disease. Link the clinical features above with clinical management decisions regarding mechanical ventilation. Each answer may be used once, more than once, or not at all.

1 In favour of mechanical ventilation

2 Against mechanical ventilation

3 No influence on decision to offer mechanical ventilation.

Question 32

The following statements (T/F):

A In Churg–Strauss syndrome prognosis depends upon extent of pulmonary involvement

B Hydroxycarbamide (hydroxyurea) is contraindicated in hypereosinophilic syndrome

C Acute eosinophilic pneumonia does not usually recur after corticosteroid withdrawal

D Churg–Strauss syndrome is monitored by the ESR and eosinophil count

E Sulfasalazine may cause pulmonary eosinophilia.

Question 33

A 52-year-old man presents with a 2-month history of dyspnoea and the radiograph shown in Fig. 59. He has lost 5 kg in weight.

1 List five features you would seek to clarify in the history

2 Give the four investigations most likely to lead to the diagnosis

3 In fact, the patient proves to have a mesothelioma. Give short note answers to outline a management plan.

Fig. 59 Questions 33 and 37: Chest radiograph.

Question 34

You are asked to see a patient who complains of tiredness during the day and has the oximetry trace shown in Fig. 60. He has a body mass index of 32 kg/m².

1 What is the differential diagnosis?

2 Give five areas requiring special attention in the physical examination

Fig. 60 Questions 34 and 36: Oximetry trace.

Cardiology

Answer to Question 1

T, F, F, F, F

- Approximately 30% of patients presenting with unstable angina will have elevated troponin levels, and these patients are at higher risk of death or myocardial infarction (MI).
- Transmural infarction can be diagnosed clinically only by the presence of pathological Q waves on the ECG, and is probably more accurately called Q-wave infarction.
- Creatine kinase rises after DC cardioversion, but this is the result of skeletal (not cardiac) muscle damage.
- Elevated cardiac troponin levels indicate heart muscle damage, but give no indication of the cause. Ischaemic damage is by far the most common, but myopericarditis or heart muscle contusion after a road traffic accident may also raise troponin levels.
- Cardiac troponin levels are unaffected by skeletal muscle damage and retain the advantage of high specificity.

Answer to Question 2

T, F, F, F, T

- Although most of the evidence predates routine use of aspirin and thrombolysis, more recent trials support the view that β blockers are beneficial.
- Intravenous nitrates have not been shown to confer anything more than symptomatic benefit.
- Dihydropyridine calcium antagonists (including nifedipine and amlodipine) do not improve, and may worsen, outcome.
- Sotalol is a β blocker with additional class III antiarrhythmic activity which may, paradoxically, be pro-arrhythmic after an MI.
- Intensive insulin therapy (intravenous infusion for 24 h followed by insulin subcutaneously four times daily for 3 months) reduces mortality for at least 3 years after an MI.

Answer to Question 3

1E, 2G, 3D, 4A

- A resting 12-lead ECG is the quickest way to diagnose acute MI that will benefit from prompt thrombolysis.
- Transoesophageal echocardiography is the most sensitive and specific investigation for aortic dissection—CT scan of the chest with contrast, MRI and aortography are acceptable alternatives.
- Although patients with hypertrophic cardiomyopathy often present with an abnormal ECG, echocardiography will reveal much more specific features.
- A chest radiograph should always be requested to confirm the clinical diagnosis of pulmonary oedema.

Answer to Question 4

1C, 2G, 3D, 4G

- In the UK the treatment of choice for acute MI is thrombolysis, but if facilities are available then emergency angioplasty probably achieves better results.
- Intravenous nitrates are an important part of the emergency treatment of acute pulmonary oedema because afterload (blood pressure) reduction lowers left ventricular end-diastolic pressure and therefore left atrial pressure. Angiotensin-converting enzyme (ACE) inhibitors are commenced once the patient's condition is more stable.
- Type A aortic dissection involves the ascending thoracic aorta. There is a high risk of pericardial tamponade, coronary involvement or acute aortic regurgitation. Emergency surgical repair is the treatment of choice. While this is being arranged, blood pressure is reduced with intravenous labetolol or nitroprusside.
- Initial treatment for unstable angina should be medical. Angioplasty is indicated only if ischaemia is not controlled by antianginal and antithrombotic measures. Dihydropyridine calcium antagonists such as nifedipine should be avoided in acute coronary syndromes.

Answer to Question 5

1B, 2D, 3G, 4C

- Coronary vasospasm is best managed medically. High doses of calcium antagonists may be needed. Nicorandil may also be useful. β Blockers make spasm worse.
- The prognosis for left main-stem stenosis is greatly improved by cardiac surgery.
- Type B (descending) aortic dissection should be managed medically, with β blockers to lower blood pressure.
- Congestive cardiac failure caused by restrictive cardiomyopathy is treated with diuretics. Calcium antagonists should be avoided.

Answer to Question 6

1 Aortic dissection with aortic regurgitation and incipient tamponade. Blood loss from a self-sealing aortic rupture may produce syncope as a result of postural hypotension, which may be exacerbated by new aortic regurgitation and intrapericardial haemorrhage.

2 Urgent transoesophageal echocardiography, CT scan of the chest with contrast or aortography.

3 Lower blood pressure (systolic <120 mmHg) with intravenous labetolol or sodium nitroprusside, until emergency repair of the dissection can be arranged.

Answer to Question 7

1 Restrictive cardiomyopathy caused by cardiac amyloid. The dilated atria with normal-size ventricles seen on echocardiography strongly suggest a restrictive process.

Amyloid is one of the most common causes, and is particularly likely in a patient with a long history of active inflammatory disease, such as rheumatoid arthritis.

2 Intravenous loop diuretics with fluid restriction.

3 Review of the echocardiogram may reveal the brightly speckled myocardium characteristic of amyloid infiltration. Amyloid may be confirmed by biopsy of the anterior abdominal wall or rectum. Cardiac biopsy is not indicated. Measure 24-h urinary protein because the nephrotic syndrome commonly accompanies amyloidosis and may contribute to oedema.

Answer to Question 8

F, T, T, F, T

The three prognostically important catheter parameters are cardiac index, right atrial pressure and mixed venous oxygen saturations. Although appetite-suppressant use is a risk factor for the development of primary pulmonary hypertension, it has no bearing on prognosis.

Answer to Question 9

A2, B6, C1, D3

A Non-invasive, quick and can also rule out differential diagnoses. If the pulmonary embolus (PE) is big enough to have caused the clinical presentation, there is likely to be right ventricular dysfunction.

B Pneumothorax is more likely than PE. If the chest radiograph is negative, the next investigation is 3 because emphysematous lungs are associated with $\dot{V}/\dot{Q}$ abnormality, reducing the scan's effectiveness in the diagnosis of PE.

C This is a good indication for $\dot{V}/\dot{Q}$, with clinical probability taken into account.

D A likely candidate for a PE, but left ventricular failure also causes $\dot{V}/\dot{Q}$ abnormality.

Answer to Question 10

F, F, F, F, T

People with diabetes benefit more from all the standard interventions (A, C, D) after a myocardial infarction; they should only be denied them for significant reasons. The risk of damage to sight with thrombolysis is extremely small even if proliferative retinopathy is present, and ACE inhibitors are independently indicated for diabetic renal disease with proteinuria. Unfortunately, although glycaemic control is important, the risk remains above normal because of the associated metabolic abnormalities.

Answer to Question 11

B, D, F, 1, 4

• Lesions with high-pressure jets. In Eisenmenger's syndrome the pressures have equalized and a surgically ligated PDA will have no residual flow.

• Procedures that induce transient bacteraemia.

Answer to Question 12

• Autoantibodies and lupus anticoagulant, liver enzymes, ESR, rheumatoid factor

• Chest radiograph, pulmonary function tests, sleep study

• Echocardiography

• $\dot{V}/\dot{Q}$ scan or spiral CT

Answer to Question 13

T, T, T, F, F

• In the Wolff–Parkinson–White syndrome, δ waves are secondary to conduction antegradely down the accessory pathway. These δ waves cause a broad complex. AVRT secondary to concealed accessory pathways conduct antegradely through the AV node and retrogradely through the accessory pathway, and so do not have δ waves.

• VT with a right bundle-branch block morphology will most probably originate from the left ventricle and vice versa with left bundle-branch morphology.

• Fusion beats are an intermediate morphology of the QRS complex between the broad complex of VT and the narrow complex of sinus rhythm. Fusion beats are found in about 5% of VTs.

• Adenosine exerts its action on the AV node. The majority of VTs do not include the AV node in its re-entry mechanism and thus will not terminate the rhythm. However, in AVRT/AVNRT with aberrant conduction, adenosine is highly effective.

• Most of the large prospective studies comparing amiodarone with ICDs (e.g. AVID) have shown a clear superiority of ICDs in preventing death in patients with VT.

Answer to Question 14

F, T, T, F, F

• Temporary pacing for bifascicular (and possibly trifascicular) block should be considered only in patients who give a history of presyncope or syncope.

• Complete heart block, albeit transient, in the context of an acute anterior myocardial infarction should always be treated seriously. The patient should have a temporary pacing lead *in situ*.

• Of course! Ablation of the AV node will leave the patient in either complete heart block or ventricular standstill. In most cases a temporary pacing lead is inserted before the ablation; then a permanent system is implanted as soon as the ablation is completed or the permanent system is implanted before the ablation.

• Try to avoid, at all costs, placing a temporary pacing lead in patients who are bradycardic as a result of hypothermia. The ventricles are often 'irritable' and ventricular fibrillation is easily induced. The mainstay of treatment is slow rewarming.

• A 3.0-s pause is usually taken as the criterion for pacing in carotid sinus hypersensitivity.

Answer to Question 15
T, F, F, F, T
• Vehicular accidents are by far the most common cause.
• The creatine kinase will inevitably be raised with skeletal muscle injury. The CK-MB fraction may provide more useful information, but may still be raised in massive trauma. Consider troponin assays in this situation because they are more cardiospecific.
• The ligamentum arteriosum is the most common site for aortic trauma because this is where the aorta is tethered to other mediastinal structures. Thus, in trauma this is the site of the greatest shearing forces.
• Thrombolytic therapy is contraindicated because it may lead to catastrophic bleeding. Consider emergency coronary angiography and angioplasty.
• Postpericardiotomy syndrome is a well-documented sequel of traumatic heart disease and may result in pericardial effusion with or without tamponade.

Answer to Question 16
F, T, F, F, F
• In fact, both have equal risks postoperatively of myocardial infarction. Local anaesthesia is preferable to spinal/general anaesthesia.
• Patients with peripheral vascular disease often (30%) have significant coronary artery disease. Their vascular symptoms often limit mobility/exertion, and thus can mask the degree of coronary artery disease. Vascular procedures such as abdominal aortic aneurysm repair often require vessel clamping, which causes increases in myocardial afterload that produce increased cardiovascular demands.
• Coronary events occur most frequently in the first few days with most occurring at 48 h.
• Elective surgery is best left for 3–6 months after the myocardial infarction.
• It is generally thought that patients with carotid and coronary artery disease should have a combined procedure.

Answer to Question 17
F, F, T, F, T
• A reduction in haemodynamic performance with exercise may represent significant coronary artery disease and should be investigated further.
• Generally, a heart rate greater than 85% of the predicted is accepted as a target to achieve. However, exercise tests should not be routinely stopped at this level if the patient is asymptomatic and there are no ECG changes.
• ST-segment changes seen with digoxin therapy make the interpretation of the exercise test difficult. However,

close attention should be paid to haemodynamic responses to exercise and patient symptoms.
• Caution should be exercised in patients with previous arrhythmias. However, some patients will develop arrhythmias only with exercise; so, with a carefully supervised test, it can prove to be an invaluable tool.

Answer to Question 18
F, T, T, T, T
• Adenosine may help in establishing the diagnosis but not in treating the arrhythmias. Blocking AV conduction may reveal underlying flutter waves, confirming the diagnosis.
• If there is variable AV block.
• Rates with 2 : 1 conduction are characteristically 150/min, but this is not always the case.
• Certain types of atrial flutter (common atrial flutter) may be treated by ablating the tricuspid isthmus. AV node ablation should be used only as a last line of therapy.
• Restoration of sinus rhythm is always the main aim of treatment.

Answer to Question 19
T, T, F, T, F
• AV dissociation results in beat-to-beat variation in blood pressure.
• Typically the ventricular escape rate is 35–40/min.
• Complete heart block does not invariably respond to atropine and isoprenaline. Infusions of either should not be given as the treatment of choice in a compromised patient in transvenous pacing.
• A widened pulse pressure with complete heart block may result in a collapsing pulse.

Answer to Question 20
T, T, T, F, T
• In symptomatic patients with the Wolff–Parkinson–White syndrome, this is the treatment of choice.
• Certain forms of atrial flutter are readily cured by radiofrequency ablation.
• VT can be ablated by locating the exact location in the left or right ventricle from which the tachycardia is originating.
• Ventricular fibrillation (VF) cannot be ablated as such. However, in some patients in whom VT degenerates into VF, prevention of the VT by ablation can prevent VF.
• AVNRT is readily cured with radiofrequency ablation. However, because ablation close to the AV node is required, there is a risk of complete AV block and the need for a pacemaker in about 1%.

Answer to Question 21
F, F, F, F, F

The treatment of choice in patients with carotid sinus syncope is dual-chamber pacemaker implantation.

Answer to Question 22

T, T, T, F, T

- The causes of atrial fibrillation (AF) are many. Although thyrotoxicosis is commonly quoted, it is not seen that often.
- Any thoracic surgery can cause AF. In some studies the incidence is said to be as high as a third after CABG.
- Pericarditis is associated with AF.
- As atrial dilatation is unusual, AF in congenital VSD is uncommon. In acquired VSDs, AF is most probably secondary to ischaemia.
- Myocardial ischaemia is probably the most common cause.

Answer to Question 23

T, T, T, T, F

Common changes are a right axis deviation, right bundle-branch block and sinus tachycardia. Although cases of S1Q3T3 are commonly quoted, they are rarely seen in pulmonary embolism. Changes will often resolve in a few days.

Answer to Question 24

T, F, F, F, F

- Statins reduce mortality by about 30% over 5 years.
- Randomized trials to date have failed to confirm the apparent beneficial effects of HRT seen in observational studies.
- An early trial appeared to show reduction in non-fatal MI, but this was not confirmed in a much larger (10 000 patient) trial which showed no effect.
- Long-acting nitrates have not been shown to improve prognosis.
- PTCA is an effective treatment for stable angina that is not controlled medically, but no improvement in life expectancy has been demonstrated.

Answer to Question 25

F, F, F, F, F

- ECG should be the first test.
- The decision to thrombolyse should be based on the finding of ST elevation or new bundle-branch block on the ECG. Troponin levels do not rise until 4 h after heart muscle damage, and thrombolysis has not been shown to benefit troponin-positive patients in the absence of these ECG criteria.
- A negative troponin test indicates low short-term risk of MI or death, but gives no information about coronary anatomy.
- The exercise test is useful for screening, but coronary angiography is the gold standard for risk stratification.

- If aortic dissection is suspected on clinical grounds, detailed imaging (transoesophageal echocardiography, CT of the chest or aortography) must be undertaken urgently.

Answer to Question 26

1E, 2A, 3D, 4G

- Mutations in eight different genes, all of which encode contractile proteins, have been found in hypertrophic cardiomyopathy.
- Dilated cardiomyopathy is idiopathic in most cases, but familial cases caused by cytoskeletal protein gene mutations are increasingly being identified.
- Patients with Marfan's syndrome have a defect in the fibrillin gene and are at risk of aortic dissection.
- Long QT syndrome is the result of mutations in cardiac potassium or sodium channels, and the genotype is increasingly being used to determine the prognosis.

Answer to Question 27

T, F, T, F, F

- The positive predictive value of a finding of basal crackles is very poor, and a chest radiograph is needed to confirm the presence of pulmonary oedema.
- The clinical diagnosis of congestive cardiac failure turns out to be correct in only about one-third of cases.
- Digoxin improves symptoms and reduces the need for hospital admission in patients with more severe heart failure and sinus rhythm.
- β Blockers are an important part of the treatment of heart failure, but should be introduced only when heart failure is stabilized on diuretics and an ACE inhibitor.
- Improved ejection fraction is well documented after treatment with ACE inhibitors and β blockers.

Answer to Question 28

T, F, T, F, T

- Myofibres should be distinguished from myofibrils, which are bundles of contractile elements within cardiac myocytes.
- Thick filaments are comprised of myosin.
- Influx of extracellular calcium stimulates the release of intracellular calcium.
- Energy is supplied by a calcium-sensitive ATPase.
- The sarcoplasmic reticulum is the store for intracellular calcium.

Answer to Question 29

F, F, F, T, T

- Aortic regurgitation leads to volume overload, and therefore to eccentric hypertrophy.
- Hypertrophic cardiomyopathy typically produces asymmetrical (or focal) left ventricular hypertrophy.
- Regression of hypertrophy in treated hypertension is well recognized.

- Recent studies also show that prognosis can be improved by treatments that result in regression of hypertrophy.
- In pressure overload, the apex beat is prominent but not displaced and is referred to as concentric hypertrophy. Displacement of the apex beat occurs as a result of ventricular dilatation in volume overload (eccentric hypertrophy).

Answer to Question 30
F, F, T, T, T
- Coronary stenting should not be undertaken in patients who would benefit prognostically from CABG.
- The initial treatment should be medical, with invasive investigation reserved for high-risk patients or those who continue to have pain.
- Stenting can produce good results in diseased coronary grafts and often obviates the need for further surgery.
- Stenting significantly reduces re-stenosis, but when re-stenosis does occur within a stent it can be difficult to treat.
- Occlusive coronary dissection during angioplasty can usually be dealt with by stenting without recourse to surgery.

Answer to Question 31
T, F, T, F, F
The increase in blood volume causes anaemia (dilution), systolic flow murmurs and a third heart sound. It also contributes to the increase in cardiac output, which counteracts the decrease in systemic vascular resistance, leaving blood pressure largely unchanged. Most palpitations in pregnancy are caused by ectopics, although supraventricular tachycardias also occur.

Answer to Question 32
D
In general the ability of a patient with a cardiac lesion to tolerate pregnancy is related to pre-pregnancy functional status, the haemodynamic significance of the lesion and the presence of cyanosis and/or pulmonary hypertension. Cyanotic congenital heart disease without pulmonary hypertension is associated with a high rate of fetal loss (40%), but may be reasonably well tolerated by the mother. Patients with Marfan's syndrome are at high risk of aortic dissection, especially if the pre-pregnancy aortic root diameter is >4.5 cm.

Answer to Question 33
T, T, F, F, T
Cardiac MRI gives very good anatomical definition, but its use in functional studies is currently restricted to ventricular function and myocardial perfusion. Although most prosthetic valves are safe in the magnet, they cause significant artefact. MRI is not currently used to image

coronary arteries in clinical practice, but with improved definition this is likely to be a future use.

Answer to Question 34
B
The autoimmune rheumatic diseases are commonly associated with pericarditis. Uraemic pericarditis in renal failure is now rare, but if it occurs it is an absolute indication for dialysis.

Answer to Question 35
T, F, T, T, F, T, F, T, T

Respiratory Medicine

Answer to Question 1
T, T, F, T, F
Painless pleural effusion was the presentation in 33% of cases; only 87% of cases has clinical or histological evidence of asbestos exposure. In fact, metastasis (most commonly to the contralateral lung or peritoneum) occurs in 55%. The ratio of right lung disease to left lung disease is 1.6 : 1. The mean latency is 41 years with no cases <30 years.

 Yates DH, Corrin B, Stidolph PN, Browne K. Malignant mesothelioma in south-east England: clinicopathological experience of 272 cases. *Thorax* 1997; 52: 507–512.

Answer to Question 2
Questions: occupational history, drug (amiodarone) exposure, exposure to birds.

Investigations: pulmonary function, high-resolution CT, blood tests including ACE and avian precipitins.

Answer to Question 3
A2, B1, C5, D2, E3, F1, G6, H4, I6

G and I reflect inadequate sleep and do not discriminate between the different causes. Morning headache specifically suggests overnight carbon dioxide retention.

Answer to Question 4
D
Clinically the patient has a high probability for pulmonary embolism. Therefore to answer the question the candidate needs to know that the D-dimer level can be elevated (according to assay) by disorders other than pulmonary embolism, that V/Q scans may give false-negative results for pulmonary embolism (approximately 50% of patients with 'intermediate probability' V/Q scans

actually have pulmonary emboli), and that helical CT may miss segmental pulmonary emboli.

Answer to Question 5

T, F, F, F, T

Withdrawing or withholding mechanical ventilation (when it is indicated on physiological grounds) imply that the patient's condition will deteriorate with potentially fatal consequences. Therefore, ethically, the issues are the same. It goes without saying that, in practice, patient and para-medical staff will often accept that failing to initiate mechanical ventilation is reasonable; this is not usually the case with respect to withdrawing ventilation. Hence some ICUs adopt intermediate procedures such as ventilating on room air or a 'terminal wean' of mechanical ventilation; these practices are not ethically superior to just switching the ventilator off (provided symptoms are relieved by pre-scription of appropriate medication). A physician is not obliged to offer mechanical ventilation if it is felt that the prognosis is hopeless (i.e. that the treatment would be 'futile'). A competent adult patient may elect to have mechanical ventilation withdrawn because this is a medical therapy.

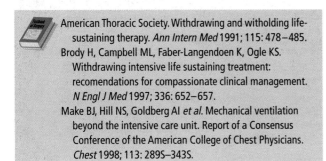

American Thoracic Society. Withdrawing and witholding life-sustaining therapy. *Ann Intern Med* 1991; 115: 478–485.
Brody H, Campbell ML, Faber-Langendoen K, Ogle KS. Withdrawing intensive life sustaining treatment: recomendations for compassionate clinical management. *N Engl J Med* 1997; 336: 652–657.
Make BJ, Hill NS, Goldberg AI *et al.* Mechanical ventilation beyond the intensive care unit. Report of a Consensus Conference of the American College of Chest Physicians. *Chest* 1998; 113: 289S–343S.

Answer to Question 6

1 C

2 Resuscitate the patient, ABC, intubate and ventilate.

This patient has presented in type II respiratory failure with hypercapnia and hypoxia. She had tuberculosis before the introduction of antituberculous chemotherapy and was treated with a left thoracoplasty, which involved lobectomy and rib resection. Many patients who had this surgery and were cured of their tuberculosis often remained well for many years but slowly developed a restrictive lung defect as a result of the chest wall deform-ity caused by the surgery and pulmonary fibrosis resulting from the infection. Many present years later having slipped insidiously into chronic type II respiratory failure which can be precipitated into acute problems by an upper respiratory chest infection. High-flow oxygen in the ambulance has caused her to depress her respiratory state even further. Any patient with a Glasgow Coma Score this low and these blood gases will require intuba-tion and ventilation on the ICU. The main problem will

be weaning her off the ventilator; she probably normally runs a high PCO$_2$ and a low PO$_2$, so she should not be 'overventilated' to try and achieve 'normal' blood gases. Once she is extubated her PCO$_2$ level should be monitored both during the day and at night for significant episodes of hypercapnia and hypoxia. She will require long-term follow-up by a respiratory team and may require home oxygen concentrator and/or non-invasive ventilatory sup-port in the future.

Answer to Question 7

1E, 2D, 3A, 4D, 5C

A simple cost-effective method of assessing patients' sleep disturbance and snoring for possible sleep apnoea is overnight oximetry; patients with positive results (see Section 2.1, p. 188) can then be referred for a formal sleep study. Although a CT scan of the thorax is useful in assessing patients with suspected lung cancer, especially for metastatic disease, bronchoscopy, to judge the extent of tumour spread and to obtain histo-logical specimens, continues to be the diagnostic invest-igation of choice. The same is true for *Pneumocystis carinii* pneumonia where sputum examination has a poor diagnostic yield and bronchoscopic lavage is the preferred investigation. Drug-induced pulmonary fibrosis is best assessed by CT scan of the thorax with prone and supine films. A diagnosis of asthma can be confirmed by pre- and postbronchodilator lung function tests looking for evidence of reversibility.

Answer to Question 8

F, F, F, F, T

Asbestos-related fibrosis is irreversible; steroids will only help if the patient has an element of reversible airway dis-ease such as COPD. Necrosing cavities are not typical of the disease, but are seen in the massive pulmonary fibrosis of coal worker's pneumoconiosis. The pleural plaques of asbestos exposure are widespread, and plaques adhered to the diaphragm are often seen. All forms of asbestos-related lung disease may be entitled to compensation from previous employers, and patients should be advised to seek legal advice from either a reliable solicitor or their trade union. Doctors should routinely discuss all deaths from industrial lung disease with the coroner.

Answer to Question 9

1 Right ventricular strain pattern

2 Pulmonary embolus

3 D.

This patient had a grand mal fit because he was hypoxic secondary to pulmonary emboli. His chest radiograph shows evidence of enlarged pulmonary vessels and his ECG shows the classical pattern of right heart strain. A *V/Q* scan (Fig. 61) showed multiple pulmonary emboli; he was later found to have an hereditary thrombophilia.

(a)

(b)

Fig. 61 Answer 9: Ventilation–perfusion scan of patient, showing multiple pulmonary emboli, particularly in the right upper and left mid zones. (a) Anterior; (b) posterior.

Answer to Question 10

F, T, F, F, T

CFA affects men and women equally with a peak incidence between 45 and 65 years. Cough occurs in 75% of the patients and CFA has been reported within families. The main symptom is progressive breathlessness, and the median survival from the onset of the symptoms is around 5 years. Finger clubbing is commonly seen and chest radiograph usually reveals bilateral, symmetrical, diffuse, small, irregular opacities with loss of lung volume. Pleural effusions are rarely seen. The late inspiratory 'Velcro' crackles which disappear on bending forward are characteristic.

Answer to Question 11

T, T, F, F, T

Pulmonary embolism is associated with a pleural effusion in up to 50% of the patients. Very rarely the effusion may be a transudate. Anticoagulants prevent new clot formation but do not dissolve the old clots. A blood-stained effusion indicates pulmonary infarct and is not a contraindication to anticoagulation. Thrombolytics should be given as early as possible; however, they appear to be effective for up to 14 days.

Answer to Question 12

A4, B1, C2, D5, E1, F5, G5, H3, I5

F and G represent clear examples of VQ mismatch. The plug represent a reduced inspired oxygen because, although O2 is added it can't get past the plug. Acid maltase is an adult onset myopathy which causes hypoventilation if severe. Pulmonary AVM's (telangectasia) and the hepatopulmonary syndrome cause right to left shunting. Amiodarone lung causes a diffusion problem; PCP probably more represents VQ mismatch.

Answer to Question 13

This woman has pulmonary sarcoidosis, which may simply present as a persistent dry cough; not infrequently, ethnicity must be taken into account when assessing patients. Irish women are 10 times more likely to present with pulmonary sarcoidosis than their English conterparts. Investigations of choice would be a bronchoscopy and transbronchial biopsy and lavage, and a high-resolution CT scan of the thorax (Fig. 62).

> **!** Do not forget to warn patients about the 10% risk of pneumothorax following transbronchial biopsy.

Fig. 62 Answer 13: High-resolution computed tomography scan of the thorax of this patient. Pulmonary sarcoidosis produces nodules adjacent to the major fissures, peribronchovascular and subpleural regions. The nodules are generally microscopic granulomas and their characteristic appearance on computed tomography scan is known as 'beading', which can be seen particularly in the right lung on this patient's scan. Sarcoidosis may also produce pulmonary fibrosis.

Answer to Question 14

C

The most likely diagnosis is that of asthma, which not infrequently presents with a chronic nocturnal cough. She should have lung function tests, including spirometry and flow–volume loops before and after inhaled bronchodilator such as salbutamol. She should be asked to keep a peak flow diary at home, with recordings in the morning and the evening to look for morning dips. First-line treatment is twice-daily inhaled corticosteroids.

Do not forget to tell the patient to rinse their mouth out after using a corticosteroid inhaler.

Answer to Question 15
F, F, F, T, F

Answer to Question 16
T, F, F, F, T
(The Kveim test may no longer be used in the UK.)

Answer to Question 17
A5, B1, C3, D4, E4

Opiates can cause bronchoconstriction and in higher doses or overdose, respiratory depression. Montelukast is a leukotriene-receptor antagonist that can be used when high-dose inhaled steroids and β agonists fail to control symptoms and as prophylaxis of exercise-induced asthma. Methotrexate is occasionally used to treat severe steroid-dependent asthma but this is not what the question asks. Dapsone is used to treat leprosy, as well as with trimethaprin as a second-line treatment for PCP. Ipratrapium is an anticholinergic used as an adjuvant treatment for COPD and asthma, but is not licensed specifically for exercise-induced asthma.

Answer to Question 18
E

In this situation he is competent and the physician has a duty to help him fulfil his wishes which he cannot do himself because he is tetraplegic; A and B are therefore wrong. Because he depends on mechanical ventilation, C and D are also wrong because it is predictable that dyspnoea will ensue if mechanical ventilation is stopped, just as pain is predictable if surgery is performed. It is logical to give drugs to relieve dyspnoea prior to stopping mechanical ventilation and be prepared to give further doses if they fail to control symptoms.

Answer to Question 19
F, T, F, F, T

Answer to Question 20
1H, 2E, 3C, 4A

Workers exposed to silica have a greatly increased risk of tuberculosis. Cement does not cause pneumoconiosis.

Answer to Question 21

1 D—The defect is restrictive because TLC is reduced and the gas transfer, even when adjusted for lung volume, is diminished so this merits comment.
2 D—Although A and E give restrictive defects the K_{CO} is normal or supernormal. Asthma is obstructive. Sarcoid is slightly preferred over fibrosing alveolitis because the K_{CO} is, relatively, preserved.

Answer to Question 22
T, F, F, T, T

Features of severe asthma are one or more of the following:
• PEF of ≤50% of predicted or best
• cannot complete sentences in one breath
• respiration ≥25 breaths/min
• pulse >110 beats/min.

Features of life-threatening asthma:
• PEF <33% predicted or best
• silent chest, cyanosis, or feeble respiratory effort
• bradycardia or hypotension
• exhaustion, confusion or coma.

B and C are features of life-threatening asthma. Severe hypoxia, Pa_{O_2} <8 kPa (60 mmHg) irrespective of treatment with oxygen is a marker of very severe life-threatening asthma. First-line treatment, as long as the patient does not require intubation and ventilation should be nebulized β agonist.

Both conditions require immediate admission to hospital. If you are the medical admissions officer, do not attempt to manage these patients alone beyond the initial phase; refer to the medical team as soon as you have assessed them and commenced treatment. If you are the medical senior house officer, make sure that you tell your on-site senior colleague about the patient as well as the ICU team.

Answer to Question 23
T, T, T, F, T

Sarcoidosis is a multi-system granulomatous disorder which is more common in females. It results in non-caseating granulomas and over 90% of patients will have liver granulomas on biopsy. It can result in polyuria and polydipsia caused either by hypercalcemia or secondary diabetes insipidus (as a result of hypothalamic–pituitary involvement). It is frequently accompanied by arthralgia, and haemoptysis may be caused by a mycetoma colonizing a pre-existing cavity. Retinopathy and chorioretinitis may occur and result in serious visual disability.

Answer to Question 24
F, F, F, F, F

Hypothyroidism is a recognized risk factor. UVPP is not advised in severe disease because it may make nasal CPAP more difficult to apply. The patient should be advised to inform the DVLA but the clinician should not unless he has reason to believe the patient is continuing to drive contrary to a DVLA decision. The question of cardio-vascular mortality remains open; the main reason for treatment is to relieve daytime somnolence. Oxygen therapy may prolong the duration of obstruction.

Answer to Question 25

T, F, T, T, T

Although the other diagnoses (not A) may have chest radiograph abnormalities, left upper lobe collapse cannot by definition have a normal radiograph. The OCP predisposes to thromboempolism.

Answer to Question 26

F, T, T, T, T

Answer to Question 27

1I, 2H, 3B, 4E, 5G

Answer to Question 28

T, F, F, F, T

Churg–Strauss syndrome is a multi-system small-vessel angiitis and may result in gastrointestinal bleed, intestinal obstruction and abdominal pain. It is associated with asthma, rhinitis and nasal polyps. Pleural effusions are seen in 30% of the patients. It may result in focal segmental glomerulonephritis and this can progress to renal failure. It is treated with high-dose systemic corticosteroids and the ESR and eosinophil count are markers of disease activity.

Answer to Question 29

• Is there a remediable cause? Check the ECG for rhythm disturbance, chest radiograph for pneumothorax or lobar pneumonia and routine blood tests (as well as physical examination).

• Is he a candidate for endotracheal intubation? If so this may be indicated immediately but if not the patient will require admission to a specialist ward such as the ICU/ HDU. The wife will contribute information crucial to make this decision.

• Premorbid disease severity (e.g. how far can he walk, can he dress himself).

• Major intercurrent illness, e.g. lung cancer.

• Has the patient expressed preferences about intubation/ICU? Is there an advance directive?

• Is there evidence of maximal therapy (e.g. LTOT, home nebulizer)?

• Is there a possibility of an overdose?

Answer to Question 30

F, F, T, T, F

Answer to Question 31

A1, B1, C2, D1, E1, F2, G1, H1, I3

A and D suggest the possibility of an overdose which should be in favour of mechanical ventilation unless the patient has received a psychiatric evaluation and was found to be perfectly competent. B suggests a reversible chest infection and by the same token pleuritic chest pain may suggest pulmonary embolism, pneumothorax or an infection which also would be in favour of mechanical ventilation. G and H also suggest a potentially reversible cause. F suggests established chronic renal failure and is against successful outcome from mechanical ventilation. Forgetfulness could suggest blood gas derangement or a reversible problem (e.g. hypothyroidism) and is not a reason to withhold mechanical ventilation without appropriate evaluation.

Answer to Question 32

F, F, T, T, T

Answer to Question 33

1 Choose from:

• smoking history

• presence/absence chest pain

• presence/absence haemoptysis

• asbestos exposure

• foreign travel

• features suggestive of chest infection, e.g. purulent phlegm, night sweats

• systematic enquiry, e.g. does he have a connective tissue disorder.

2 Blood tests may show abnormalities but these will be non-specific.

• Aspiration of pleural fluid. The fluid should be sent for conventional Gram stain and culture as well as a Ziehl–Nielsen stain and acid-fast bacillus culture. It should also be sent for measurement of protein and pH and cytological examination.

• Percutaneous pleural biopsy. At least one specimen should be sent for acid-fast bacillus culture as well as histology.

• CT scan of the thorax. This may demonstrate underlying lung disease or cancer as well as pleural neoplasm or thickening.

• Fibreoptic bronchoscopy. This may show an endobronchial cancer. If not washing of the lung underlying the effusion may yield an infectious agent.

3 Management needs to be considered under the following areas:

• conveying the diagnosis in an appropriate way

• management of the effusion to control symptom of dyspnoea. Consider surgical pleurodesis

• irradiation of chest drain sites

• assess and manage pain

• compensation advice.

Answer to Question 34

1

• Obstructive sleep apnoea syndrome

• Obesity hypoventilation syndrome

• Type II respiratory failure (e.g. caused by restrictive or neuromuscular disease).

The Medical Masterclass series

Clinical Skills

General Clinical Issues

Pain Relief and Palliative Care

Medicine for the Elderly

Emergency Medicine

Infectious Diseases and Dermatology

Infectious Diseases

Cardiology and Respiratory Medicine

Cardiology

Neurology, Ophthalmology and Psychiatry

Neurology

Nephrology

Rheumatology and Clinical Immunology

Index